Prevention in Mental Health: Lifespan Perspective

Guest Editors

DILIP V. JESTE, MD
CARL C. BELL, MD, DLAPA, FACPsych

PSYCHIATRIC CLINICS OF NORTH AMERICA

www.psych.theclinics.com

March 2011 • Volume 34 • Number 1

SAUNDERS an imprint of ELSEVIER, Inc.

W.B. SAUNDERS COMPANY
A Division of Elsevier Inc.

1600 John F. Kennedy Boulevard • Suite 1800 • Philadelphia, PA 19103-2899

http://www.theclinics.com

PSYCHIATRIC CLINICS OF NORTH AMERICA Volume 34, Number 1
March 2011 ISSN 0193-953X, ISBN-13: 978-1-4557-0498-9

Editor: Sarah E. Barth
Developmental Editor: Jessica Demetriou

Psychiatric Clinics of North America (ISSN 0193-953X) is published quarterly by Elsevier Inc., 360 Park Avenue South, New York, NY 10010-1710. Months of issue are March, June, September, and December. Business and Editorial Offices: 1600 John F. Kennedy Blvd., Suite 1800, Philadelphia, PA 19103-2899. Periodicals postage paid at New York, NY and additional mailing offices. Subscription prices are $265.00 per year (US individuals), $473.00 per year (US institutions), $131.00 per year (US students/residents), $321.00 per year (Canadian individuals), $589.00 per year (Canadian Institutions), $399.00 per year (foreign individuals), $589.00 per year (foreign institutions), and $194.00 per year (international & Canadian students/residents). Foreign air speed delivery is included in all *Clinics'* subscription prices. All prices are subject to change without notice. **POSTMASTER:** Send address changes to *Psychiatric Clinics of North America*, Elsevier Health Sciences Division, Subscription Customer Service, 3251 Riverport Lane, Maryland Heights, MO 63043. Customer Service: 1-800-654-2452 (US). From outside the United States, call 1-314-447-8871. Fax: 1-314-447-8029. E-mail: journalscustomerservice-usa@elsevier.com (for print support) and journalsonlinesupport-usa@elsevier.com (for online support).

Reprints. For copies of 100 or more, of articles in this publication, please contact the Commercial Reprints Department, Elsevier Inc., 360 Park Avenue South, New York, New York 10010-1710. Tel.: (212) 633-3813, Fax: (212) 462-1935, E-mail: reprints@elsevier.com.

Psychiatric Clinics of North America is covered in *MEDLINE/PubMed (Index Medicus), Current Contents/Social and Behavioral Sciences, Social Science Citation Index, Embase/Excerpta Medica,* and PsycINFO.

Printed and bound by CPI Group (UK) Ltd, Croydon, CRO 4YY
Transferred to Digital Print 2011

Contributors

GUEST EDITORS

DILIP V. JESTE, MD
Estelle and Edgar Levi Chair in Aging; Director, Sam and Rose Stein Institute for Research on Aging; Distinguished Professor of Psychiatry and Neurosciences, University of California, San Diego, San Diego, California

CARL C. BELL, MD, DLAPA, FACPsych
President/CEO, Community Mental Health Council, Inc; Director, Institute for Juvenile Research; Professor of Psychiatry, Department of Psychiatry, College of Medicine; Professor of Public Health, School of Public Health, University of Illinois at Chicago, Chicago, Illinois

AUTHORS

STEVEN M. ALBERT, PhD, MSPH
Department of Behavioral and Community Health Sciences, Graduate School of Public Health, University of Pittsburgh, Pittsburgh, Pennsylvania

ALINNE Z. BARRERA, PhD
Pacific Graduate School of Psychology, Palo Alto University, Palo Alto, California

WILLIAM R. BEARDSLEE, MD
Director, Baer Prevention Initiatives and Chairman Emeritus, Department of Psychiatry, Children's Hospital; Gardner/Monks Professor of Child Psychiatry, Harvard Medical School; Judge Baker Children's Center, Boston, Massachusetts

CARL C. BELL, MD, DLAPA, FACPsych
President/CEO, Community Mental Health Council, Inc; Director, Institute for Juvenile Research; Professor of Psychiatry, Department of Psychiatry, College of Medicine; Professor of Public Health, School of Public Health, University of Illinois at Chicago, Chicago, Illinois

CINNAMON S. BLOSS, PhD
Assistant Professor, Scripps Translational Science Institute and Scripps Health, La Jolla, California

ELIZABETH CHATTILLION, BA
Department of Psychiatry, University of California, San Diego, La Jolla, California

COLIN A. DEPP, PhD
Sam and Rose Stein Institute for Research on Aging; Department of Psychiatry, University of California, San Diego, La Jolla, California

MARY AMANDA DEW, PhD
Department of Psychiatry, Western Psychiatric Institute and Clinic, University of Pittsburgh, School of Medicine, Pittsburgh, Pennsylvania

KOBIE DOUGLAS, MD
Staff Psychiatrist, Community Mental Health Council, Inc, Chicago, Illinois

DENNIS D. EMBRY, PhD
President/Senior Scientist, PAXIS Institute, Tucson, Arizona

ROHAN GANGULI, MD, FRCP
Professor and Canada Research Chair, Center for Addiction and Mental Health, University of Toronto, Toronto, Ontario, Canada; Adjunct Professor, Western Psychiatric Institute and Clinic, University of Pittsburgh, Pittsburgh, Pennsylvania

TRACY R.G. GLADSTONE, PhD
Research Scientist, The Robert S. and Grace W. Stone Primary Prevention Initiatives, Wellesley Centers for Women, Wellesley College, Wellesley; Department of Psychiatry, Children's Hospital; Judge Baker Children's Center, Boston, Massachusetts

GENE GRIFFIN, JD, PhD
Assistant Professor, Mental Health Services and Policy Program, Northwestern University Feinberg School of Medicine, Chicago, Illinois

FAWZI HINDI, BA
Department of Psychiatry, Western Psychiatric Institute and Clinic, University of Pittsburgh, School of Medicine, Pittsburgh, Pennsylvania

DILIP V. JESTE, MD
Estelle and Edgar Levi Chair in Aging; Director, Sam and Rose Stein Institute for Research on Aging; Distinguished Professor of Psychiatry and Neurosciences, University of California, San Diego, San Diego, California

HARISH KAVIRAJAN, MD
Department of Psychiatry and Biobehavioral Sciences, University of California, Los Angeles, Costa Mesa, California

ELIZABETH M. LARUSSO, MD
Instructor, Department of Psychiatry, Dartmouth Medical School, Dartmouth Hitchcock Medical Center, Lebanon, New Hampshire

FRANCIS E. LOTRICH, MD, PhD
Department of Psychiatry, Western Psychiatric Institute and Clinic, University of Pittsburgh, School of Medicine, Pittsburgh, Pennsylvania

NICHOLAS MAHONEY
Section of General Internal Medicine, Department of Medicine, The University of Chicago, Chicago, Illinois

RINA MAZO
Section of General Internal Medicine, Department of Medicine, The University of Chicago, Chicago, Illinois

DOMINICA F. MCBRIDE, PhD
Co-Founder, Co-President, and Program Evaluation Consultant, The HELP Institute, Inc, Huntsville, Alabama

GARY M. MCCLELLAND, PhD
Mental Health Services and Policy Program, Northwestern University Feinberg School of Medicine, Chicago, Illinois

ERWIN MCEWEN, AM
Director, Illinois Department of Children and Family Services, Chicago, Illinois

WILLIAM R. MCFARLANE, MD
Professor of Psychiatry, Tufts University Medical School, Boston, Massachusetts;
Director, Center for Psychiatric Research, Maine Medical Center Research Institute,
Maine Medical Center, Portland, Maine

DAVID A. MERRILL, MD, PhD
Assistant Clinical Professor of Psychiatry and Biobehavioral Sciences, Division of
Geriatric Psychiatry; Associate Director of Ambulatory Care, Semel Institute for
Neuroscience and Human Behavior, David Geffen School of Medicine at the University
of California, Los Angeles, Los Angeles, California

LAURA J. MILLER, MD
Lecturer, Harvard Medical School; Vice Chair for Academic Clinical Services; Director,
Women's Mental Health, Department of Psychiatry, Brigham and Women's/Faulkner
Hospitals, Boston, Massachusetts

RICARDO F. MUÑOZ, PhD
Department of Psychiatry, San Francisco General Hospital, University of California,
San Francisco, California

ERIN E. O'CONNOR, BA
Research Assistant, Judge Baker Children's Center, Boston, Massachusetts

RONALD C. PETERSEN, PhD, MD
Professor of Neurology, College of Medicine; Cora Kanow Professor of Alzheimer's
Disease Research; Director, Department of Neurology, Mayo Clinic Study of Aging, Mayo
Alzheimer's Disease Research Center, Mayo Clinic, Rochester, Minnesota

MURRAY RASKIND, PhD
Director, Mental Illness Research, Education and Clinical Center, Veterans Affairs
Puget Sound Health Care System, Seattle Division; Professor and Vice-Chairman,
Department of Psychiatry and Behavioral Sciences, University of Washington
School of Medicine; Director, Alzheimer's Disease Research Center, University
of Washington, Seattle, Washington

JUANITA L. REDD, MPA, MBA
Senior Vice President; Director of Strategic Leadership, Community Mental Health
Council, Chicago, Illinois

CHARLES F. REYNOLDS III, MD
Department of Behavioral and Community Health Sciences, Graduate School of Public
Health; Department of Psychiatry, Western Psychiatric Institute and Clinic, University
of Pittsburgh, School of Medicine, Pittsburgh, Pennsylvania

BRYAN H. SAMUELS, MPP
Commissioner for Administration on Children, Youth, and Families, Administration
on Children, Youth and Families, Washington, DC

RODOLFO SAVICA, MD, MSc
Department of Neurology, Mayo Clinic, Rochester, Minnesota

NICHOLAS J. SCHORK, PhD
Professor, Molecular and Experimental Medicine, The Scripps Research Institute;
and Director of Biostatistics and Bioinformatics, Scripps Translational Science Institute,
La Jolla, California

CHRISTOPHER P. SIEMER, BS
Section of General Internal Medicine, Department of Medicine, The University of Chicago, Chicago, Illinois

GARY W. SMALL, MD
Parlow-Solomon Professor on Aging; Professor of Psychiatry and Biobehavioral Sciences; Director, UCLA Center on Aging; Director, Memory and Aging Research Center; Director, Geriatric Psychiatry Division, Semel Institute for Neuroscience and Human Behavior, David Geffen School of Medicine at the University of California, Los Angeles, Los Angeles, California

HEATHER M. SONES, BS
Doctoral Student, Joint Doctoral Program in Clinical Psychology, San Diego State University and University of California, San Diego, San Diego, California

MARTIN STRASSNIG, MD
Assistant Professor, Center for Addiction and Mental Health, University of Toronto, Toronto, Ontario, Canada

HAYWARD SUGGS, MS, MBA
Senior Vice President; Director of Organization Development, Community Mental Health Council, Chicago, Illinois

STEVEN R. THORP, PhD
Research Psychologist, Center of Excellence in Stress and Mental Health, Veterans Affairs San Diego Healthcare System, San Diego; Assistant Professor, Department of Psychiatry, The University of California, San Diego, Medical Center, La Jolla, California

BENJAMIN W. VAN VOORHEES, MD, MPH
Section of General Internal Medicine, Department of Medicine; Section of Child and Adolescent Psychiatry, Department of Psychiatry; Section of Developmental and Behavioral Pediatrics, Department of Pediatrics, The University of Chicago, Chicago, Illinois

IPSIT V. VAHIA, MD
Sam and Rose Stein Institute for Research on Aging; Department of Psychiatry, University of California, San Diego, La Jolla, California; Sun Valley Behavioral Medical Center, Imperial, California

Contents

Preface: Prevention in Mental Health: Lifespan Perspective　　　　　　xiii

Dilip V. Jeste and Carl C. Bell

Dedication　　　　　　xvii

Dilip V. Jeste and Carl C. Bell

**Behavioral Vaccines and Evidence-Based Kernels: Nonpharmaceutical Approaches
for the Prevention of Mental, Emotional, and Behavioral Disorders**　　　　　　1

Dennis D. Embry

> In the United States the rates for some mental, emotional, and behavioral
> problems (MEBs) have objectively increased over the past 20 to 50 years.
> The attributes of a public health approach to the treatment of MEBs are de-
> fined in this article. Multiple examples of how public health approaches
> might reduce or prevent MEBs using low-cost evidence-based kernels,
> which are fundamental units of behavior, are discussed. Such kernels
> can be used repeatedly, which then act as "behavioral vaccines" to reduce
> morbidity or mortality and/or improve human wellbeing. The author calls
> for 6 key policy actions to improve MEBs in young people.

The Prevention of Adolescent Depression　　　　　　35

Tracy R.G. Gladstone, William R. Beardslee, and Erin E. O'Connor

> This article provides a conceptual framework for research and outlines
> several new directions for the same on the prevention of depression in
> youth and reviews the recent literature on prevention efforts targeting chil-
> dren and adolescents. Prevention efforts should target both specific and
> nonspecific risk factors, enhance protective factors, use a developmental
> approach, and target selective and/or indicated samples. A review of the
> literature indicates that prevention programs using cognitive-behavioral
> and/or interpersonal approaches and family-based prevention strategies
> are the most helpful. Overall, it seems that there is reason for hope
> regarding the role of interventions in preventing depressive disorders in
> youth.

Preventing Postpartum Depression　　　　　　53

Laura J. Miller and Elizabeth M. LaRusso

> Major depression is a frequent complication of the postpartum period.
> Untreated postpartum depression increases the risk of maternal suicide
> and can impair parenting capability with resultant adverse effects on
> offspring development. A number of factors influence a woman's vulnera-
> bility to postpartum depressive episodes. This article summarizes pro-
> cesses for assessing these risk factors and implementing primary
> preventive interventions, and summarizes methods of early detection to
> promote secondary and tertiary prevention.

Preventing Depression in Later Life: State of the Art and Science Circa 2011   67

Fawzi Hindi, Mary Amanda Dew, Steven M. Albert, Francis E. Lotrich, and Charles F. Reynolds III

Unipolar major depression is among the leading contributors to the global burden of illness-related disability, and is predicted to be the greatest contributor to illness burden by 2030. It is a matter of public health significance to identify people at high risk for depression and/or already mildly symptomatic, and to discover ways of implementing timely and rational risk reduction strategies to preempt major depression. In this article, the published literature is reviewed to summarize what is known about depression prevention in older adults, and, ultimately, to inform future research.

Prevention of Posttraumatic Stress Disorder   79

Heather M. Sones, Steven R. Thorp, and Murray Raskind

Traumatic events are common, but the psychological distress that may follow usually subsides naturally. For some individuals, distress develops into posttraumatic stress disorder (PTSD). PTSD lends itself to the application of prevention strategies for at-risk individuals. The identification of a causal event may make prevention efforts for PTSD more feasible and effective than for other psychological disorders. For PTSD, these efforts target those traumatized persons who are beginning to exhibit symptoms of PTSD. These interventions could also target individuals meeting criteria for acute stress disorder with the goal of preventing chronic PTSD.

Prevention of the First Episode of Psychosis   95

William R. McFarlane

Long a desired goal but increasingly a focus of research on clinical practice, prevention of psychosis has emerged as one of the most promising and effective areas of investigational interest and effort in psychiatry. Spurred by long-term studies that have associated outcome with duration of untreated psychosis, current research is focused on improving the accuracy of prediction based on clinical and neurocognitive measures and on refining treatments of the earliest symptoms of the psychoses. Both efforts are bearing success, although there remains ambiguity as to the most effective preventive interventions. This article reviews the leading studies of, and remaining issues for, this important enterprise.

Prevention of Metabolic Syndrome in Serious Mental Illness   109

Rohan Ganguli and Martin Strassnig

The interaction of lifestyle, socioeconomic status, genetic factors, and treatment with antipsychotic medications likely accounts for the high risk of metabolic syndrome, diabetes, heart disease, and premature mortality in people with serious mental illness. Given the high risk of developing diabetes and cardiovascular disease in persons with serious mental illness, psychiatrists who treat these individuals need to ensure they are familiar with these risks, monitor metabolic parameters in their patients, and educate their patients (and caregivers) about the risks and how to prevent them.

Prevention of Dementia   127

Rodolfo Savica and Ronald C. Petersen

Dementia is a neurological condition that is characterized by decline in multiple cognitive domains and is accompanied by a functional impairment. It is important to identify the factors that may delay the onset, slow the progression, or prevent cognitive decline. This review highlights the protective and risk factors of dementia, suggesting that physical activity, intellectual activity, and social engagement may reduce Alzheimer disease and cognitive decline and may be also helpful for enhancing quality of life.

Genomics for Disease Treatment and Prevention   147

Cinnamon S. Bloss, Dilip V. Jeste, and Nicholas J. Schork

The enormous advances in genetics and genomics of the past decade have the potential to revolutionize health care, including mental health care, and bring about a system predominantly characterized by the practice of genomic and personalized medicine. This article briefly reviews the history of genetics and genomics and assesses the extent to which the results of genetic and genomic studies are currently being leveraged clinically for disease treatment and prevention. Relevant social, economic, and policy issues relevant to genomic medicine are also reviewed, and priority research areas in which further work is needed are identified.

Internet-Based Depression Prevention over the Life Course: A Call for Behavioral Vaccines   167

Benjamin W. Van Voorhees, Nicholas Mahoney, Rina Mazo, Alinne Z. Barrera, Christopher P. Siemer, Tracy R.G. Gladstone, and Ricardo F. Muñoz

Technology-based approaches for the prevention of depression offer considerable benefits including easy access, patient autonomy, and "nonconsumable" services that are autonomous from traditional (face-to-face) interventions. The authors have previously worked to develop Internet interventions based on the frameworks for conventional, face-to-face effective community-based interventions, and propose to integrate these models into a "behavioral vaccine model" aptly applicable to technology-based delivery. This article reviews the literature on Internet-based depression prevention programs using this behavioral vaccine development model, reviewing literature relevant to each component of the model in turn.

Infusing Protective Factors for Children in Foster Care   185

Gene Griffin, Erwin McEwen, Bryan H. Samuels, Hayward Suggs, Juanita L. Redd, and Gary M. McClelland

This article looks at an example of infusing protective factors into a child welfare system. Focusing on Illinois and its state child welfare agency, the article reviews some of the research on the relationship between risk behaviors and protective factors of traumatized youth. Next, it looks at adapting treatment and evidence-based early intervention practices to local child welfare settings. These interventions are placed in the wider context of a state plan to enhance protective factors. The article reviews how the state and local plans have been influenced by federal policies and how the Illinois experience might help refine future policy.

Youth Homicide Prevention   205

Kobie Douglas and Carl C. Bell

> Homicide continues to be a problematic public health concern, but homi-
> cide rates have dropped considerably since the mid-1980s. This article
> proposes that the decrease in violence was caused by a large number
> of national and local violence prevention initiatives. Homicide and violence
> data are reviewed and the developmental dynamics of violence and homi-
> cide are discussed, noting the different tracks youth take toward violence.
> The risk factors that lead youth toward a violent lifestyle are compared with
> the protective factors that shield them from it. The principles involved in the
> prevention of violent behavior such as homicide are also discussed.

Human Immunodeficiency Virus Prevention with Youth   217

Dominica F. McBride and Carl C. Bell

> For years, the HIV pandemic was seemingly mysterious and uncontrol-
> lable. However, it is now known that with technology, this virus can be
> stopped from becoming fatal, and with prevention further infection can
> be stopped. With the application of certain principles and knowledge,
> this pandemic can be turned into something much less nocuous and per-
> vasive. Various researchers and programs have effectively demonstrated
> this reality, showing the possibilities of ameliorating the propagation of
> this virus through prevention. This article reviews the risk and protective
> factors associated with HIV-related behaviors and describes various effec-
> tive prevention programs.

Psychological Protective Factors Across the Lifespan: Implications for Psychiatry   231

Ipsit V. Vahia, Elizabeth Chattillion, Harish Kavirajan, and Colin A. Depp

> Although there are many challenges in operationally defining and measur-
> ing positive psychological constructs, there is accumulating evidence that
> optimism, resilience, positive attitudes toward aging, and spirituality are
> related to reduced risk for morbidity and mortality in older age. This article
> reviews the definition, measurement, associations, and putative mecha-
> nisms of selected positive psychological constructs on subjective and ob-
> jective indicators of health with a focus on the latter half of the lifespan.

Prevention in Psychiatry: Effects of Healthy Lifestyle on Cognition   249

David A. Merrill and Gary W. Small

> People are living longer than ever. With greater longevity, a critical ques-
> tion becomes whether or not our memories endure across the life span.
> This article reviews the common forms of age-related memory change
> and the emerging evidence related to putative risk and protective factors
> for brain aging. With increasing awareness of Alzheimer disease and
> related dementias, patients, families, and clinicians are eager for concise
> and accurate information about the effects and limitations of preventative
> strategies related to lifestyle choices that may improve cognitive health.

Index   263

FORTHCOMING ISSUES

June 2011
Geriatric Psychiatry
George S. Alexopoulos, MD and
Dimitris Kiosses, MD, *Guest Editors*

September 2011
Psychosomatic Medicine
Joel Dimsdale, MD, *Guest Editor*

December 2011
Obesity and Eating Disorders
Thomas A. Wadden, PhD, G. Terrence
Wilson, PhD, Robert I. Berkowitz, MD and
Albert J. Stunkard, MD, *Guest Editors*

RECENT ISSUES

December 2010
Traumatic Brain Injury: Defining Best Practice
Silvana Riggio, MD and
Andy Jagoda, MD, FACEP, *Guest Editors*

September 2010
Cognitive Behavioral Therapy
Bunmi O. Olatunji, PhD, *Guest Editor*

June 2010
Women's Mental Health
Susan G. Kornstein, MD and
Anita H. Clayton, MD, *Guest Editors*

RELATED INTERESTS

Primary Care: Clinics in Office Practice, December 2008 (Vol. 35, No. 4)
Wellness and Prevention
Vincent Morelli, MD and Roger Zoorob, MD, MPH, *Guest Editors*

Child and Adolescent Psychiatric Clinics of North America, April 2007
(Vol. 16, No. 2)
Resilience
Normand Carrey, MD, FRCP(C), ABPN and Michael Ungar, PhD, *Guest Editors*

THE CLINICS ARE NOW AVAILABLE ONLINE!

Access your subscription at:
www.theclinics.com

Preface

Prevention in Mental Health: Lifespan Perspective

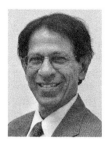 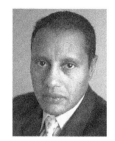

Dilip V. Jeste, MD   Carl C. Bell, MD, DLAPA, FACPsych
                         Guest Editors

The goal of this monograph is to inform the mental health community that prevention of several psychiatric disorders is not a futuristic fantasy but is possible and even practical today. Obviously, the state of science in this arena varies considerably across disorders. Thus, there are more data available on prevention of several types of depression than on prevention of schizophrenia. Nonetheless, the evidence base for preventive interventions is becoming increasingly robust, and use of these interventions should be considered not only ethical but also cost-effective for the overall health care.

The two of us came to the field of prevention in different ways. One of us (DVJ) has been interested for the past several years in successful cognitive and emotional aging. His literature reviews as well as the work done by his group at the University of California, San Diego have demonstrated the value of preventive strategies in enhancing the likelihood of positive aging. CCB did his first formal scientific prevention research with Dr Brian Flay in 1992 when the Aban Aya research team began to study how to prevent

Psychiatr Clin N Am 34 (2011) xiii–xvi
doi:10.1016/j.psc.2011.01.001
0193-953X/11/$ – see front matter © 2011 Elsevier Inc. All rights reserved.

violence, drug use, and early sexual debut in Chicago Public Schools. He then went on to do HIV prevention research with Drs Roberta Paikoff and Mary McKay that led to his R-01 HIV prevention research in Durban, South Africa. In the early 2000s, CCB's work on violence prevention got him involved with Dr David Satcher's Youth Violence Prevention Report and the Institute of Medicine (IOM)'s report on reducing suicide. CCB was one of the authors of the 2009 IOM report on *Preventing Mental, Emotional, and Behavioral Disorders among Young People: Progress and Possibilities* that guided the prevention initiatives found in the Patient Protection and Affordable Care Act. In sum, CCB's work had focused on children, adolescents, and young adults, whereas DVJ's primary research and clinical interest was in middle-aged and older adults. This issue thus represents a combined and rather unique lifespan approach to prevention in psychiatry.

Embry's article highlights some of the prevention strategies in the 2009 IOM prevention report and his concept of "kernels" –easy, doable strategies to support prevention of mental health problems. This is followed by a number of articles on prevention of specific disorders including depression in different groups of patients, PTSD, first-episode psychosis, metabolic syndrome, and dementia. The adolescent depression prevention article reminds us of Jane Knitzer's (author of "Unclaimed Children") admonishment that, if you are an adult psychiatrist treating depressed adults and you ignore the risk these patients' children have for the development of depression and all you do is to treat the parent without making an effort to prevent the patients' offspring from being depressed, something is seriously wrong with your practice of psychiatry. The prevention strategies in the postpartum depression prevention article constitute what one may consider some of the "low hanging fruit" in public health as the technology needed to identify mothers with postpartum depression is well established and the prevention intervention for this disorder is not difficult to accomplish. Hindi and colleagues discuss the strengths and limitations of the current modalities of prevention of depression in later life. A better understanding of the pathophysiological risk factors for depression that help to identify when and how to intervene in at-risk patients, along with a mastery of the Internet as a powerful dissemination tool, may pave the way to making depression prevention a widely practiced and effective intervention.

Because PTSD results from a specific, identifiable event, the disorder lends itself to the application of prevention strategies for at-risk individuals; yet PTSD prevention research is only in its infancy. Sones and colleagues describe how PTSD presents a formidable challenge as well as a clear opportunity. Having spent a considerable amount of our careers treating schizophrenia, it is clear that if psychiatry could develop the political will needed to implement interventions for prevention of schizophrenia, we would prevent a great deal of morbidity and mortality in our society, with enormous financial savings. Ganguli reviews the role of genetic factors, treatment with antipsychotic medication, socioeconomic status, and lifestyle in the risk of metabolic syndrome, diabetes, heart disease, and premature mortality in people with serious mental illness. Mental health treatment facilities, including community mental health centers, need to offer their patients/clients access to evidence-based lifestyle interventions and to adequate primary care. We must follow these recommendations to reduce the 20- to 25-year mortality gap between people with serious mental illness and the rest of the population that exists today. Finally, Savica and Petersen discuss suggestions for prevention of dementias of different types.

The next series of articles focus, not on individual psychiatric disorders, but rather on broader bio-psycho-social and behavioral strategies that have implications for a variety of mental illnesses. Bloss and coworkers highlight exciting areas where genetic and genomic discoveries are already being used in the clinic to improve health care, including mental health care (eg, pharmacogenomics). However, while the pace of genetic and genomic science, technology, and discovery has been rapid, more work is needed to fully realize the potential for impacting disease treatment and prevention, especially in mental health. The article on internet-based depression prevention shows how modern technology has the possibility of making it easy to disseminate and implement evidence-based prevention techniques in a way that has fidelity to the original efficacious intervention and is also inexpensive. Having explored the impact of exposure to violence since 1976, CCB is especially heartened to see the child protective services field take a protective factor, strength-based approach to children in foster care. Thanks to Dr Satcher's Youth Violence report and CCB's research and naturalistic studies in Chicago Public Schools, the article on the prevention of youth homicide cuts through the myths of youth violence and provides science and real-life experience in preventing this major social issue. The contribution of HIV prevention in youth owes a great deal to Dr Willo Pequegnat and the NIMH Center for Mental Health Research on AIDS –Consortium on Families and HIV/AIDS.

Vahia and coworkers show that major strides have been made in refining constructs related to positive psychological traits and suggest that these traits may have an independent positive effect on health, especially in older adults. Merrill and Small discuss how healthy lifestyle choices have numerous potential benefits that may prevent cognitive decline.

We would like to express our gratitude to several special people. It was truly a pleasure to work with all the authors of the individual articles—international prevention experts—not only due to their knowledge of psychiatric prevention interventions, but also because of the reliability and timeliness with which they completed their work for this monograph. Special thanks to Dr Dominica F. McBride for her help with the editing of several articles. The staff of Elsevier has been extraordinarily professional and skilled in their assistance. We thank Dr David Satcher, Rosalyn Carter, and A. Kathryn Power of the SAMHSA for their leadership in mental health advocacy and guidance of our efforts. Last, we owe a lot to our colleagues, trainees, and staff at the University of California, San Diego and at the Community Mental Health Council, Inc, as well as the Institute for Juvenile Research in the Department of Psychiatry, College of Medicine, University of Illinois at Chicago for their invaluable work and support.

Although definitive large-scale randomized controlled trials of prevention present a major challenge for scientists in the coming years, clinicians in practice need not wait to encourage patients and their family members who come into the office to discuss healthy lifestyle choices and guide them in practical approaches to integrating them into their daily lives. Prevention is not restricted to the youth. As psychiatry prepares to deal with the impending growth in the older population, a future research agenda in this area should include broadening our understanding of psychological and biological mechanisms that underlie positive psychological traits and to devise and assess interventions aimed at promoting them. More immediately, psychiatric clinicians should dedicate time and effort to incorporating means to reinforce these traits in ongoing psychiatric treatment.

One of the core tenets of the community psychiatry is to provide consultation and education in the hopes that public health prevention strategies can be applied to psychiatry. After all, mental retardation secondary to phenylketonuria had once been a serious cause of mental health impairment but, due to prevention, this problem is no longer seen in the United States. Let us hope that, in the near future, preventive strategies in psychiatry will make many psychiatric disorders a thing of the past.

Dilip V. Jeste, MD
University of California, San Diego
9500 Gilman Drive #0664
San Diego, CA 92093, USA

Carl C. Bell, MD, DLAPA, FACPsych
Community Mental Health Council, Inc
8704 South Constance Avenue
Chicago, IL 60617, USA

Institute for Juvenile Research
Department of Psychiatry
College of Medicine
School of Public Health
University of Illinois at Chicago
1747 West Roosevelt Road, Room 155
Chicago, IL 60608-1264, USA

E-mail addresses:
djeste@ucsd.edu (D.V. Jeste)
carlcbell@pol.net (C.C. Bell)

Dedication

I would like to dedicate this volume to my colleagues and staff at UCSD, and my family (Sonali, Shafali, Richard, Neelum, Nischal, and Kiran). –DVJ

I would like to dedicate this volume to my three children (Cristin Carole, Briatta H. Bell, William Yancy Bell, IV), my grandson Benjamin Winter Bell, the staff at the Community Mental Health Council, Inc, and my "Be-ing" who have made it possible for me to do my work. –CCB

Psychiatr Clin N Am 34 (2011) xvii
doi:10.1016/j.psc.2011.01.002
0193-953X/11/$ – see front matter © 2011 Elsevier Inc. All rights reserved.

psych.theclinics.com

Behavioral Vaccines and Evidence-Based Kernels: Nonpharmaceutical Approaches for the Prevention of Mental, Emotional, and Behavioral Disorders

Dennis D. Embry, PhD

KEYWORDS

- Evidence-based kernels • Behavioral vaccines • Prevention
- Public health

The Institute of Medicine Report on the Prevention of Mental, Emotional and Behavioral Disorders Among Young People[1] (IOM Report) provides a powerful map for how the United States might significantly prevent mental illnesses and behavioral disorders like alcohol, tobacco, and other drug use among America's youth. This document is already shaping United States policies, and will almost certainly affect Canada and other countries' policies. Mental, emotional, and behavioral disorders (MEBs) among America's youth and young adults present a serious threat to the country's national security[2] and to our economic competitiveness compared with 22 other rich countries.[3–7] Such MEBs are also the leading preventable cost center for local, state, and the federal governments.[1,4] Further, safe schools, healthy working environments, and public events or places are seriously compromised by MEBs as well.

A grant from the National Institute on Drug Abuse (DA028946) for the Promise Neighborhood Research Consortium provided support to the author for work on this article.
Financial disclosure and conflict of interest obligations: D.D.E. is an employee and stockholder of PAXIS Institute, which receives fees and royalties for research, products, consulting and other services related evidence-based kernels and behavioral vaccines. He is also stockholder and officer in a web-based company, SimpleGifts.com, designed to make evidence-based kernels accessible to individuals and organizations.
PAXIS Institute, PO Box 31205, Tucson, AZ 85751, USA
E-mail address: dde@paxis.org

Psychiatr Clin N Am 34 (2011) 1–34
doi:10.1016/j.psc.2010.11.003
0193-953X/11/$ – see front matter © 2011 Elsevier Inc. All rights reserved.

The IOM Report opines:

Behavioral health could learn from public health in endorsing a population health perspective. (IOM[p19])
   Families and children have ready access to the best available evidence-based prevention interventions, delivered in their own communities...in a respectful non-stigmatizing way.[p387]
   Preventive interventions are provided as a routine component of school, health, and community service systems...[p387]
   Services are coordinated and integrated with multiple points of entry for children and their families...[p387]
   ...Prevention strategies contribute to narrowing rather than widening health disparities...[p388]

WHY A PUBLIC HEALTH APPROACH TO PREVENTION IS NEEDED

The first scientific public health approach to prevention was by John Snow, who removed the Broad Street water pump handle. He stopped the deadly cholera epidemic in London. His analysis and identification of water-borne disease from a single pump is an action metaphor for our own contemporary multiple, related epidemics (ie, syndemics)[8-11] of MEBs that cause so many afflictions and consequences for North American societies. Why is a public health approach to the prevention of MEBs (which includes all addictions) necessary in the United States and other countries? A few simple facts make the point:

- Every family in America has one or more family members who have been touched with MEBs during a given year, based on prevalence estimates.[12-14] Common MEBs (eg, childhood attention-deficit/hyperactivity disorder [ADHD]) have adverse effects on child rearing, marriages, income, domestic violence, and health.[15-24]
- Every American business has one or more employees who are directly or indirectly affected by MEBs, which have multiple documented adverse impacts on health, costs, and productivity.[25-27] Worse still, the lack of health care for the employees in small businesses in America has a large negative impact on the productivity of small businesses in the United States as compared with rich countries with national health care.[3]
- Schools, health care carriers, and communities across America are struggling with the costly burdens of these disorders via special education and behavioral difficulties.[28-35]
- Some of these disorders are rising in prevalence in the United States,[7,36,37] particularly the more disturbing costly problems such as conduct disorders.[7]
- The United States has more of these problems that many other rich countries,[5,6] and there are increasingly clear epidemiological reasons why this might be so.[38-44]

Previous investigators have used these statistics to call for more mental health professionals.[45] However, this fails a public health approach in 2 ways: (1) treatment by professionals is perceived as stigmatizing, and many of the most vulnerable groups do not seek "treatment" because of such perceived stigma[46]; and (2) focusing only on expanding treatment ignores that MEBs can be prevented by very low-cost procedures delivered by existing persons in communities.[47-60] While expanding mental health professionals might be helpful in treatment issues, it is a "downstream" rather than "upstream" model. A public health "upstream" model is a logical alternative.

HOW IS A PUBLIC HEALTH APPROACH DIFFERENT?

A public health approach to the prevention of MEBs would look much different than the existing "rationing" approaches. It would be more like that of European countries (*IOM Report*[pp388–95]), or like some Canadian provinces where access is far more universal. The benefits are evident in the Netherlands, for example, where the utilization of psychotropic drugs among children and youth is half of that of the United States.[61] The Netherlands, for example, widely promotes two of the most highlighted universal access prevention approaches in the IOM Report—Triple P (a multilevel parenting support system)[62,63] and the Good Behavior Game.[52,64,65] The United Kingdom, which has lower rates of MEBs,[7,36,37] even provided the parenting tips found in Triple P in the context of an 8-week TV show, which significantly reduced disturbing and disruptive behaviors of children whose parents followed the show.[66–68] Another United Kingdom study remedied dietary deficiency widely linked to psychiatric disorders[38,69,70] during the normal course of school[44,71]; this resulted in fewer problematic behaviors and improvements in academic success.[44,71] These types of preventive strategies can be delivered as a matter of course or choice, rather than limiting access by families, schools, or neighborhoods based on a "rationing model" of prevention in which only those who have positive "screening" at an individual, family, school, or neighborhood level receive prevention services.

A public health model of preventing MEBs might resemble the implementation of medical vaccines for childhood illnesses. Governments or private insurance subsidize such vaccines to reduce mortality or morbidity. Governments and private insurance companies also subsidize "behavioral" vaccines such as car safety seats for children or hand washing. *A behavioral vaccine is a repeated simple behavior that reduces morbidity or mortality and increases wellbeing.*[52,72,73] Like medical vaccines, behavioral vaccines can provide "herd immunity" as protection against behavioral contagion—a phenomenon well documented in behavioral and epidemiological science.[74–83]

What defines a public health approach? The author and his colleagues I propose some parameters:

1. *Universality of Harm:* A public health approach predicates that the risk of the problem or disease is widely distributed, and that vulnerability is common because of national, regional, or even basic human vulnerabilities. Thus, car safety seats are needed because any child can be in a serious car crash, and any child can fall victim to almost any of the serious childhood illnesses prevented by medical vaccines. Similarly, the adverse impact of tobacco can harm any person—including those exposed to tobacco second-hand or through social costs. MEBs pass that test, given that 20% to 25% of the population[25] experiences one or more in any given year.[13,45]

2. *Personal or Group Risk is Common:* Although some individuals or groups may have higher levels of vulnerability because of genetics, social conditions, or history, the overall risk of the problem or disorder is widely distributed; this means that attempts to isolate or identify the individuals or groups at risk are inefficient and prone to error. While it is true that some children and their families, for example, are more likely to be victims of car crashes, morbidity and mortality risk of such crashes is as widespread as MEBs. For example, substantiated child-maltreatment or childhood ADHD are clearly associated with risk factors such as poverty,[84–87] yet identification of such risks does not per se result in earlier treatment or prevention.[88] Indeed, an emphasis on static predictors can mask the opportunity to have a population-level, cost-efficient impact on serious issues such as child

maltreatment, mental health outcomes, and conduct disorders.[47,49,51,57,89] When a successful public health approach has been taken, the individuals or groups who need more intensive support are easier to indentify than when access is rationed.[49,90]

3. *Protection of the Whole Population:* Protection against car crashes, against contagious life-threatening diseases, against second-hand effects of tobacco, or against crime are examples of a public health approach. The burden of MEBs fits this framing with so many children, adolescents, and adults affected. In some cases, a broad approach is needed even when a smaller number of people with the problem have very costly consequences—such as a child with lifetime conduct disorders. This can cost between 2 and 4 million dollars per child, affecting public safety, health care, social services, school and workplace productivity, and so forth.[91] As mentioned earlier, a public health approach can confer "herd immunity" for the population.[92-95]

4. *Stigmatizing Persons or Groups At Risk Reduces Prevention:* When policies or practices focus only or mostly on presumed persons or groups at risk, such individuals or groups decline to participate because of perceived stigmatization.[96] This is especially true when it involves racial or ethnic groups.[88]

5. *Cost Efficiency:* Population-level or public health approaches are often more cost effective in terms of preventive results than costly processes of identifying those at risk, recruiting participation of persons at risk, and dealing with the adverse effects of stigma. Often, just making the preventive strategy widely available is the most efficient way of "case finding" for at-risk populations. The tobacco control efforts clearly demonstrate the benefits of a public health approach (eg, clean indoor air or restricted access to tobacco)[97-101] versus a risk-selection only approach.[98]

COST EFFECTIVENESS AND PREVALENCE REDUCTION WITH A PUBLIC HEALTH APPROACH

Can a public health approach work for the prevention of MEBs? The author and colleagues say "yes", especially with a "consumer" approach that allows individuals or groups to participate easily in proven strategies. Let us examine the evidence and rationale.

It is important to begin with an obvious, but not well-recognized detail about evidence-based prevention strategies for mental, emotional, and behavior disorders (including alcohol and other drugs) in the United States. That is, not a single evidence-based prevention tool on the National Registry of Effective Programs and Practices (NREPP) for mental, emotional, or behavioral disorders is available at Amazon (the largest bookstore), Walmart (the largest retail chain), or iTunes (the largest "apps" store) in North America or in Europe for that matter.

Consumer Prevention Product Logic

Compare the aforementioned to the prevention of childhood diseases or the prevention of childhood injuries. Most people can obtain a "walk-in" vaccination for children's illnesses at "minute clinics" at Walgreens, CVS, or Shoppers Drug Mart (Canada) dotting major intersections all across North America. Most families can obtain injury prevention devices (car seats, bike helmets, fall gates, electric socket protectors, medicine cabinet safety latches, and so forth) at Walgreens, CVS, Target, Walmart, Loblaw (Canada), Sobeys (Canada), or Amazon within minutes. Some people may need free vaccines or car seats. Some people may need special supports to use or apply the strategies. Some groups, including schools, may need special marketing or cultural adaptations to succeed. Nevertheless, the reach, adoption, and maintenance of these prevention products far outstrip the reach, adoption, and maintenance of prevention strategies for MEBs in the United States. In North America no parent, concerned family members, or concerned community person can easily purchase or obtain any evidence-based prevention strategy for MEBs. It is even difficult for any normal citizen (parent, teacher, or community person) to obtain the scientific journal articles about such prevention tools that would enable citizens to "roll their own" prevention strategies successfully.

Although the proven strategies that can prevent MEBs are not easily accessible in North America, the things that we are trying to prevent are very easy to obtain directly as consumers. Ironically, alcohol, tobacco, and illegal drugs are accessible to students on virtually every school campus. Prescription drugs that are widely abused are, too frequently, promoted on TV channels, in print, on the Internet, in movies, and on the radio. Your doctor gets free samples delivered to his or her office every week, by pharmaceutical sales staff. Paradoxically, things that are scientifically documented to increase the prevalence rates of MEBs are easy to get. Devices or entertainment that increase sleep deprivation and worsen multiple MEBs[102-104] are a mouse-click away. Child-targeted foods that cause deficiency in essential brain nutrients involved in with MEB rates in America are advertised on children's TV.[40,41,105]

Cost-Offsetting Consequences

With no easy consumer access to proven prevention tools, the consumers (parents, teachers, businesses, and so forth) engage in shifting prevention, intervention, and treatment costs to third-party payers. Consider these examples:

1. *Parent Example:* When a parent receives a teacher's complaint about a child's inattentive or disturbing behaviors, most parents have no viable remedy except medication (cost offset to health insurance) or an Individualized Educational Plan (IEP; cost offset to school district).
2. *Teacher Example:* When a teacher faces a child with mental, emotional, or behavioral symptoms in the classroom, he or she has almost no options except to influence the parent to start the child on medication, or insist that the child have an IEP.
3. *Business or Organizational Example:* Business or organizational leaders face similar dilemmas of cost offsetting with a lack of options. A business or organization will rarely perceive actionable alternatives that do not involve either increased health care or service costs or employee turnover.

These cost-shifting issues are easily predictable from behavioral economics and common pool resources.[106-108] Indeed, without easy to access consumer-based choices, the documented spiraling costs of psychotropic medications and special education in the United States are a foregone conclusion. The fact that businesses have no clear option to expensive offsets causes businesses to raise deductibles or restrict benefits or other strategies that hurt the common pool (eg, the wellbeing of children, youth, families, and communities).

Evidence for a Public Health, Consumer-Focused Approach to Prevention

Is there high-quality evidence—meeting the standards of evidence by the Society for Prevention Research[109]—that population-level, public health consumer approaches can prevent or reduce MEBs? Yes; here are a few examples, in which science-based prevention was not rationed but made widely available:

- *Triple P Parenting Support System (IOMp[167]):* There are now 3 population-level studies providing universal access to a system of parenting support so that families (not professionals) are able to determine how little or how much they want.
  1. A broadcast TV show (*Driving Mum and Dad Mad*) resulted in viewership outdrawing *Desperate Housewives* in the same time slot in the United Kingdom. Of the family viewers, some 360,000 families had children with high levels of MEBs, and 48% of those "high-risk" families were able to bring their children beneath the clinical score range using the tools from the TV show and Web site.[67]
  2. An 18-county randomized study, sponsored by the Centers for Disease Control and Prevention (CDC) using Triple P, was able to reduce 3 major population-level indicators of child maltreatment in the 9 randomly selected Triple P counties.[49] All families, rather than risk-selected families, were the target of the strategy, which was highly cost efficient at reducing maltreatment indicators, at the cost of less than $13.00 per child (ages 0–9 years) in the targeted counties.[90] Reducing exposure to adverse childhood experiences is one of the key pathways of preventing lifetime MEBs as well as high health care costs.[110–113]
  3. A multi-city comparison study, called "Every Family", was conducted in Australia. The target population was all parents of 4- to 7-year-old children residing in 10 geographical areas in Brisbane (Triple P), compared with 10 control matched areas in Sydney and Melbourne (Children are Unbeatable [CAU]). After intervention there were significantly greater reductions in the number of children with clinically elevated and borderline behavioral and emotional problems in the Triple P communities compared with the CAU communities. Similarly, parents in Triple P communities reported a greater reduction in the prevalence of depression, stress, and coercive parenting. Findings show the feasibility of targeting dysfunctional parenting practices in a cost-effective manner. Triple P is the first parenting system to demonstrate longitudinal, population-level effects for parents and children on MEBs.
- *Safe-Playing Injury Control Studies:* In late 1970s and through the mid-1980s, pedestrian injuries were one of the top 5 causes of death to preschool children 3 to 5 years old in the United States and many Organization of Economic Development (OECD) countries. Whereas fatal injuries were statistically uncommon per child, dangerous or risky behaviors such as dashing into the street before a car on a Bigwheel or chasing a ball or playmate were not. About half of any given sample of observed children entered the street every hour in the course of outdoor play without any parental awareness during baseline.[114–118] When parents in North America and New Zealand were offered easy access to simple behavioral prevention tools, as much as 50% of community samples adopted and implemented the evidence-based recipe to alter children's safety behaviors.[116,118]
- *Tobacco Prevention:* The following paragraph is from a recent publication on involving communities with sustainable prevention strategies[97]:

Project SixTeen is an example of a multimodal community intervention trial aimed at preventing youth tobacco use by random assignment. Eight Oregon communities received an intervention that included classroom-based prevention curricula, media advocacy, youth anti-tobacco activities, family communication activities, and a systematic campaign to reduce tobacco sales to underage youth[100]; another eight schools received classroom curricula only (ie, Project PATH).[119]

At one and five years post intervention, communities receiving the comprehensive intervention showed a significantly lower prevalence of cigarette use compared to those receiving the school-based intervention alone. At two years, ninth-grade boys in the comprehensive intervention, compared to those in the school intervention, reported lower use of smokeless tobacco. Over a span of four years, alcohol and marijuana use increased less rapidly in intervention communities than in the school-only communities.

A recently completed systematic replication took elements from Project SixTeen[100,101] and applied it across 2 whole states, showing population-level reductions for those states on Youth Risk Behavior Survey (YRBS) data for any 30-day and everyday tobacco use, resulting in a NREPP designation as "environmental policy" with a valid experimental design.[120]

- *School-Based Violence Prevention:* In the 1990s, youth violence rates significantly increased, and schools experienced a notable increase in school-based violence. PeaceBuilders was one of the first evidence-based strategies with both theoretical roots and demonstrable effects.[121] In Pima County, some 85 elementary schools signed up in 1 year to participate in a community-wide effort of teaching, reinforcing, and promoting peaceful behavior.[121,122] Within those schools, 8 sites were randomly assigned to a wait-list control that received extensive evaluation of 4-hour in-service, materials, and technical supports. The independent evaluation revealed that the schools receiving PeaceBuilders had fewer violent injuries coded by nurses.[123] The prevention strategy also had medium effect sizes on social competence and aggressive behavior as reported by teachers using psychometrically valid tools,[124] especially for the most disturbed and aggressive boys.[125]

These examples actually have several features in common, which are not transparent when reading the published articles. One needs to examine the actual strategies to appreciate how these examples embody a consumer approach to prevention. Here are some common features:

1. *Small Units of Change:* Each example emphasizes small units of behavior change (ie, active ingredients) that can be adopted by the consumers (eg, children, teachers, parents, and so forth) via simple verbal explanations, demonstrations, or symbolic modeling. For example, in the Safe Playing initiative, parents read a storybook to the child with his or her name as the actor, which then depicted the caregiver setting a timer, giving simple stickers on a chart, and sharing surprise rewards for playing safely (ie, not going into the street or crossing other demarked boundaries).[117] In the case of PeaceBuilders, adults and students created a chart of what they would see, hear, and do in a peaceful school, and those charts were posted throughout the site.[121] Then adults learned to write "praise notes" to students for doing those "peacebuilding behaviors"; the students wrote similar notes to each other that were publicly posted, and they wrote praise notes to adults for building peace.[126] Consumer-based prevention typically does not require extensive training or face-to-face educational programs for the child or adult; rather, such strategies more resemble easy-to-use appliances or software.

2. *Proximal Benefits:* Consumer-friendly prevention "products" tend to produce easily noticed proximal benefits or "early wins" in the organizational change literature. For example, the Safe Playing intervention typically yields immediate change in less risky and safer behavior.[116,117] Similarly, the various "praise notes" used in Peace-Builders have effects that are noticeable among students or adults within a day or two, and tend to accelerate as more of the notes are used.[127,128]

3. *Testing in ABA Studies:* MEBs are not abstractions or "just labels" to families, teachers, or even the young people affected by those disorders. Rather, the disorders entail noticeable events that can happen many times in a day or an hour. For example, a child with oppositional defiance disorder may easily engage in oppositional, disturbing, or disruptive behavior 10 to 50 times per hour at home or in the classroom, depending on the antecedents or behavior of parents, teachers, siblings, or peers.[129,130] Therefore, consumer-friendly prevention products for oppositional defiance must have behavioral benefits that can be easily proven by direct observation and with consumer satisfaction. This proof is best done in reversal or multiple-baseline (ABA) studies that use repeated measures of the "symptoms" in real time.[131,132] That is, the intervention can reliably demonstrate, within subjects, behavior change in symptoms. This feature is a critical one for dissemination and diffusion because it means that most consumers who adopt it will experience benefit for themselves—not just between group differences. That is, consumers can see, hear, feel, or otherwise notice differences directly. The subjects do not care whether 25% of the treatment group gets better; they care about their own situation getting better. The benefits are not abstract or delayed in time to consumers. It is useful to note that many of the most powerful prevention programs and practices listed in the IOM Report such as the Good Behavior Game or Triple P had some 60 or more ABA studies[52,62] long-before any of major randomized trials, providing a thorough understanding of active ingredients, problems of use, and linkages to measureable benefits achieved quickly and reliably. Testing strategies used in ABA studies means that a developer must pay attention to producing measurable benefit to the consumer, rather than obfuscating weak strategies by blaming the consumer for denial, resistance, laziness, or other attributions. These proximal benefits, sensitive to an ABA design, are not limited to just home or classroom interventions. For example, in the case of the tobacco prevention effort, the community measures of reduced illegal sales of tobacco were easily measured in weeks at a community or even state level.[100,101,120] Such designs can detect many community actions.[133–137]

A USEFUL ADDITION TO PUBLIC HEALTH PREVENTION NOMENCLATURE: EVIDENCE-BASED KERNELS AND BEHAVIORAL VACCINES

The etiology and epidemiology of MEBs challenges the notion that prevention, intervention, and treatment require complex evidence-based programs. Consider a few examples that can be found of such etiology and epidemiology in the Institute of Medicine Report on Prevention.[1]

- Dishion and colleagues (IOM[p270]) proved deviant adolescent behavior follows the Matching Law,[138,139] predicting delinquency rates over time.[140] Strategies, however, that deliberately manipulate the Matching Law to increase peer social reinforcement for nondeviant behaviors and reduce accidental attention to deviant behavior prevent such delinquent or risky behavior in the short and long term.[54,57,59,124,125] This effect can be demonstrated experimentally in a single classroom.[127] Strategies such as Good Behavior Game[52] or Peace-Builders[141] explicitly make use of the Matching Law.
- Hibbeln and colleagues have clearly demonstrated that deficiency of omega-3 in the American diet is associated with MEBs (IOM[pp213–4]). Randomized, placebo-controlled trials show that the provision of omega-3 reduces MEBs in children and adolescents.[47,48,142]

- Multiple references in the IOM Report[pp182,189,216] cite aggression at school as a significant and malleable predictor of MEBs. While such aggression can be clearly reduced by various programs and curricula, aggressive or disruptive behavior can be averted by multiple examples of interventions that do not rise to the level of programs or curricula. Here are a few simple strategies that have experimental demonstrations to reduce aggression at school, even among very high-risk children or teens: (1) positive notes home[128,143–145]; (2) beat the timer in the classroom to reduce dawdling and disruption[146,147]; (3) group public feedback with group rewards[148]; (4) reduction of TV viewing and video game use at home reduces aggression at school[149]; and (5) cooperative games on the playground.[150,151]
- Parental substance abuse has many adverse effects on mental, emotional, and behavioral disorders among infants, children, and adolescents (IOM[pp161,422]). Home-visiting programs such as the Nurse Family Partnership (NFP) have argued that much of NFP effects stem from reducing tobacco use in pregnant mothers.[152,153] There is good epidemiological evidence to support this assertion, as reviewed by Biglan and colleagues.[4] Can such impact on maternal smoking be achieved more cost efficiently? The answer is clearly yes. Multiple experiments have shown that straightforward contingency management systems have more robust impact on cessation rates of tobacco among high-risk women,[154] as well as for alcohol or illegal drugs, than home-visiting programs alone.[155–157] A major reason for the substantial attrition rates in home-visiting programs (25%–75%) and poor outcomes are addictions and associated domestic violence.[158–160] Thus, using simple cost-efficient tools such as contingency management has considerable public health or safety benefits in reducing addictions among women child-bearing age and men.[156,161–170]

These and other examples of simple behavioral strategies in the prevention of MEBs have historically lacked any kind of a taxonomy or synthesis. Such examples are widespread in the scientific literature, but seldom rise in major awareness in policy and practice initiatives. The IOM Report, however, highlights an emerging nomenclature for such preventive, intervention, and treatment strategies[pp210,420]: evidence-based kernels and behavioral vaccines, defined as follows.

- *Evidence-based kernels* are fundamental units of behavioral influence.[171] Every kernel must have peer-reviewed, published experimental studies demonstrating effects. In an earlier article,[171] Biglan and the author offered this definition:

An evidence-based kernel is an indivisible procedure empirically shown to produce reliable effects on behavior, including psychological processes.[72] The unit is indivisible in the sense that it would be ineffective upon elimination of any of its components. Examples of kernels include timeout, written praise notes, self-monitoring, framing relations among stimuli to affect the value of a given stimulus, and increasing Omega-3 fatty acids in the diet in order to influence behavior. A kernel may increase the frequency of a behavior or it may make a behavior less likely. It can have its impact by altering antecedent or consequent events in the psychological environment of the person or it can affect behavior by directly manipulating a physiological function. Kernels, by definition, target a single behavior, whereas programs typically target multiple behaviors.

- *Behavioral vaccines* are a repeated use of kernel or a simple recipe of kernels that prevent or reduce morbidity or mortality or improve wellbeing. Hand washing or buckling a seatbelt are clear health examples of behavioral vaccines. The Good Behavior Game (IOM[p184]) is a behavioral vaccine, which involves several kernels in a recipe used several times a day to reduce disturbing and disruptive behavior in a classroom and has large immediate effects on such behaviors.[52] The Good Behavior Game has major long-term outcomes for multiple MEBs in longitudinal randomized control trials.[54,55,57,59] The Substance Abuse and Mental Health Services Administration is funding a 10-school district demonstration of the Good Behavior Game in 2010 (RFA SM-10-017).

Can evidence-based kernels (or, behavioral vaccines) be used for major public health and public safety benefit in the prevention of MEBs? The author argues affirmatively, yes.

Consider a proof of concept based on Biglan's earlier work on Reward and Reminder (R&R).[100,101] R&R consists of 3 basic evidence-based kernels: (1) a relational frame about prosocial behavior of not selling tobacco to minors, (2) mystery shoppers who reward and recognize clerks/stores who do not sell tobacco to minors, and (3) public posting of the stores/clerks who do not sell. This recipe, which is repeated in communities or states, has immediate effects on reducing illegal sales of tobacco. When the kernel recipe is repeated in states for a year or so, there are related declines in any self-reported tobacco use by minors in the last 30 days and tobacco use every day in the last month.[120]

There are other examples that suggest the use of kernels might have some impact on selected, indicated, and universal prevention, as shown in **Table 1**, which is adapted from the 2008 article by Embry and Biglan on kernels.[171] **Table 1** provides an example from the 4 types of evidence-based kernels: reinforcement, relational, physiological, and antecedent.

Multiple kernels can be used for indicated, selected, and universal prevention, as illustrated in **Table 1**. Many can be used in homes, schools, organizations, clinical practice, and even the mass media for varying levels of intensity, as depicted in **Fig. 1**. **Fig. 1** also shows that kernels and related behavioral vaccines have potential impact across every human developmental stage.

These features have many advantages for policy and practice. First, this means that training of communities and individuals can be far more cost efficient. Second, the widespread utility means that it will be far easier to maintain outcomes in organizations or communities over time. Third, the modular nature of kernels means that community providers and organizations will be better able to respond effectively to new prevention or treatment issues, because new threats arise all the time for which there will be no evidence-based program per se, such as the methamphetamine epidemic. Such multilevel models are clearly more cost efficient, and are likely to be more effective in terms of Quality-Adjusted Life Years (QALYS).[51,90]

For kernels or kernel recipes (or policy or program, for that matter) to have population-level effects on public health or public safety (eg, whole communities, counties, states, or provinces), it is necessary for the RE-AIM formula to be applied.[172,173] RE-AIM stands for Reach, Efficacy, Adoption, Implementation, and Maintenance. This formula proposes that a large number of people must buy or select ("Adopt") the strategy, typically around 20% or more to have a major impact. More than 20% (say 30%–50%) will have to be "Reached" to get 20% to adopt the strategy. The adoption rate is moderated by the "Efficacy" of the strategy: the bigger the effect size, the fewer people required to impact population-level numbers. If a very large number of people adopt a weak strategy, there can still be population impact. "Implementation" means the percentage of people who actually use the adopted strategy. "Maintenance" refers to percentage of people who continue to use a strategy, if that is required to sustain effects.

Table 1
Example of kernel utility for selected, indicated, and universal prevention

Evidence-Based Kernel	Selected Prevention	Indicated Prevention	Universal Prevention
Prize bowl/mystery motivator (reinforcement kernel)	Reduce alcohol, tobacco or drug use[161,163,164] Improve engagement in treatment goals[169,170]	Reduce problem behavior in high-risk children or youth[222–224]	Improve engaged learning of whole class and reduce disruptions of whole class[225–227]
Goal/node mapping (relational frame kernel)	Reduce relapse or recidivism rates[228,229] Improve recovery[230]	Prevent use rates of alcohol, tobacco, and other drugs[228,231] Improve attainment of therapeutic goals[231,232]	Increase academic success or cognitive processes[233–236]
Omega-3 fatty acid supplementation (physiological kernel)	Treat depression, borderline and/or bipolar disorder[70] Reduce autism symptoms[71,142]	Prevent emergence of psychotic episodes in prodromal adolescents[47]	Improve children's cognitive performance and prevent behavioral disorders[69,237–239]
Public posting (antecedent kernel)	Reduce community illegal behaviors[100,101,120]	Improve problematic behavior in therapeutic settings[240,241]	Reduce impulsive or risky behaviors in general population[242,243] Improved academics[244–246] Promoting participation or community goods[247,248]

POLICY ACTIONS

The IOM Report[pp388–92] notes that other rich countries are far more advanced in applying prevention science, with the irony that most of the research for these efforts comes from the United States, and is even true for northern neighbors Canada. For example, the province of Manitoba established the Healthy Child Committee of Cabinet, which

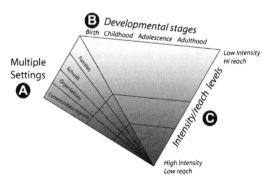

Fig. 1. Potential reach of evidence-based kernels for public health prevention effects. (*Courtesy of* PAXIS Institute, Tuscon, AZ; with permission. Available at: www.paxis.org.)

brought universal parenting support for the whole province as a true population-level, public health model using the Triple P model highlighted in the IOM Report. Norway has implemented the original parenting behavioral vaccine discovered in North America[174–176] throughout the entire country,[177] which is probably one of the reasons why Norway has a lower national incidence of MEBs compared with other countries, as noted in the IOM Report.[5] As injury-control research on car safety seats was translated into broad public policy years ago, so can prevention science involving evidence-based kernels for MEBs. A few policy actions exist that could make a big impact:

1. *Unleash Consumer Access:* Expand the scope of CDC and other health and/or prevention agencies, to deliver and promote evidence-based kernels or behavioral vaccine recipes, just as they promote medical vaccines for common childhood diseases. These agencies could facilitate and enable direct consumer access (eg, parents, teachers, business owners) to scientifically proven kernels or behavioral vaccines that can be easily adopted and implemented in homes, classrooms, and community settings. This process would follow along the same lines as those involving injury-control products that are now easily accessible consumer products and have clearly reduced injuries and deaths—from car seats, to latches, to nonslip rugs, to protective helmets, and so forth. The expansion of behavioral vaccines could include special calls for Small Business Innovation Research awards (SBIR) initiatives as well as special private sector incentives or state/local initiatives. Of note, not a single evidence-based program/practice on the NREPP is available at Amazon.com—the largest book store in the world.
2. *Create Third-Party Reimbursements:* HealthCare.gov (www.healthcare.gov/law/provisions/preventive/index.htm) notes some important inclusions and coverage about prevention in the Health Care Reform Act:

   "Counseling from your health care provider on such topics as quitting smoking, losing weight, eating better, treating depression, and reducing alcohol use…" Multiple evidence-based kernels cited in the Embry and Biglan 2008 article have such prevention effects.[171] Thus, providers' time taken to prescribe and recommend such kernels and the actual goods/materials/instructions ought to be reimbursable or otherwise covered.

   "Counseling and guidance from your doctor about your child's health development…" Because multiple evidence-based kernels and related behavioral vaccines actually improve the health outcomes, such kernels and services of the provider are logically reimbursable or otherwise covered.

   "Special, pregnancy-tailored counseling from a doctor that will help pregnant women quit smoking and avoid alcohol use…" Again, multiple evidence-based kernels have clear evidence of those effects, noted in the review by Embry and Biglan. The time and related prescription for behavior change need to be covered, because these kernels are highly cost effective.

   "Screenings and counseling to prevent, detect, and treat common childhood problems…" The IOM Report and the Embry and Biglan review clearly document low-cost kernels or behavioral vaccines that prevent or treat common childhood problems such as ADHD, oppositional defiance, anxiety, phobias, depression, aggression, and learning disabilities. By logic and legislative intent, such low-cost strategies when based in solid evidence ought to be fully covered and reimbursable.

   "Immunizations like an annual flu vaccine and many other childhood vaccinations and boosters, from the measles to polio…" There are equally powerful

"behavioral vaccines," and such behavioral vaccines are substantially less expensive and/or cost effective[51,58,90] than any listed medical vaccine on the CDC Web site.

Make selected kernels or behavioral vaccines reimbursable in health-care reform just as childhood medical vaccines are. The United States government presently recommends that all children receive approximately $2400 worth of medical vaccines (see www.cdc.gov/vaccines/programs/vfc/cdc-vac-price-list.htm), excluding the cost of promotion and delivery. The total costs of these medical vaccines to almost every child in the United States are paid for largely by third-party sources in the form of government or privately funded health care. In summary, cost-efficient kernels or behavioral vaccines in the IOM Report like Triple P, the Good Behavior Game, or supplementation of omega-3 deficiency can clearly prevent or reduce costly problems such as ADHD,[51,64] oppositional defiance,[51,64] conduct disorder,[51,178] or psychotic disorders.[47,48] Therefore, these cost-effective strategies must become reimbursable in the context of the reconciliation bill for Health-Care Reform passed by the US Senate. Quick deployment of these incentives gives patients and physicians or licensed caregivers additional, low-cost options, which could significantly affect health care costs quickly, as well as improve public indicators of wellbeing. It is useful to note that no prescription psychotropics, which are largely reimbursed by third parties, have been scientifically documented to prevent MEBs in children or adolescents. However, several evidence-based kernels or behavioral vaccines described herein have been scientifically proven in peer-reviewed, high-quality journals to prevent costly MEBs.[47,49,54,55,57,59,64] Preventive childhood "behavioral vaccines" need to be on reimbursement parity with childhood medical vaccines, as do the kernels or behavior vaccines that are proven to reduce, abate, or stop the symptoms of MEBs. These kernels or behavioral vaccines need to be on parity with prescription medications for the same disorders, because there is compelling emerging evidence that such kernels or behavioral vaccines are often substantially more cost effective. Further, they are more correlated to positive outcomes with fewer measured adverse medical events (eg, sudden cardiac death, psychosis, suicidality, metabolic disorders, abuse of prescription drugs by others or self).[38,51,55,58,59,90,179]

3. *Initiate Public/Private Prevention Mobilizations:* Key leaders (eg, governors, mayors, first spouses of high elected officials, CEOs, corporate boards, and other leaders) could convene these partnerships to facilitate focused community mobilization prevention efforts. When communities mobilize around clear, simple evidence-based prevention strategies for many or all, there is consistent evidence that rapid change in major outcomes can happen. This evidence comes from multiple sources including parenting literature,[49,50,180,181] tobacco control literature,[99,100,120] alcohol prevention efforts for communities,[182-184] youth substance abuse,[180,181] and health disparities efforts[185] as well as charitable activities such as United Way and Toys for Tots. Focused community mobilizations or projects are different than broad-capacity building or needs assessments efforts. Focused mobilizations or projects have clear objective goals and behavior-change strategies, rather than emphasizing developmental processes or attitudinal change. Successful focused mobilizations also avoid overt or accidental stigmatization by appealing to the broader good and not isolating those at risk or implying blame. Focused models are especially powerful when the risks are widely distributed and the harms or benefits are widespread, such as for the prevalence of most MEBs (including addictions) among children and youth. These public/private

partnerships leverage resources to contain the nation's most expensive problems, and reinforce and strengthen self-sufficiency rather than dependency.

4. *Use Proven, Powerful Marketing Campaign Strategies:* Collegiate and professional sports use powerful marketing strategies to engage many people, and these same strategies have powerful analogs in public health approaches for prevention. Media campaigns must urge people to join in common clear actions, rather than promote stigma, blame, fear, or mere "awareness." Campaigns must have highly publicized "scoreboards" of people joining and participating as well as goals being achieved. The campaigns must:

- Create a sense of belonging to something bigger and socially desirable
- Emphasize outcomes and measures that are visible or understandable to most citizens, not obtuse or infrequent measures
- Use "soft" competition between communities or groups to boost engagement in the goals
- Give everybody something to do that makes a difference (which can include cheering, wearing alignment symbols, and so forth).

Within the efforts, there are many opportunities for groups (businesses, individuals, organizations, and so forth) to be "sponsors" of the efforts. Further, such campaigns provide frequent rewards and recognition for change. These "social marketing" principles for prevention have been outlined in successful behavior-change studies.[72,120] The campaigns must use powerful techniques that have previously demonstrated success, including:

- Testimonials[186]
- "Tupperware" type events or "tell 2 friends"—which, interestingly, has even been used to market new tobacco products that the author and colleagues are trying to prevent[187]
- "Mobbing" or "viral" methods with Internet media.[187–190]

When these principles are used in prevention campaigns, very high levels of participation and behavior change are possible.[50,72,118,120]

5. *Create Cost-Saving Estimators:* Every business plan includes a break-even analysis and a profit-and-loss analysis, but this simply does not happen with the prevention of MEBs (including addictions). It is true that the IOM Report includes a discussion of the benefits and costs of prevention (Chapter 9[pp241–62]), as do other documents such as the *Shoveling UP Report*,[191] which details the state-level burden of substance abuse. However, these documents are not sufficient for policy planning any more than reading an accounting textbook is sufficient for predicting the profitability of any given business per se, in the absence of a specific financial audit. While QALYS are used in academic literature, they are less useful for elected officials and the multiple agencies they govern when it comes to figuring out how to balance federal, state, county, or local budgets affected by MEBs. Policy makers need straightforward spreadsheet estimators (like one would find in a software package for a business plan) to show what the positive impact (costs averted or savings) might be across governmental agency budgetary silos. These spreadsheet estimators need to have sliders, which policy makers or their staff can easily adjust to examine different assumptions. These estimators are vital when considering prevention strategies because there are proximal, immediate, and distal benefits across budgetary silos.

Can this be done? The answer is yes. The population-level study of the effects of the Triple P study (see IOM[p167] for description) funded by the CDC[49] provides an excellent platform for illustration. First, the effect sizes for child maltreatment are at a population level, meaning that one only needs to input population data and matching prevalence rates for any selected political jurisdiction—all of which are federally collected. Second, the costs of implementation are established in a peer-reviewed publication.[90] Third, collateral benefits across silos have been demonstrated in a peer-reviewed publication.[51] Fourth, cost savings from problems prevented by Triple P have independent assessments.[91] Accordingly, a demonstration of such an estimator has been created showing 3 benefit domains for each state, with adjusters for some assumptions. This estimator is visible and downloadable at www.paxis.org/triplep. **Figs. 2–4** illustrate a series of screen snapshots showing the impact on 3 specific outcomes associated with MEBs and the costs averted or saved using federally reported data: reduced substantiated cases of child maltreatment, reduced out-of-home placements of dependent children, and averted lifetime cases of conduct disorders (estimated from studies).

Businesses routinely develop profit-and-loss estimates and break-even analyses for new products that have not even been sold. It is also quite possible and realistic to develop similar estimators for proven and tested prevention strategies to guide policy and practice.

The estimator shows that the predicted prevention effects could avert many cases and save a great deal of money in the immediate term, with compounded long-term savings. The savings from reduced out-of-home placement alone would more than pay for the marginal costs of implementation. The impact on lifetime conduct disorders would solely have a major impact of billions of dollars on California public finances within 5 to 10 years.[91]

6. *Measuring Population-Level Impact of Major Public Health Initiatives:* Academic and scientific journals are now filled with evidence-based prevention trials, almost all of them efficacy trials of individuals or schools. An efficacy trial, however, is deliberately designed to insulate both the strategy and subjects (persons or settings) from the vicissitudes of real-world conditions (policies, program staffing,

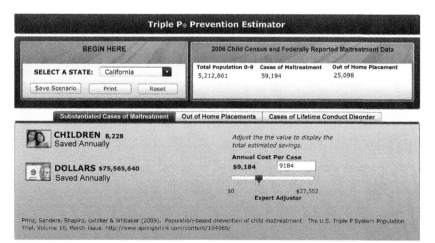

Fig. 2. Impact estimator on substantiated child maltreatment. (*Courtesy of* PAXIS Institute, Tuscon, AZ; with permission. Available at: www.paxis.org.)

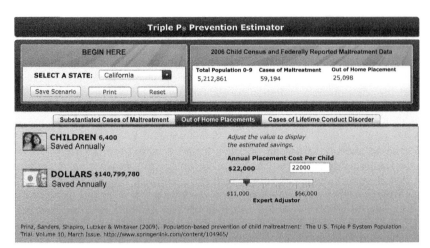

Fig. 3. Impact estimator for out-of-home placements. (*Courtesy of* PAXIS Institute, Tuscon, AZ; with permission. Available at: www.paxis.org.)

resources, management issues, and so forth) that might affect the main factors being tested. That said, stunning results in exquisite efficacy trials do not guarantee similar or desired results in other effectiveness trials, which has been demonstrated in a variety of controlled prevention studies.[192,193] Efficacy trials of prevention protocols may show proximal changes on knowledge, attitudes, and some behaviors, yet not show any impact on "big-ticket" outcomes sought by policy makers when put in a large-scale effectiveness trial.[194] There are many sound reasons for this frequent finding:

> Early randomized trials with simple pre- and post-test data alone will seriously underestimate natural and structural sources of variability associated with effectiveness. For example, efficacy trials often buy off in-service days, give teachers cash incentives, and offer exemptions from normal organization requirements. A few measures will not allow the investigators to see

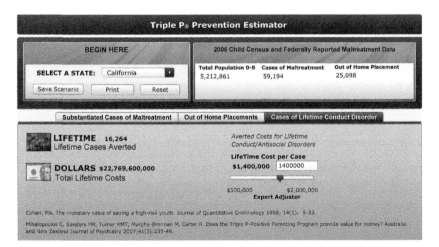

Fig. 4. Impact estimator on lifetime conduct disorders. (*Courtesy of* PAXIS Institute, Tuscon, AZ; with permission. Available at: www.paxis.org.)

confounding influences, such as new policies, rules, or other events. Thus, the experimental design masks important externalities and contingencies. Failure in the "real world" is then almost certain.

Studies using repeated measures (eg, hourly, daily, weekly, or monthly) in reversal or multiple baseline experimental designs, however, do allow identification of naturally occurring contingencies and externalities. Virtually all of the best preventive interventions in the IOM Report (eg, Triple P, Good Behavior Game, Incredible Years, Parent Management Training) all have very powerful histories of reversal designs or multiple baselines BEFORE they were evaluated in randomized trials. These designs are not well covered in most textbooks in graduate schools, and are often labeled as inferior by labels such as "quasi-experimental." There is, however, a fundamental truth: if you cannot demonstrate experimental effects in an interrupted time-series design (reversal, multiple-baseline, multicomponent, or multi-probe design),[195–198] a randomized trial will almost certainly show no effects, weak effects or, worse, adverse effects. There are sound logical, epidemiological, methodological, and practical reasons to measure early effects by such designs—especially when the ultimate intent is for large public health approaches.[131,133,199] After such proof, efficacy trials are more likely to have robust effects when brought to scale.

Interrupted time-series designs (which can also be randomized) reemerge when it comes time to test big effects across big political units (eg, counties, states, or provinces). Such political units of analysis are important for public health and policies. It is theoretically possible to randomize such political units, but obviously difficult. In some cases, it will be impossible for legal or ethical reasons. One can then turn to interrupted time-series designs for measuring prevention outcomes at population levels. Wagenaar and colleagues proved the utility of such designs for community-level alcohol use prevention.[134–137,200,201] Anthony Biglan and the author have used such designs for a multiple-baseline study across states using archival data collected under the direction of the Federal Government.

In **Fig. 5**, one can see the effects of R&R for not selling tobacco in Wyoming and Wisconsin. The author's group replicated this earlier in an interrupted time-series and randomized trial in small communities in Oregon.[100,101] In **Fig. 6**, one can also see the correlated impact of R&R on cigarette smoking, measured by the CDC's YRBS survey, among Wyoming and Wisconsin adolescents. The time series design also allows for an analysis of other contextual events, such as the $1 per pack tax increase in Wisconsin on smoking every day (but not on any smoking in the last 30 days). Because governments and agencies can rarely roll out a program in every large jurisdiction effectively, the use of interrupted time-series designs allows for a reasonable contextual approach to evaluating public health approaches to prevention. Another advantage of these designs is that the results are easy to convey to elected officials, policy makers, the general public, and the media.

ECONOMIC IMPACT

The United States and Canadian federal governments, state or provincial governments, local governments, businesses, and citizens or taxpayers have much to gain by widespread implementation of behavioral vaccines and kernels. For example, most states could recover the cost of implementation in 2 years by reducing expenditure for child maltreatment.[51,90] In the course of 2 to 5 years, there should be lower

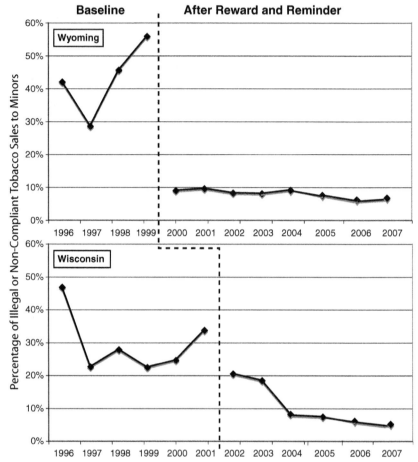

Fig. 5. Impact of reward and reminder on illegal tobacco sales across states. (*Courtesy of* PAXIS Institute, Tuscon, AZ; with permission. Available at: www.paxis.org.)

rates of DSM-IV (*Diagnostic and Statistical Manual of Mental Disorders* Fourth Edition, Text Revised) diagnoses and prescription for psychotropic medications in the pediatric population.[47,51,64,70,178,202] Over the course of a decade, school districts could potentially cut their special education expenditures by one third, because fewer children would need such services.[44,47,51,54,69,71,142] Over the course of the same decade, the juvenile and adult criminal justice system would see lower drug-related crimes and violent crime rates, including homicides.[38,39,51,57,59,203–206] Communities would see lower rates of tobacco use in youth in 5 to 7 years[60,207,208] as well as reductions in alcohol and illegal drug use by adolescents and young adults in 5 to 10 years.[56,57,59,209,210] All of these changes translate into reductions of short-, medium-, and long-term health care, education, social service, and public safety costs.

Costs of Risky Behaviors

By any calculation imaginable, the costs associated with risky human behaviors from childhood through adulthood are the deepest well of private and public expenditures in the United States (IOM[pp251–3]) and many industrialized nations. This well of despair

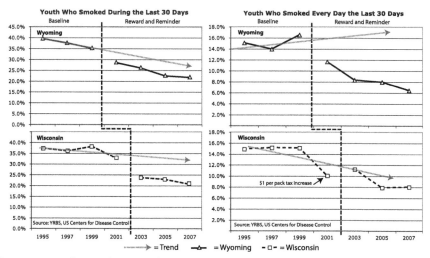

Fig. 6. Impact of reward & reminder on youth tobacco use across states. (*Courtesy of* PAXIS Institute, Tuscon, AZ; with permission. Available at: www.paxis.org.)

includes violence, addictions, mental illnesses, obesity, many cancers, cardiovascular diseases, unintentional injuries, and more. Consider just this one quotation from the IOM report[p252]:

> Miller (in Biglan, Brennan, and colleagues, 2004) provides a much higher estimate of $435.4 billion in 1998 ($557.3 in 2007 dollars) for the costs of problem behaviors among youth, defined as underage drinking, heroin or cocaine abuse, high-risk sex, youth violence, youth smoking, high school dropout, and youth suicide acts. More than half was attributable to suffering and quality of life, with the balance consisting of work losses, medical spending, and other resource costs. Averaged across all youth, this would be an average cost of $12,300 per youth ages 12–20 ($15,744 in 2007 dollars).

The IOM gives an alternative, lower estimate (IOM[p251]), suggesting that the total annual economic costs for MEBs of people younger than 25 are roughly $247 billion as of 2007 (in 2007 dollars), or about $2380 per person younger than 25 years. This per-person total includes about $500 in health service costs and $1900 in health, productivity, and crime-related costs.

Total Annual Cost Burden

The total cost burden of MEBs therefore almost certainly ranges from $250 to $500 billion per year for young people in the United States alone. This situation is not good for North America's future and global competitiveness, when one considers that base rates for many such disorders are worse than other rich countries that compete against the United States. This burden is particularly acute for the more expensive problems involving disturbing, disruptive, aggressive, and criminal behaviors.[7,36,37]

Cost-Burden Silo Example

Let us examine the cost of just one of the MEB "silos", ADHD. Children who manifest early ADHD (about 3%–7% of children in the United States) have high probability of school failure or learning disabilities[211,212]; intentional and unintentional injuries[213,214];

conduct disorders, crime, and delinquency[215]; alcohol, tobacco, and drug addictions[216]; development of other serious mental illnesses such as bipolar disorder or other mental illnesses[217]; increased cancer risk[218]; sudden cardiac death[219]; work-related problems[220]; and difficult social relationships in marriage and child-rearing as adults. The behavioral footprints of ADHD help explain its fiscal footprints.

In the United States in 2003, the direct cost of Medicaid attributable to children with ADHD was $2.15 billion dollars annually—about 2% of all health care costs for children.[221] However, this is an underestimate of national costs. An analysis by a private insurance company suggests the total excess cost of ADHD in the United States in 2000 was $31.6 billion. Of this total, $1.6 billion was for the ADHD treatment of patients, $12.1 billion was for all other health care costs of persons with ADHD, $14.2 billion was for all other health care costs of family members of persons with ADHD, and $3.7 billion was for the work loss cost of adults with ADHD and adult family members of persons with ADHD. Pelham and colleagues,[15] using a conservative prevalence rate of 5%, computed the annual societal cost of illness for ADHD in childhood and adolescence at $42.5 billion, with a range between $36 billion and $52.4 billion. Their estimates are preliminary because the literature is incomplete; many potential costs have not been assessed in extant studies.

There are now multiple behavioral vaccines and evidence-based kernels that prevent, reduce the symptoms, or avert the sequelae of ADHD,[43,51,54,59,60,64,71,171] at a far lower cost and risk of adverse medical consequences. Those behavior vaccines or kernels, all together, do not rise to the cost of 1 or 2 months of therapy on any of the psychotropic drugs being used with ADHD-diagnosed children or youth.

SUMMARY

Policy and practice for the prevention of MEBs (which includes addictions) must include a public health approach to reach all children, families, and communities; this is one of the key messages of the IOM Report. The response to unique individual, family, school, neighborhood, or community risk factors will be most cost efficient, if the "pump handle of John Snow" for the contaminated well that serves all is removed first. This action must happen before implementation of special interventions that might be needed for those more vulnerable to the contaminated water.

The IOM Report[1] clearly outlines that we have a public health problem of MEBs, and a public health approach to affect all children and youth is required to move the population-level indicators. The population-level public health approach often remediates the most difficult problems and difficult instances in controlled studies,[49,50] which then lessens the costs of reaching higher-risk groups. In this spirit, the IOM Report wisely calls on America to move from a "treatment-oriented" approach to prevention to a true public health approach, wherein prevention is available for every child, family, school, or community to prevent MEBs, including addictions. Evidence-based kernels and behavioral vaccines offer a unique opportunity for the prevention of MEBs to happen at a public health level. The fact that kernels can be used for universal, selected, and indicated prevention represents considerable cost efficiencies. Psychiatrists, physicians, mental health professionals, school counselors, juvenile justice professionals, and others can clearly make use of evidence-based kernels for selected or indicated prevention. An even larger number of parents, teachers, and others can use kernels to improve the odds for children, youth, and young adults.

The time to act is now: the IOM Report outlines the compelling reasons to expand prevention in North America.[1] There is an urgent need for the health of the nation, given epidemiological trends. There is an economic necessity for safety and security of the

Republic. While our most potent economic competitors are already acting for their immediate and long-term benefit, there are promising pathways for action via health care reform and related initiatives. The true wealth of a nation derives from the health of all the minds, bodies, spirits, and behaviors of its children and youth. Let us act for all our futures.

REFERENCES

1. O'Connell ME, Boat T, Warner KE, editors. Preventing mental, emotional, and behavioral disorders among young people: progress and possibilities. Washington, DC: Institute of Medicine; National Research Council; 2009. Committee on the Prevention of Mental Disorders and Substance Abuse Among Children, Youth and Young Adults: Research Advances and Promising Interventions.
2. McMichael WH. Most U.S. youths unfit to serve, data show. Army Times November 5, 2009.
3. Schmitt J, Lane N. Small-business employment in 22 rich economies. Int J Health Serv 2010;40(1):151–63.
4. Biglan A, Brennan PA, Foster SL, et al. Helping adolescents at risk: prevention of multiple problem behaviors. New York: Guilford Press; 2004.
5. Heiervang E, Goodman A, Goodman R. The Nordic advantage in child mental health: separating health differences from reporting style in a cross-cultural comparison of psychopathology. J Child Psychol Psychiatry 2008;49(6):678–85.
6. Heiervang E, Stormark KM, Lundervold AJ, et al. Psychiatric disorders in Norwegian 8- to 10-year-olds: an epidemiological survey of prevalence, risk factors, and service use. J Am Acad Child Adolesc Psychiatry 2007;46(4):438–47.
7. Collishaw S, Maughan B, Goodman R, et al. Time trends in adolescent mental health. J Child Psychol Psychiatry 2004;45(8):1350–62.
8. Krieger N. Theories for social epidemiology in the 21st century: an ecosocial perspective. Int J Epidemiol 2001;30(4):668–77.
9. Krieger N. A glossary for social epidemiology. J Epidemiol Community Health 2001;55(10):693–700.
10. Singer M, Clair S. Syndemics and public health: reconceptualizing disease in bio-social context. Med Anthropol Q 2003;17(4):423–41.
11. Trochim WM, Cabrera DA, Milstein B, et al. Practical challenges of systems thinking and modeling in public health. Am J Public Health 2006;96(3):538–46.
12. Hudson CG. Validation of a model for estimating state and local prevalence of serious mental illness. Int J Meth Psychiatr Res 2009;18(4):251–64.
13. Young AS, Klap R, Shoai R, et al. Persistent depression and anxiety in the United States: prevalence and quality of care. Psychiatr Serv 2008;59(12):1391–8.
14. Kessler RC, Wang PS. The descriptive epidemiology of commonly occurring mental disorders in the United States. Annu Rev Public Health 2008;29:115–29.
15. Pelham WE, Foster EM, Robb JA. The economic impact of attention-deficit/hyperactivity disorder in children and adolescents. J Pediatr Psychol 2007;32(6):711–27.
16. Kelleher KJ. Use of services and costs for youth with ADHD and related conditions. Attention deficit hyperactivity disorder: state of the science-best practices. Kingston (NJ): Civic Research Institute; 2002. p. 27–14.
17. Wymbs BT, Pelham WE Jr. Child effects on communication between parents of youth with and without attention-deficit/hyperactivity disorder. J Abnorm Psychol 2010;119(2):366–75.
18. Wymbs BT. Does disruptive child behavior cause interparental discord? An experimental manipulation, US ProQuest Information & Learning. Buffalo (NY): State University of New York; 2009.

19. Smith DH. Review of ADHD in adults: what the science says. Can J Psychiatr Rev Canad Psychiatr 2009;54(6):423–4.
20. Heckel LD, Clarke AR, Barry RJ, et al. The relationship between divorce and children with AD/HD of different subtypes and comorbidity: results from a clinically referred sample. J Divorce & Remarriage 2009;50(6):427–43.
21. Heckel L, Clarke A, Barry R, et al. The relationship between divorce and the psychological well-being of children with ADHD: differences in age, gender, and subtype. Emotional & Behavioural Difficulties 2009;14(1):49–68.
22. Wymbs BT, Pelham WE Jr, Molina BSG, et al. Rate and predictors of divorce among parents of youths with ADHD. J Consult Clin Psychol 2008;76(5):735–44.
23. Semiz UB, Basoglu C, Oner O, et al. Effects of diagnostic comorbidity and dimensional symptoms of attention-deficit-hyperactivity disorder in men with antisocial personality disorder. Aust N Z J Psychiatry 2008;42(5):405–13.
24. Sartor CE, Lynskey MT, Heath AC, et al. The role of childhood risk factors in initiation of alcohol use and progression to alcohol dependence. Addiction 2007; 102(2):216–25.
25. Kessler RC, Aguilar-Gaxiola S, Alonso J, et al. The global burden of mental disorders: an update from the WHO World Mental Health (WMH) Surveys. Epidemiol Psichiatr Soc 2009;18(1):23–33.
26. Pilette PC. Presenteeism & productivity: two reasons employee assistance programs make good business cents. Ann Am Psychother Assoc 2005;8(1):12–4.
27. Biederman J. Impact of comorbidity in adults with attention deficit/hyperactivity disorder. J Clin Psychiatry 2004;65(Suppl 3):3–7.
28. Borsuk AJ. Cost of special education noted: MPS chief sees voucher inequities. Milwaukee-WIsconsin Journal Sentinel 2008.
29. Morrison I, Clift SM, Stosz LM. Supported further education provision for people with long-term mental health needs: findings from a survey of further education colleges and primary care trusts across the south east of England. Perspect Public Health 2010;130(2):78–85.
30. Marks DJ, Mlodnicka A, Bernstein M, et al. Profiles of service utilization and the resultant economic impact in preschoolers with attention deficit/hyperactivity disorder. J Pediatr Psychol 2009;34(6):681–9.
31. Gould E. Childhood lead poisoning: conservative estimates of the social and economic benefits of lead hazard control. Environ Health Perspect 2009; 117(7):1162–7.
32. Nyden A, Myren KJ, Gillberg C. Long-term psychosocial and health economy consequences of ADHD, autism, and reading-writing disorder: a prospective service evaluation project. J Atten Disord 2008;12(2):141–8.
33. Sices L, Harman JS, Kelleher KJ. Health-care use and expenditures for children in special education with special health-care needs: is dual classification a marker for high use? Public Health Rep 2007;122(4):531–40.
34. Pelham WE, Foster EM, Robb JA. The economic impact of attention-deficit/ hyperactivity disorder in children and adolescents. Ambul Pediatr 2007; 7(Suppl 1):121–31.
35. Rawe J. Who pays for special ed? Time 2006;168(13):62–3.
36. Costello EJ, Foley DL, Angold A. 10-year research update review: the epidemiology of child and adolescent psychiatric disorders: II. Developmental epidemiology. J Am Acad Child Adolesc Psychiatry 2006;45(1):8–25.
37. Costello EJ, Egger H, Angold A. 10-year research update review: the epidemiology of child and adolescent psychiatric disorders: I. Methods and public health burden. J Am Acad Child Adolesc Psychiatry 2005;44(10):972–86.

38. Hibbeln JR, Nieminen LR, Blasbalg TL, et al. Healthy intakes of n-3 and n-6 fatty acids: estimations considering worldwide diversity. Am J Clin Nutr 2006; 83(Suppl 6):1483S–93S.
39. Hibbeln JR, Nieminen LR, Lands WE. Increasing homicide rates and linoleic acid consumption among five Western countries, 1961–2000. Lipids 2004; 39(12):1207–13.
40. Howard AL, Robinson M, Smith GJ, et al. ADHD is associated with a 'western' dietary pattern in adolescents. J Atten Disord 2010. [Epub ahead of print].
41. Oddy WH, Robinson M, Ambrosini GL, et al. The association between dietary patterns and mental health in early adolescence. Prev Med 2009;49(1): 39–44.
42. McNeil DA, Wilson BN, Siever JE, et al. Connecting children to recreational activities: results of a cluster randomized trial. Am J Health Promot 2009; 23(6):376–87.
43. Sinn N, Bryan J. Effect of supplementation with polyunsaturated fatty acids and micronutrients on learning and behavior problems associated with child ADHD. J Dev Behav Pediatr 2007;28(2):82–91.
44. Richardson AJ, Montgomery P. The Oxford-Durham Study: a randomized, controlled trial of dietary supplementation with fatty acids in children with developmental coordination disorder. Pediatrics 2005;115(5):1360–6.
45. Thomas KC, Ellis AR, Konrad TR, et al. County-level estimates of mental health professional shortage in the United States. Psychiatr Serv 2009;60(10):1323–8.
46. Jagdeo A, Cox BJ, Stein MB, et al. Negative attitudes toward help seeking for mental illness in 2 population-based surveys from the United States and Canada. Can J Psychiatr Rev Canad Psychiatr 2009;54(11):757–66.
47. Amminger GP, Schafer MR, Papageorgiou K, et al. Long-chain {omega}-3 fatty acids for indicated prevention of psychotic disorders: a randomized, placebo-controlled trial. Arch Gen Psychiatry 2010;67(2):146–54.
48. Sinn N, Milte C, Howe PR. Oiling the brain: a review of randomized controlled trials of omega-3 fatty acids in psychopathology across the lifespan. Nutrients 2010;2(2):128–70.
49. Prinz RJ, Sanders MR, Shapiro CJ, et al. Population-based prevention of child maltreatment: the U.S. Triple P System Population Trial. Prev Sci 2009;10:1–12.
50. Sanders MR, Ralph A, Sofronoff K, et al. Every family: a population approach to reducing behavioral and emotional problems in children making the transition to school. J Prim Prev 2008;29(3):197–222.
51. Mihalopoulos C, Sanders MR, Turner KMT, et al. Does the Triple P-Positive Parenting Program provide value for money? Aust N Z J Psychiatry 2007; 41(3):239–46.
52. Embry DD. The good behavior game: a best practice candidate as a universal behavioral vaccine. Clin Child Fam Psychol Rev 2002;5(4):273–97.
53. Domitrovich CE, Bradshaw CP, Greenberg MT, et al. Integrated models of school-based prevention: logic and theory. Psychol Sch 2010;47(1):71–88.
54. Bradshaw CP, Zmuda JH, Kellam S, et al. Longitudinal impact of two universal preventive interventions in first grade on educational outcomes in high school. J Educ Psychol 2009;101(4):926–37.
55. Wilcox HC, Kellam S, Brown CH, et al. The impact of two universal randomized first- and second-grade classroom interventions on young adult suicide ideation and attempts [special issue]. Drug Alcohol Depend 2008;95(Suppl 1):S60–73.
56. Poduska JM, Kellam SG, Wang W, et al. Impact of the Good Behavior Game, a universal classroom-based behavior intervention, on young adult service

use for problems with emotions, behavior, or drugs or alcohol. Drug Alcohol Depend 2008;95(Suppl 1):S29–44.

57. Petras H, Kellam S, Brown CH, et al. Developmental epidemiological courses leading to antisocial personality disorder and violent and criminal behavior: effects by young adulthood of a universal preventive intervention in first- and second-grade classrooms [special issue]. Drug Alcohol Depend 2008;95(Suppl 1):45–59.

58. Miller TR, Hendrie D. Substance abuse prevention dollars and cents: a cost-benefit analysis. Substance Abuse and Mental Health Administration. Washington, DC: Center for Substance Abuse Prevention; 2008. Available at: http://download.ncadi.samhsa.gov/prevline/pdfs/SMA07-4298.pdf. Accessed November 11, 2010.

59. Kellam S, Brown CH, Poduska J, et al. Effects of a universal classroom behavior management program in first and second grades on young adult behavioral, psychiatric, and social outcomes [special issue]. Drug Alcohol Depend 2008; 95(Suppl 1):S5–28.

60. Huizink AC, van Lier PA, Crijnen AA. Attention deficit hyperactivity disorder symptoms mediate early-onset smoking. Eur Addict Res 2008;15(1):1–9.

61. Zito JM, Safer DJ, Berg LT, et al. A three-country comparison of psychotropic medication prevalence in youth. Child Adolesc Psychiatry Ment Health 2008; 2(1):26.

62. Sanders MR, Cann W, Markie-Dadds C. The triple P-positive parenting programme: a universal population-level approach to the prevention of child abuse. Child Abuse Rev 2003;12(3):155–71.

63. Bor W, Sanders MR, Markie-Dadds C. The effects of the Triple P-positive Parenting Program on preschool children with co-occurring disruptive behavior and attentional/hyperactive difficulties. J Abnorm Child Psychol 2002;30(6): 571–87.

64. van Lier PA, Muthen BO, van der Sar RM, et al. Preventing disruptive behavior in elementary schoolchildren: impact of a universal classroom-based intervention. J Consult Clin Psychol 2004;72(3):467–78.

65. Witvliet M, van Lier PA, Cuijpers P, et al. Testing links between childhood positive peer relations and externalizing outcomes through a randomized controlled intervention study. J Consult Clin Psychol 2009;77(5):905–15.

66. Sanders MR, Montgomery DT, Brechman-Toussaint ML. The mass media and the prevention of child behavior problems: the evaluation of a television series to promote positive outcome for parents and their children. J Child Psychol Psychiatry 2000;41(7):939–48.

67. Sanders M, Calam R, Durand M, et al. Does self-directed and web-based support for parents enhance the effects of viewing a reality television series based on the Triple P-Positive Parenting Programme? J Child Psychol Psychiatry 2008;49(9):924–32.

68. Calam R, Sanders MR, Miller C, et al. Can technology and the media help reduce dysfunctional parenting and increase engagement with preventative parenting interventions? Child Maltreat 2008;13(4):347–61.

69. Hibbeln J, Davis JM, Steer C, et al. Maternal seafood consumption in pregnancy and neurodevelopmental outcomes in childhood (ALSPAC study): an observational cohort study. Lancet 2007;369(9561):578–85.

70. Freeman MP, Hibbeln JR, Wisner KL, et al. Omega-3 fatty acids: evidence basis for treatment and future research in psychiatry. J Clin Psychiatry 2006;67(12): 1954–67.

71. Richardson AJ. Omega-3 fatty acids in ADHD and related neurodevelopmental disorders. Int Rev Psychiatry 2006;18(2):155–72.

72. Embry DD. Community-based prevention using simple, low-cost, evidence-based kernels and behavior vaccines. J Community Psychol 2004;32(5):575.
73. L'Abate L, editor. Low-cost approaches to promote physical and mental health: theory, research and practice. New York: Springer; 2007.
74. Baker A, Lewin T, Reichler H, et al. Evaluation of a motivational interview for substance use within psychiatric in-patient services. Addiction 2002;97(10): 1329–37.
75. Landback J, Prochaska M, Ellis J, et al. From prototype to product: development of a primary care/internet based depression prevention intervention for adolescents (CATCH-IT). Community Ment Health J 2009;45(5):349–54.
76. Martino S, Carroll KM, Nich C, et al. A randomized controlled pilot study of motivational interviewing for patients with psychotic and drug use disorders. Addiction 2006;101(10):1479–92.
77. Monti PM, Colby SM, Barnett NP, et al. Brief intervention for harm reduction with alcohol-positive older adolescents in a hospital emergency department. J Consult Clin Psychol 1999;67(6):989–94.
78. Mun EY, White HR, Morgan TJ. Individual and situational factors that influence the efficacy of personalized feedback substance use interventions for mandated college students. J Consult Clin Psychol 2009;77(1):88–102.
79. Thush C, Wiers RW, Moerbeek M, et al. Influence of motivational interviewing on explicit and implicit alcohol-related cognition and alcohol use in at-risk adolescents. Psychol Addict Behav 2009;23(1):146–51.
80. Van Voorhees BW, Fogel J, Pomper BE, et al. Adolescent dose and ratings of an Internet-based depression prevention program: a randomized trial of primary care physician brief advice versus a motivational interview. J Cogn Behav Psychother 2009;9(1):1–19.
81. Van Voorhees BW, Vanderplough-Booth K, Fogel J, et al. Integrative Internet-based depression prevention for adolescents: a randomized clinical trial in primary care for vulnerability and protective factors. J Can Acad Child Adolesc Psychiatry 2008;17(4):184–96.
82. Walters ST, Neighbors C. Feedback interventions for college alcohol misuse: what, why and for whom? Addict Behav 2005;30(6):1168–82.
83. White HR, Mun EY, Pugh L, et al. Long-term effects of brief substance use interventions for mandated college students: sleeper effects of an in-person personal feedback intervention. Alcohol Clin Exp Res 2007;31(8):1380–91.
84. Bussing R, Fernandez M, Harwood M, et al. Parent and teacher SNAP-IV ratings of attention deficit hyperactivity disorder symptoms: psychometric properties and normative ratings from a school district sample. Assessment 2008;15(3):317–28.
85. Perry-Burney G. Poverty, special education, and ADHD. Mental health care in the African-American community. New York: Haworth Press; 2007. p. 139–53.
86. Bigelow BJ. There's an elephant in the room: the impact of early poverty and neglect on intelligence and common learning disorders in children adolescents, and their parents. Developmental Disabilities Bulletin 2006;34(1–2):177–215.
87. Lanier P, Jonson-Reid M, Stahlschmidt MJ, et al. Child maltreatment and pediatric health outcomes: a longitudinal study of low-income children. J Pediatr Psychol 2010;35(5):511–22.
88. Bussing R, Zima BT, Gary FA, et al. Barriers to detection, help-seeking, and service use for children with ADHD symptoms. J Behav Health Serv Res 2003;30(2):176–89.
89. Raviv T, Wadsworth ME. The efficacy of a pilot prevention program for children and caregivers coping with economic strain. Cognit Ther Res 2010;34(3):216–28.

90. Foster EM, Prinz R, Sanders M, et al. Costs of a public health infrastructure for delivering parenting and family support. Child Youth Serv Rev 2007;30:493–501.
91. Cohen M, Piquero A. New evidence on the monetary value of saving a high risk youth. J Quant Criminol 2009;25(1):25–49.
92. Christakis NA. Social networks and collateral health effects: have been ignored in medical care and clinical trials, but need to be studied. BMJ 2004;329(7459): 185–6.
93. Lloyd A, Patel N, Scott DA, et al. Cost-effectiveness of heptavalent conjugate pneumococcal vaccine (Prevenar) in Germany: considering a high-risk population and herd immunity effects. Eur J Health Econ 2008;9(1):7–15.
94. Moran NE, Shickle D, Munthe C, et al. Are compulsory immunisation and incentives to immunise effective ways to achieve herd immunity in Europe? Ethics and infectious disease. Malden (MA): Blackwell Publishing; 2006. p. 215–31.
95. Siegal G, Siegal N, Bonnie RJ. An account of collective actions in public health. Am J Public Health 2009;99(9):1583–7.
96. González HM, Vega WA, Williams DR, et al. Depression care in the United States: too little for too few. Arch Gen Psychiatry 2010;67(1):37–46.
97. Biglan A, Hinds E. Evolving prosocial and sustainable neighborhoods and communities. Annu Rev Clin Psychol 2009;5:169–96.
98. Biglan A, Taylor TK. Why have we been more successful in reducing tobacco use than violent crime? Am J Community Psychol 2000;28(3):269–302.
99. Biglan A, Ary D, Yudelson H, et al. Experimental evaluation of a modular approach to mobilizing antitobacco influences of peers and parents. Am J Community Psychol 1996;24(3):311–39.
100. Biglan A, Ary D, Koehn V, et al. Mobilizing positive reinforcement in communities to reduce youth access to tobacco. Am J Community Psychol 1996;24(5): 625–38.
101. Biglan A, Henderson J, Humphrey D, et al. Mobilising positive reinforcement to reduce youth access to tobacco. Tob Control 1995;4(1):42–8.
102. O'Brien LM. The neurocognitive effects of sleep disruption in children and adolescents. Child Adolesc Psychiatr Clin N Am 2009;18(4):813–23.
103. Roberts RE, Roberts CR, Duong HT. Sleepless in adolescence: prospective data on sleep deprivation, health and functioning. J Adolesc 2009;32(5): 1045–57.
104. Mednick SC, Christakis NA, Fowler JH. The spread of sleep loss influences drug use in adolescent social networks. PLoS One 2010;5(3):e9775.
105. O'Sullivan TA, Robinson M, Kendall GE, et al. A good-quality breakfast is associated with better mental health in adolescence. Public Health Nutr 2009;12(2): 249–58.
106. Ostrom E. Policies that crowd out reciprocity and collective action. Moral sentiments and material interests: the foundations of cooperation in economic life. Cambridge (MA): MIT Press; 2005. p. 253–75.
107. Ostrom E. The value-added of laboratory experiments for the study of institutions and common-pool resources. J Econ Behav Organ 2006;61(2):149–63.
108. Ostrom E, Burger J, Field CB, et al. Revisiting the commons: local lessons, global challenges. Evolutionary perspectives on environmental problems. Piscataway (NJ): Transaction Publishers; 2007. p. 129–40.
109. Flay BR, Biglan A, Boruch RF, et al. Standards of evidence: criteria for efficacy, effectiveness and dissemination. Prev Sci 2005;6(3):151–75.
110. Alemayehu B, Warner KE. The lifetime distribution of health care costs. Health Serv Res 2004;39(3):627–42.

111. Anda RF, Brown DW, Felitti VJ, et al. Adverse childhood experiences and prescribed psychotropic medications in adults. Am J Prev Med 2007;32(5): 389–94.
112. Pilowsky DJ, Keyes KM, Hasin DS. Adverse childhood events and lifetime alcohol dependence. Am J Public Health 2009;99(2):258–63.
113. Tam TW, Zlotnick C, Robertson MJ. Longitudinal perspective: adverse childhood events, substance use, and labor force participation among homeless adults. Am J Drug Alcohol Abuse 2003;29(4):829–46.
114. Embry DD, Malfetti JM. Reducing the risk of pedestrian accidents to preschoolers by parent training and symbolic modeling for children: an experimental analysis in the natural environment. Falls Church (VA): American Automobile Association Foundation for Traffic Safety; 1980.
115. Embry DD, Malfetti JM. The safe-playing program: final report on nation-wide process field test. Falls Church (VA): Ameican Automobile Foundation for Traffic Safety; 1982.
116. Embry DD. The safe-playing program: a case study of putting research into practice. In: Paine S, Bellamy B, editors. Human services that work: from innovation to standard practice. Baltimore (MD): Brookes Co.; 1984. p. 624.
117. Embry DD, Rawls JM, Hemingway W. My safe playing book: an experimental evaluation of a bibliotherapuetic approach to reduce the risk of pedestrian accidents to 4-year old children. Wellington (New Zealand): Ministry of Transport, Road Safety Division; 1985.
118. Embry DD, Peters L. A three-city evaluation of the diffusion of a pedestrian-safety injury control intervention. In: Division RS, editor. Wellington (New Zealand): New Zealand Ministry of Transport; 1985.
119. Biglan A, James LE, LaChance P, et al. Videotaped materials in a school-based smoking prevention program. Prev Med 1988;17(5):559–84.
120. Reward and reminder: an environmental strategy for population-level prevention. Substance Abuse and Mental Health Administration; 2009. Available at: www.nrepp.samhsa.gov. Accessed February 3, 2010.
121. Embry DD, Flannery DJ, Vazsonyi AT, et al. PeaceBuilders: a theoretically driven, school-based model for early violence prevention. Am J Prev Med 1996;12(Suppl 5):91.
122. Miller S, Sheff-Cahan V. Give peace a chance: psychologist Dennis Embry helps to transform schoolyard bullies into angels. People. Los Angeles (CA): Time, Inc; 1999. p. 151–4.
123. Brener ND, Krug EG, Dahlberg LL, et al. Nurses' logs as an evaluation tool for school-based violence prevention programs. J Sch Health 1997;67(5): 171–4.
124. Flannery DJ, Vazsonyi AT, Liau AK, et al. Initial behavior outcomes for the PeaceBuilders universal school-based violence prevention program. Dev Psychol 2003;39(2):292–308.
125. Vazsonyi AT, Belliston LM, Flannery DJ. Evaluation of a school-based, universal violence prevention program: low-, medium-, and high-risk children. Youth Violence Juv Justice 2004;2(2):185–206.
126. Embry DD. Does your school have a peaceful environment? Using an audit to create a climate for change and resiliency. Intervention in School and Clinic 1997;32:217–22.
127. Skinner CH, Cashwell TH, Skinner AL. Increasing tootling: the effects of a peer-monitored group contingency program on students' reports of peers' prosocial behaviors. Psychol Sch 2000;37(3):263–70.

128. Kelley ML, Carper LB, Witt JC, et al. Home-based reinforcement procedures. Handbook of behavior therapy in education. New York: Plenum Press; 1988. p. 419–38.

129. Wahler RG. Some structural aspects of deviant child behavior. J Appl Behav Anal 1975;8(1):27–42.

130. Wahler RG, Vigilante VA, Strand PS. Generalization in a child's oppositional behavior across home and school settings. J Appl Behav Anal 2004;37(1):43–51.

131. Embry DD. Things Cook and Campbell never told you. Or, practical and methodological issues in large-scale safety research. 1984 Traffic Seminar, vol. 2. Wellington (New Zealand): Traffic Research Council and Ministry of Transport; 1984. p. 40.

132. Baer DM, Wolf MM, Risley TR. Some current dimensions of applied behavior analysis. J Appl Behav Anal 1968;1(1):91–7.

133. Biglan A, Ary D, Wagenaar AC. The value of interrupted time-series experiments for community intervention research. Prev Sci 2000;1(1):31–49.

134. Wagenaar AC, Murray DM, Wolfson M, et al. Communities mobilizing for change on alcohol: design of a randomized community trial [special issue]. J Community Psychol 1994;79–101.

135. Holder HD, Wagenaar AC. Mandated server training and reduced alcohol-involved traffic crashes: a time series analysis of the Oregon experience. Accid Anal Prev 1994;26(1):89–97.

136. Wagenaar AC, Maybee RG, Sullivan KP. Mandatory seat belt laws in eight states: a time-series evaluation. J Safety Res 1988;19(2):51–70.

137. Wagenaar AC. Preventing highway crashes by raising the legal minimum age for drinking: an empirical confirmation. J Safety Res 1982;13(2):57–71.

138. Herrnstein RJ. On the law of effect. J Exp Anal Behav 1970;12:243–66.

139. Herrnstein RJ. Formal properties of the matching law. J Exp Anal Behav 1974; 21(1):159–64.

140. Dishion TJ, Spracklen KM, Andrews DW, et al. Deviancy training in male adolescents friendships. Behav Ther 1996;27(3):373–90.

141. Embry DD, Flannery DJ. Two sides of the coin: multi-level prevention and intervention to reduce youth violent behavior. In: Flannery DJ, Huff CR, editors. Youth violence: prevention, intervention and social policy. Washington, DC: American Psychiatric Press; 1999. p. 47–72.

142. Amminger GP, Berger GE, Schäfer MR, et al. Omega-3 fatty acids supplementation in children with autism: a double-blind randomized, placebo-controlled pilot study. Biol Psychiatry 2007;61(4):551–3.

143. McCain AP, Kelley ML. Improving classroom performance in underachieving preadolescents: the additive effects of response cost to a school-home note system. Child Fam Behav Ther 1994;16(2):27–41.

144. McCain AP, Kelley ML. Managing the classroom behavior of an ADHD preschooler: the efficacy of a school-home note intervention. Child Fam Behav Ther 1993;15(3):33–44.

145. Jurbergs N, Palcic J, Kelley ML. School-home notes with and without response cost: increasing attention and academic performance in low-income children with attention-deficit/hyperactivity disorder. Sch Psychol Q 2007;22(3):358–79.

146. Wurtele SK, Drabman RS. "Beat the buzzer" for classroom dawdling: a one-year trial. Behav Ther 1984;15(4):403–9.

147. Wolf MM, Hanley EL, King LA, et al. The timer-game: a variable interval contingency for the management of out-of-seat behavior. Except Child 1970;37(2): 113–7.

148. Christ TJ, Christ JA. Application of an interdependent group contingency mediated by an automated feedback device: an intervention across three high school classrooms. School Psych Rev 2006;35(1):78–90.
149. Robinson TN, Wilde ML, Navracruz LC, et al. Effects of reducing children's television and video game use on aggressive behavior: a randomized controlled trial [see comment]. Arch Pediatr Adolesc Med 2001;155(1):17–23.
150. Bay-Hinitz AK, Peterson RF, Quilitch HR. Cooperative games: a way to modify aggressive and cooperative behaviors in young children. J Appl Behav Anal 1994;27(3):435–46.
151. Murphy HA, Hutchison JM, Bailey JS. Behavioral school psychology goes outdoors: the effect of organized games on playground aggression. J Appl Behav Anal 1983;16(1):29.
152. Olds DL, Henderson CR Jr, Tatelbaum R. Prevention of intellectual impairment in children of women who smoke cigarettes during pregnancy. Pediatrics 1994; 93(2):228–33 [Erratum appears in Pediatrics 1994;93(6 Pt 1):973].
153. Olds DL, Henderson CR Jr, Tatelbaum R. Intellectual impairment in children of women who smoke cigarettes during pregnancy. Pediatrics 1994;93(2):221–7 [Erratum appears in Pediatrics 1994;93(6 Pt 1):973].
154. Donatelle RJ, Prows SL, Champeau D, et al. Randomised controlled trial using social support and financial incentives for high risk pregnant smokers: significant other supporter (SOS) program. Tob Control 2000;9(Suppl 3): III67–9.
155. Olmstead TA, Sindelar JL, Petry NM. Cost-effectiveness of prize-based incentives for stimulant abusers in outpatient psychosocial treatment programs. Drug Alcohol Depend 2007;87(2–3):175–82.
156. Peirce JM, Petry NM, Stitzer ML, et al. Effects of lower-cost incentives on stimulant abstinence in methadone maintenance treatment: a National Drug Abuse Treatment Clinical Trials Network study. Arch Gen Psychiatry 2006; 63(2):201–8.
157. Sindelar J, Elbel B, Petry NM. What do we get for our money? Cost-effectiveness of adding contingency management. Addiction 2007;102(2):309–16.
158. Bartu A, Sharp J, Ludlow J, et al. Postnatal home visiting for illicit drug-using mothers and their infants: a randomised controlled trial. Aust N Z J Obstet Gynaecol 2006;46(5):419–26.
159. Black MM, Nair P, Kight C, et al. Parenting and early development among children of drug-abusing women: effects of home intervention. Pediatrics 1994;94(4 Pt 1): 440–8.
160. Doggett C, Burrett S, Osborn DA. Home visits during pregnancy and after birth for women with an alcohol or drug problem. Cochrane Database Syst Rev 2005;4:CD004456.
161. Stitzer M, Petry N. Contingency management for treatment of substance abuse. Annu Rev Clin Psychol 2006;2(1):411–34.
162. Roll JM, Petry NM, Stitzer ML, et al. Contingency management for the treatment of methamphetamine use disorders. Am J Psychiatry 2006;163(11):1993–9.
163. Petry NM, Peirce JM, Stitzer ML, et al. Effect of prize-based incentives on outcomes in stimulant abusers in outpatient psychosocial treatment programs: a National Drug Abuse Treatment Clinical Trials Network Study. Arch Gen Psychiatry 2005;62(10):1148–56.
164. Petry NM, Tedford J, Austin M, et al. Prize reinforcement contingency management for treating cocaine users: how low can we go, and with whom? Addiction 2004;99(3):349–60.

165. Petry NM, Simcic F Jr. Recent advances in the dissemination of contingency management techniques: clinical and research perspectives. J Subst Abuse Treat 2002;23(2):81–6.
166. Petry NM, Petrakis I, Trevisan L, et al. Contingency management interventions: from research to practice. Am J Psychiatry 2001;158(5):694–702.
167. Petry NM, Martin B, Finocche C. Contingency management in group treatment: a demonstration project in an HIV drop-in center. J Subst Abuse Treat 2001; 21(2):89–96.
168. Petry NM, Martin B, Cooney JL, et al. Give them prizes and they will come: contingency management for treatment of alcohol dependence. J Consult Clin Psychol 2000;68(2):250–7.
169. Petry NM, Tedford J, Martin B. Reinforcing compliance with non-drug-related activities. J Subst Abuse Treat 2000;20(1):33–44.
170. Petry NM, Bickel WK, Tzanis E, et al. A behavioral intervention for improving verbal behaviors of heroin addicts in a treatment clinic. J Appl Behav Anal 1998;31(2):291–7.
171. Embry DD, Biglan A. Evidence-based kernels: fundamental units of behavioral influence. Clin Child Fam Psychol Rev 2008;11(3):75–113.
172. Lafferty CK, Mahoney CA. A framework for evaluating comprehensive community initiatives. Health Promot Pract 2003;4(1):31–44.
173. Glasgow RE, Vogt TM, Boles SM. Evaluating the public health impact of health promotion interventions: the RE-AIM framework. Am J Public Health 1999;89(9): 1322–7.
174. Patterson GR, Capaldi DM. Antisocial parents: unskilled and vulnerable. Family transitions. England. Hillsdale (NJ): Lawrence Erlbaum Associates, Inc; 1991. p. 195–218.
175. Patterson GR, DeGarmo D, Forgatch MS. Systematic changes in families following prevention trials. An official publication of the International Society for Research in Child and Adolescent Psychopathology. J Abnorm Child Psychol 2004;32(6):621–33.
176. Patterson GR, Dishion TJ, Bank L. Family interaction: a process model of deviancy training. Aggress Behav 1984;10(3):253–67.
177. Ogden T, Forgatch MS, Askeland E, et al. Implementation of parent management training at the national level: the case of Norway. J Soc Work Pract 2005;19(3):317–29.
178. Ialongo N, Poduska J, Werthamer L, et al. The distal impact of two first-grade preventive interventions on conduct problems and disorder in early adolescence. J Emot Behav Disord 2001;9(3):146–60.
179. British Associate Parliamentary Food and Health Forum. The links between diet and behaviour: the influence of nutrition on mental health. London; 2008. p. 43. Available at: www.fhf.org.uk/inquiry. Accessed December 9, 2010.
180. Spoth R, Redmond C, Shin C, et al. Substance-use outcomes at 18 months past baseline: the PROSPER community-university partnership trial. Am J Prev Med 2007;32(5):395–402.
181. Redmond C, Spoth RL, Shin C, et al. Long-term protective factor outcomes of evidence-based interventions implemented by community teams through a community, a university partnership. J Prim Prev 2009;30(5):513–30.
182. Månsdotter AM, Rydberg MK, Wallin E, et al. A cost-effectiveness analysis of alcohol prevention targeting licensed premises. Eur J Public Health 2007;17(6):618–23.
183. Midford R, Wayte K, Catalano P, et al. The legacy of a community mobilisation project to reduce alcohol related harm. Drug Alcohol Rev 2005;24(1):3–11.

184. Shults RA, Elder RW, Nichols JL, et al. Effectiveness of multicomponent programs with community mobilization for reducing alcohol-impaired driving. Am J Prev Med 2009;37(4):360–71.
185. Collie-Akers V, Schultz JA, Carson V, et al. Evaluating mobilization strategies with neighborhood and faith organizations to reduce risk for health disparities. REACH 2010: Kansas City, Missouri. Health Promot Pract 2009;10(Suppl 2): 118S–27S.
186. Buller DB, Young WF, Fisher KH, et al. The effect of endorsement by local opinion leaders and testimonials from teachers on the dissemination of a web-based smoking prevention program. Health Educ Res 2007;22(5):609–18.
187. Anderson SJ, Ling PM. "And they told two friends.and so on": RJ Reynolds' viral marketing of eclipse and its potential to mislead the public. Tob Control 2008; 17(4):222–9.
188. Gosselin P, Poitras P. Use of an internet "viral" marketing software platform in health promotion. J Med Internet Res 2008;10(4):e47.
189. Yancey AK. The meta-volition model: organizational leadership is the key ingredient in getting society moving, literally! Prev Med 2009;49(4):342–51.
190. Cruz D, Fill C. Evaluating viral marketing: isolating the key criteria. Market Intell Plann 2008;26(7):743–58.
191. Shoveling Up II: the impact of substance abuse on federal, state and local budgets. New York: The National Center on Addiction and Substance Abuse at Columbia University; 2009.
192. Hallfors D, Cho H, Sanchez V, et al. Efficacy vs effectiveness trial results of an indicated "model" substance abuse program: implications for public health. Am J Public Health 2006;96(12):2254–9.
193. Jorm AF, Kitchener BA, O'Kearney R, et al. Mental health first aid training of the public in a rural area: a cluster randomized trial [ISRCTN53887541]. BMC Psychiatry 2004;4:33.
194. Kendrick D, Coupland C, Mason-Jones AJ, et al. Home safety education and provision of safety equipment for injury prevention [systematic review]. Cochrane Database Syst Rev 2009;1:CD005014.
195. Johnston MV, Smith RO. Single subject designs: current methodologies and future directions. OTJR: Occupation, Participation and Health 2010;30(1):4–10.
196. Perdices M, Tate RL. Single-subject designs as a tool for evidence-based clinical practice: are they unrecognised and undervalued? Neuropsychol Rehabil 2009;19(6):904–27.
197. Satake EB, Jagaroo V, Maxwell DL. Handbook of statistical methods: single subject design. San Diego (CA): Plural Publishing; 2008.
198. Rapoff M, Stark L. Editorial: Journal of pediatric psychology: statement of purpose: section on single-subject studies. J Pediatr Psychol 2008;33(1):16–21.
199. Biglan A. Contextualism and the development of effective prevention practices. Prev Sci 2004;5(1):15–21.
200. Wagenaar AC. Aggregate beer and wine consumption: effects of changes in the minimum legal drinking age and a mandatory beverage container deposit law in Michigan. J Stud Alcohol 1982;43(5):469–87.
201. Wagenaar AC. Effects of the raised legal drinking age on motor vehicle accidents in Michigan. HSRI Research Review 1981;11(4):8.
202. Ialongo NS, Werthamer L, Kellam SG, et al. Proximal impact of two first-grade preventive interventions on the early risk behaviors for later substance abuse, depression, and antisocial behavior. Am J Community Psychol 1999;27(5): 599–641.

203. Buydens-Branchey L, Branchey M, McMakin DL, et al. Polyunsaturated fatty acid status and relapse vulnerability in cocaine addicts. Psychiatry Res 2003; 120(1):29–35.
204. Hibbeln JR. Seafood consumption and homicide mortality. A cross-national ecological analysis. World Rev Nutr Diet 2001;88:41–6.
205. Hibbeln JR. From homicide to happiness–a commentary on omega-3 fatty acids in human society. Cleave Award Lecture. Nutr Health 2007;19(1–2):9–19.
206. Gesch CB, Hammond SM, Hampson SE, et al. Influence of supplementary vitamins, minerals and essential fatty acids on the antisocial behaviour of young adult prisoners. Randomised, placebo-controlled trial. Br J Psychiatry 2002; 181:22–8.
207. Kellam SG, Anthony JC. Targeting early antecedents to prevent tobacco smoking: findings from an epidemiologically based randomized field trial. Am J Public Health 1998;88(10):1490–5.
208. Storr CL, Ialongo NS, Kellam SG, et al. A randomized controlled trial of two primary intervention strategies to prevent early onset tobacco smoking. Drug Alcohol Depend 2002;66(1):51.
209. Furr-Holden CD, Ialongo NS, Anthony JC, et al. Developmentally inspired drug prevention: middle school outcomes in a school-based randomized prevention trial. Drug Alcohol Depend 2004;73(2):149–58.
210. Kellam SG, Rebok GW, Ialongo N, et al. The course and malleability of aggressive behavior from early first grade into middle school: results of a developmental epidemiology-based preventive trial. J Child Psychol Psyc 1994;35: 259–81.
211. Schubiner H, Tzelepis A, Milberger S, et al. Prevalence of attention-deficit/hyperactivity disorder and conduct disorder among substance abusers. J Clin Psychiatry 2000;61(4):244–51.
212. Merrell C, Tymms PB. Inattention, hyperactivity and impulsiveness: their impact on academic achievement and progress. Br J Educ Psychol 2001;71(1):43.
213. DiScala C, Lescohier I, Barthel M, et al. Injuries to children with attention deficit hyperactivity disorder. Pediatrics 1998;102(6):1415–21.
214. Smith CA. Dis-attachment. Aust N Z J Psychiatry 1994;28(4):691.
215. Fletcher J, Wolfe B. Long-term consequences of childhood ADHD on criminal activities. J Ment Health Policy Econ 2009;12(3):119–38.
216. Elkins IJ, McGue M, Iacono WG. Prospective effects of attention-deficit/hyperactivity disorder, conduct disorder, and sex on adolescent substance use and abuse. Arch Gen Psychiatry 2007;64(10):1145–52.
217. Hornig M. Addressing comorbidity in adults with attention-deficit/hyperactivity disorder. J Clin Psychiatry 1998;59(Suppl 7):69–75.
218. Tercyak KP, Lerman C, Audrain J. Association of attention-deficit/hyperactivity disorder symptoms with levels of cigarette smoking in a community sample of adolescents. J Am Acad Child Adolesc Psychiatry 2002;41(7):799–805.
219. Denchev P, Kaltman JR, Schoenbaum M, et al. Modeled economic evaluation of alternative strategies to reduce sudden cardiac death among children treated for attention deficit/hyperactivity disorder. Circulation 2010;121(11):1329–37.
220. Schaeffer B, Thomas JC, Hersen M. Learning disabilities and attention deficits in the workplace. Psychopathology in the workplace: recognition and adaptation. New York: Brunner-Routledge; 2004. p. 201–24.
221. Burd L, Klug MG, Coumbe MJ, et al. Children and adolescents with attention deficit-hyperactivity disorder: 1. Prevalence and cost of care. J Child Neurol 2003;18(8):555–61.

222. Moore LA, Waguespack AM, Wickstrom KF, et al. Mystery motivator: an effective and time efficient intervention. School Psych Rev 1994;23(1):106–18.
223. Valum JL. Student-Managed Study Skills Teams: academic survival for adolescents at risk of school failure. Dissertation abstracts international section A: humanities and social sciences 1996. ProQuest Information & Learning: US. p. 3064.
224. Maus MB. Independent group contingencies for reducing disruptive behavior in preschoolers with PDD-NOS. Dissertation abstracts international: section B: the sciences and engineering 2007. ProQuest Information & Learning: US. p. 614.
225. Madaus MM, Kehle TJ, Madaus J, et al. Mystery motivator as an intervention to promote homework completion and accuracy. Sch Psychol Int 2003;24(4): 369–77.
226. Bennett MM. An interdependent group contingency with mystery motivators to increase spelling performance. Dissertation abstracts international: section B: the sciences and engineering 2007. ProQuest Information & Learning: US. p. 6040.
227. De Martini-Scully D, Bray MA, Kehle TJ. A packaged intervention to reduce disruptive behaviors in general education students. Psychol Sch 2000;37(2): 149–56.
228. Collier CR, Czuchry M, Dansereau DF, et al. The use of node-link mapping in the chemical dependency treatment of adolescents. J Drug Educ 2001;31(3):305.
229. Czuchry M, Dansereau DF. Node-link mapping and psychological problems: perceptions of a residential drug abuse treatment program for probationers. J Subst Abuse Treat 1999;17(4):321.
230. Pitre U, Dansereau DF, Newbern D, et al. Residential drug abuse treatment for probationers: use of node-link mapping to enhance participation and progress. J Subst Abuse Treat 1998;15(6):535.
231. Newbern D, Dansereau DF, Czuchry M, et al. Node-link mapping in individual counseling: treatment impact on clients with ADHD-related behaviors. J Psychoactive Drugs 2005;37(1):93.
232. Newbern D, Dansereau DF, Pitre U. Positive effects on life skills motivation and self-efficacy: node-link maps in a modified therapeutic community. Am J Drug Alcohol Abuse 1999;25(3):407.
233. Nesbit JC, Adesope OO. Learning with concept and knowledge maps: a meta-analysis. Rev Educ Res 2006;76(3):413–48.
234. O'Donnell AM, Dansereau DF, Hall RH. Knowledge maps as scaffolds for cognitive processing. Educ Psychol Rev 2002;14(1):71–86.
235. Blankenship J, Dansereau DF. The effect of animated node-link displays on information recall. J Exp Educ 2000;68(4):293–308.
236. Czuchry M, Dansereau DF. The generation and recall of personally relevant information. J Exp Educ 1998;66(4):293–315.
237. Dunstan JA, Mitoulas LR, Dixon G, et al. The effects of fish oil supplementation in pregnancy on breast milk fatty acid composition over the course of lactation: a randomized controlled trial. Pediatr Res 2007;62(6):689–94.
238. Dunstan JA, Roper J, Mitoulas L, et al. The effect of supplementation with fish oil during pregnancy on breast milk immunoglobulin A, soluble CD14, cytokine levels and fatty acid composition. Clin Exp Allergy 2004;34(8):1237–42.
239. Helland IB, Smith L, Saarem K, et al. Maternal supplementation with very-long-chain n-3 fatty acids during pregnancy and lactation augments children's IQ at 4 years of age. Pediatrics 2003;111(1):e39–44.
240. Bacon-Prue A, Blount R, Hosey C, et al. The public posting of photographs as a reinforcer for bedmaking in an institutional setting. Behav Ther 1980; 11(3):417.

241. Lyman RD. The effect of private and public goal setting on classroom on-task behavior of emotionally disturbed children. Behav Ther 1984;15(4):395.
242. Houten RV, Nau P, Marini Z. An analysis of public posting in reducing speeding behavior on an urban highway. J Appl Behav Anal 1980;13(3):383–95.
243. Kehle TJ, Bray MA, Theodore LA, et al. A multi-component intervention designed to reduce disruptive classroom behavior. Psychol Sch 2000;37(5):475.
244. Van Houten R, Morrison E, Jarvis R, et al. The effects of explicit timing and feedback on compositional response rate in elementary school children. J Appl Behav Anal 1974;7(4):547–55.
245. Van Houten R, Hill S, Parsons M. An analysis of a performance feedback system: the effects of timing and feedback, public posting, and praise upon academic performance and peer interaction. J Appl Behav Anal 1975;8(4):449–57.
246. Gross AM, Shapiro R. Public posting of photographs: a new classroom reinforcer. J Child Psychol Psyc 1981;3(1):81.
247. Stokes TF, Mathews RM, Fawcett SB. Promoting participation in a community-based educational program. J Child Psychol Psyc 1978;3(1):29–31.
248. Jackson NC, Mathews RM. Using public feedback to increase contributions to a multipurpose senior center. J Appl Behav Anal 1995;28(4):449–55.

The Prevention of Adolescent Depression

Tracy R.G. Gladstone, PhD[a,b,c], William R. Beardslee, MD[b,c,d],*,
Erin E. O'Connor, BA[c]

KEYWORDS

• Depression • Prevention • Intervention • Adolescent

Depression is the most common psychiatric disorder in the United States, with more than 16% of the US population reporting a major depressive episode (MDD) during their lifetime.[1] Depression is one of the leading causes of morbidity and mortality in the world today[2] and places a significant economic burden on the society.[3,4] Depression is among the most treatable mental disorders yet it remains a chronic illness, with 85% of people who experience a single episode of depression experiencing another episode within 15 years.[5]

In recent years, researchers and policy makers have recognized the importance of focusing on prevention efforts for depression. Prevention requires a paradigm shift from traditional disease models, in which symptoms are treated when they emerge, to a proactive focus on mental health and on maximizing protective factors while reducing risk factors for mental illness.[6] This article reviews depression prevention efforts that aim to promote mental health and prevent the onset of depressive disorder in children and adolescents. First, the authors review the epidemiology of youth depression and then outline a conceptual framework for depression prevention research. The research on depression prevention programs for youth is also reviewed. Finally, the authors discuss directions for future research and the key issues to consider when developing and evaluating depression prevention efforts.

EPIDEMIOLOGY OF YOUTH DEPRESSION

Like depression in adulthood, youth depression is quite common.[7] The 1-year prevalence rates for MDD are about 2% in childhood and range from 4% to 7% in

[a] Wellesley Centers for Women, Wellesley College, 106 Central Street, Wellesley, MA 02481, USA
[b] Department of Psychiatry, Children's Hospital, 300 Longwood Avenue, Boston, MA 02115, USA
[c] Judge Baker Children's Center, 53 Parker Hill Avenue, Boston, MA 02120, USA
[d] Harvard Medical School, 25 Shattuck Street, Boston, MA 02115, USA
* Corresponding author. 21 Autumn Street, Suite 130.2, Boston, MA.
E-mail address: william.beardslee@childrens.harvard.edu

Psychiatr Clin N Am 34 (2011) 35–52
doi:10.1016/j.psc.2010.11.015
0193-953X/11/$ – see front matter © 2011 Elsevier Inc. All rights reserved.

adolescence.[8] According to the National Comorbidity Survey,[9] the lifetime prevalence of MDD in adolescents aged 15 to 18 years is 14%, and an estimated 20% of adolescents will have had a depressive disorder by the time they are 18 years of age.[10,11] Point prevalence rates of depression during adolescence range from 4% to 7%, and the average age for the first onset of depression is 15 years.[12] Half of the first episodes of depression occur during adolescence,[13] and early-onset depression is associated with a chronic episodic course of illness.[8] Although successful treatments for youth depression have been explored, such as administration of antidepressants, cognitive-behavioral (CB) interventions, and interpersonal psychotherapy, such treatments have been found to work for only about 50% to 60% of cases under controlled research conditions.[14]

Similar to adult depression, adolescent depression frequently is persistent and recurring.[7,10,11] In 12% of children the depression relapses within 1 year; in 40%, within 2 years; and in 75%, there is a second episode within 5 years.[12,15,16] Adolescent depression is associated with negative long-term functional and psychiatric outcomes, including impairment in school, work, interpersonal relationships, and substance abuse.[17–23] Of particular note is the association between adolescent depression and suicidal behavior. Suicide is the third leading cause of death in adolescents.[24] Over a 1-year period, 13.8% of adolescents in the United States reported seriously considering suicide, 10.9% had made suicidal plans, and 6.3% reported making a suicide attempt.[25]

Evidence-based treatments for youth depression, such as CB therapy and interpersonal approaches, are associated with benefits that, for some, persist over time.[26,27] However, most depressed youth do not receive treatment of depressive symptoms or disorder.[28] When they do receive treatment, although many adolescents respond well to CB treatment approaches, about half of the depressed children who respond well have the condition within 2 years of terminating treatment.[29] Likewise, even adolescents who respond well to combined treatments for youth depression (eg, CB plus medication), often experience residual symptoms of depression. Only 37% of depressed youth who receive combined treatment are no longer depressed by 12 weeks.[30] Finally, recent data suggest that the duration of depression moderates the treatment outcome, such that the longer the duration of a depressive episode, the less likely it is to respond to evidence-based treatments.[31] Overall, while treatment of youth depression is important and can be beneficial, many who receive treatment of depression do not respond, have residual symptoms, or experience relapses of the disorder.[32–35]

Given the high prevalence and costs of youth depression, the connection between early-onset depression and recurrence of the disorder in adulthood, the impairment associated with youth depression, and the difficulty in treating the depression once it has developed, efforts to prevent depression are warranted. The importance of preventing depressive disorder through the development and evaluation of preventive interventions was highlighted by the Institute of Medicine (IOM) report[6] *Preventing Mental Disorders*[36] and has been emphasized by numerous recent expert panels.[37,38] The IOM report defined prevention as interventions that occur before the onset of the disorder and that are designed to prevent the occurrence of the disorder. Indeed, prevention may be the key to decreasing the burden of adolescent and adult depression on society and may be more cost effective and less distressing than waiting for the condition to appear and then trying to treat a full depressive episode.

CONCEPTUAL FRAMEWORK FOR DEPRESSION PREVENTION RESEARCH

In the past several decades, research on the prevention of youth depression has blossomed, and as a result, we now know much more about ways to maximize the efficacy of prevention efforts. That is, we know more about the variables to target, the timing of interventions, and the samples that will be most likely to benefit from depression prevention efforts.

RISK/PROTECTIVE FACTORS

A key early stage of prevention research involves understanding specific and nonspecific risk and protective factors for these particular disorders, as prevention efforts benefit by focusing on decreasing these risk factors while enhancing these protective factors. Understanding the risk and protective factors for depression enables researchers to make careful choices about the prevention strategies they use.

Specific Risk Factors

Specific risk factors are those factors that have been associated with increased risk for youth depression in empirical investigations. Specific risk factors for adolescent depression include having low self-esteem, being female, developing negative body image, low social support, a negative cognitive style, and ineffective coping.[39] In the case of youth depression, the strongest risk factor for the development of depression, above and beyond the variance accounted for by other risk factors, is having a parent with depressive illness.[40] Offspring of depressed parents are at about a 2- to 4-fold increased risk of developing depressive disorders, and more than half of the parents bringing their depressed adolescents for services themselves have current mood disorders.[40] Research in the past 20 years suggests that children who grow up with depressed parents have more internalizing disorders such as depression and anxiety, more externalizing disorders such as conduct disorder and attention-deficit disorder,[41] more cognitive delays and academic difficulties, and more social difficulties.[40] However, not all children of depressed parents become depressed and many children of depressed parents are resilient and do well over time.[42] Thus, many depression prevention efforts in youth have targeted either those with symptoms or those whose parents have depression.

Nonspecific Risk Factors

A comprehensive approach to the prevention of depression involves addressing both specific and nonspecific risk factors. Nonspecific risk factors are associated with increased risk for a range of disorders, including depression. Nonspecific risk factors that are documented to increase rates of youth depression include poverty, exposure to violence, social isolation, child maltreatment, and family breakup.[39] In fact, reducing the burdens of poverty, exposure to violence, child maltreatment, and other forms of family instability may play an important role in the reduction of depressive disorders in youth.[39]

For example, both poverty and child maltreatment have been associated with many negative outcomes. Specifically, a recent study of a subsample of the United States National Collaborative Perinatal Project examined the relation between lower socioeconomic status (SES) in families of young children and lifetime rates of depression.[43] The lifetime risk for depression was related to the occupational level of the parents during the birth of the children. Children with parents of lower SES backgrounds had significantly increased lifetime rates of depression. In particular, having a family history of mental illness was associated with later depression, whereas adult educational attainment and depression were inversely related. Also, in a prospective longitudinal study of 676 maltreated children and 520 nonabused and nonneglected control subjects Widom and colleagues[44] found significant relations between child physical abuse and increased risk for lifetime MDD and between child neglect and increased risk for current MDD. Research on the additive effects of child-hood risk factors suggests that addressing both specific and nonspecific risk factors together may have the best chance of preventing the disorder.[6,39]

Resilience and Protective Factors

Although the presence of both specific and nonspecific risk factors does indicate an increased risk for youth depression, it is important to remember that not all children and adolescents who are exposed to these risk factors develop the disorder. In fact, many children who are exposed to risk factors for depression also have protective factors and exhibit resilience, which means that they have characteristics that decrease the likelihood of developing depression.[39] Protective factors for youth depression include the presence of supportive adults, strong family relationships, strong peer rela-tionships, coping skills, and skills in emotion regulation.[39] In a specific study of children of depressed parents,[42] the authors studied a subset of resilient youth whose parents had experienced depression. In the youth, they found that several factors contributed to resilience, including a focus on accomplishing age-appropriate developmental tasks, on relationships, and on understanding their parents' illness, whereas in the parents, they found that resilience was associated with a commitment to parenting despite depression and a commitment to relationships.

TIMING OF INTERVENTION DELIVERY

Most mental disorders have their onsets during childhood or adolescence. In fact, 75% of all adult mental health disorders have their onset by the age of 24 years, and 50% of adult disorders have an onset by the age of 14 years.[6] Further, data on the onset of mental disorders suggests that early symptoms of a disorder emerge a few years before the full diagnostic criteria are met (**Fig. 1**).[6]

Successful prevention efforts use a developmental approach, positioning the inter-vention in the developmental epoch preceding or during the age of peak incidence.

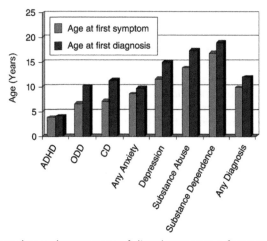

Fig. 1. Data suggests that early symptoms of disorder emerge a few years before full diag-nostic criteria are met. ADHD, attention-deficit/hyperactivity disorder; CD, conduct disorder; ODD, oppositional defiant disorder. (*From* National Research Council and Institute of Medi-cine. Prevention Committee. Preventing mental, emotional, and behavioral disorders among young people: progress and possibilities. Washington, DC: National Academies Press; 2009; with permission.)

Data on the onset of disorder suggest that, during childhood and adolescence there may be opportune developmental windows in which to intervene to maximize the benefits of intervention.[6] For example, although the mean age of first diagnosis for depression is 15 years,[12] symptoms of depression generally emerge 3 to 4 years earlier.[6] Successful depression prevention programs target the developmental window from ages 11 to15 years, when symptoms are present, but before the onset of full-blown disorder.[6]

DEFINITION OF PREVENTION AND SAMPLE DEFINITION

According to the IOM (1994) report,[6] there are 3 categories of preventive interventions: universal, selective, and indicated. Universal preventive interventions target the general public or community regardless of risk. An example of a universal prevention program is a curriculum that teaches about the dangers of substance abuse to all high-school freshmen in the community. Selective prevention programs target members of a subgroup who are at a higher risk for disorder, such as children of depressed parents. Finally, indicated prevention programs target all people who display subclinical signs or symptoms of a given disorder. An example of an indicated prevention program is a curriculum that teaches depression prevention strategies to teenagers with subclinical depressive symptoms.

Horowitz and Garber[45] conducted a meta-analysis of 30 depression prevention studies for youth and found that at postintervention, selective prevention programs, such as those focusing on children of depressed parents, were more effective than universal programs that targeted all high-school students district-wide. They also found that selective and indicated prevention programs were more effective than universal programs at the 6-month follow-up. Although targeted prevention programs appear to be more effective than universal programs, several studies have demonstrated favorable outcomes using universal programs.

REVIEW OF DEPRESSION PREVENTION EFFORTS FOR YOUTH

To date, researchers who have studied the effects of preventive interventions on depression in youth have generally based their prevention strategies on CB and/or interpersonal approaches.[46] These approaches have been found to be helpful in the treatment of depression[47] and recently have been evaluated to determine whether they may be useful in preventing youth depression. In the following sections, the authors review recent research on depression prevention efforts for youth, using the IOM categories for preventive interventions. They begin by reviewing research on universal prevention programs, and then review selective prevention programs followed by indicated prevention programs.

Universal Prevention Programs

School-based programs

One successful universal prevention program was evaluated by Spence and colleagues,[48,49] who report data from a universal school-based prevention program targeting 1500 youth aged 12 to 14 years attending high school in Queensland, Australia. Schools were assigned randomly to the Problem Solving for Life (PSFL) intervention or the school-as-usual condition (MC). Participants were evaluated for depressive symptoms as well as a range of other risk variables at baseline (preintervention), postintervention, and again at a 12-month follow-up. A group of high-risk participants was identified at baseline based on elevated scores on measures of depressive symptoms. The PSFL intervention consists of eight 45- to 50-minute weekly sessions that focus on teaching cognitive restructuring and problem solving. The program is implemented by classroom teachers who are trained in the program's theory, content, and implementation techniques during a 6-hour training session.

Overall, at postintervention, students assigned to the PSFL condition demonstrated reduced symptoms of depression, relative to students assigned to the MC condition, and a greater number of high-risk students in the PSFL condition were no longer classified as high risk. However, these group differences were not maintained. Moreover, survival analyses revealed there was no significant group difference in the incidence of depressive disorders in high-risk participants over time. This work suggests that prevention programs can be delivered by teachers with fidelity, that youth may be receptive to interventions, and that this intervention can yield short-term effects in reducing depressive symptoms in Australia. However, this work also highlights the importance of long-term follow-up and the difficulties of using a universal prevention approach to reduce depression diagnoses.

Another universal school-based program aimed at preventing depression in adolescence was evaluated by Shochet and colleagues.[50] Students in grade 9 (n = 260) were assigned to one of 3 different groups: Resourceful Adolescent Program-Adolescents (RAP-A), Resourceful Adolescent Program-Family (RAP-F), and Adolescent Watch (AW). RAP-A was part of an 11-session program as part of the school curriculum; it focused on building resilience in the students. The RAP-F was similar to RAP-A, but in RAP-F, the students' parents were invited to participate in a parent program consisting of 3 different sessions. The AW program was the comparison group in which the adolescents only completed measures of depressive symptoms and hopelessness.

Results indicated that the 2 intervention groups (RAP-A and RAP-F) did not differ from one another but did differ from the comparison group (AW). For the 2 intervention groups, there were significant reductions in depressive symptoms and hopelessness scores that were maintained at a 10-month follow-up. For the AW program, there were no significant changes in scores after intervention. These results indicate that the addition of the parent component to the RAP-A program did not significantly increase the program's efficacy.

Merry and colleagues[51] evaluated the efficacy of another school-based program, the RAP-Kiwi intervention, based on the RAP program by Shochet and colleagues,[50] as described above. This intervention is derived from CB therapy and consists of 11 sessions in which principles of CB and interpersonal therapy are incorporated. The intervention used by Merry and colleagues targeted students (n = 392) aged 13 to 15 years, and each student was randomized to the intervention (RAP-Kiwi) (n = 207) or a placebo program (n = 185). The placebo program contained elements focusing on having fun, such as arts and crafts, rather than elements that have been identified as aiding in preventing depression.

Results indicated that depressive symptoms were significantly reduced by the RAP-Kiwi program more so than the placebo program. Categorical analyses indicated that there was an absolute risk reduction of 3% for the RAP-Kiwi group. These results remained consistent at an 18-month follow-up, with the RAP-Kiwi group having a greater mean difference in depression scores (M = 1.55) than the placebo group (M = 1.31). This study indicates that a school-based universal depression prevention program administered by teachers is effective in reducing depressive symptoms in adolescents, both in the short-term and in the long-term.

CB program

Horowitz and colleagues[52] evaluated a universal group CB program for preventing depressive symptoms in adolescence, which was based on the Coping With Stress

(CWS) program of Clark and colleagues.[53] High-school students enrolled in wellness classes (n = 380) were randomly assigned to one of the 3 programs: the CB program, the Interpersonal Psychotherapy-Adolescent Skills Training Program (IPT-AST), or a no-intervention control. Eight group leaders, all of whom were trained master's-level clinical psychology graduate students or recent clinical psychology PhDs, and 8 coleaders, all of whom were clinical graduate students or undergraduate honor students, led the groups.

The results indicated that the difference between the CB and IPT-AST groups were largest for the students who had higher levels of depressive symptoms at baseline. These data indicate that the prevention programs were more effective for participants who were at risk for depression based on elevated depressive symptoms scores at baseline, consistent with an indicated prevention approach.

Selective Prevention Programs

School-based

The Penn Resiliency Program (PRP),[54] perhaps the most widely evaluated depression prevention program for youth,[55] was developed to target cognitive and behavioral risk factors for depression in school-aged children. Based on CB therapy, PRP is a school-based program that teaches participants the connection between life events, their beliefs about those events, and the emotional consequences of their interpretations. The manualized PRP curriculum is generally conducted by trained school personnel during the school day and consists of twelve 90- to 120-minute group sessions.

PRP has been evaluated empirically over several years with children and adolescents of varying ages and from varying ethnic and cultural backgrounds, both in universal and in targeted prevention studies.[55,56] Overall, these studies have found that, relative to participants in the control conditions, participants in PRP experienced reduced depressive symptoms over follow-up intervals ranging from 6 months to 2 years. In one such prevention study, conducted in primary care clinics within a Health Maintenance Organization (HMO), children aged 11 and 12 years identified as high risk based on a self-report questionnaire were invited to participate. Although PRP was found to improve explanatory style (ie, world view) for positive events and reduced depressive symptoms for girls only, no overall preventive effects of PRP were found for depression diagnoses. Gillham and colleagues[57] examined the efficacy of adding a parent intervention component to the PRP. The parent intervention component was designed to increase parents' overall resilience as well as their parenting skills. Results indicated that students in the PRP-plus-parent group reported lower levels of depressive symptoms ($P = .05$) and anxiety symptoms ($P = .01$) over the follow-up period, relative to those receiving usual care. These findings have important clinical implications. First, it seems that this intervention prevents both depressive and anxiety symptoms, which have been found to be potential risk factors for youth depression.[57] Second, these findings support the involvement of parents in preventing youth depression.

The PRP has further been evaluated with African American and Latino children who were at risk because of their low-income status.[58] The Latino children, primarily Puerto Rican, reported significantly fewer depressive symptoms ($P = .001$) than did the children in the control group, and these results were consistent at the 6-month follow-up. Furthermore, Latino children in the prevention group had fewer negative automatic thoughts ($P = .01$) and feelings of hopelessness ($P = .1$). For the African American children, however, there were no significant differences in the number of reported depressive symptoms between the intervention and control groups. Similarly, there were no significant differences in negative automatic thoughts or hopelessness between the

2 groups of African American children. Importantly however, children in the prevention group did show significant improvement over the course of the intervention, but the results were not significantly different from the no-treatment control condition. These results were found to be consistent at a 2-year follow-up.[59]

CB program

Based on research by Lewinsohn and colleagues[60] examining the risk for depression in adolescents, Clarke and colleagues[61] developed the CWS course, a manual-based psychoeducational group program targeting adolescents at risk for the development of depressive disorders. The CWS program aims to help at-risk teenagers gain control over negative moods, resolve conflicts that arise at home and with peers, and alter maladaptive thought patterns. The CWS program targets teenagers aged 13 to 17 years and is delivered by trained mental health professionals (eg, social workers and psychologists) in a group setting.

Clarke and colleagues[61] examined the effectiveness of the CWS program, relative to a Usual-Care Control (UC) condition, in a randomized controlled trial (RCT) of 94 adolescent offspring of adults treated for depression in an HMO. Eligible teenagers had to have subdiagnostic depressive symptoms and/or a history of mood disorder and a parent with a significant depressive disorder. Results indicated that, relative to teenagers assigned to the UC program, teenagers in the CWS program reported fewer depressive symptoms, fewer symptoms of suicide, and better overall functioning. At 12-month follow-up, 9.3% of the teenagers in the CWS program met diagnostic criteria for major depression compared with 28.8% of the teenagers in the UC condition ($P = .003$). Although the significant preventive effect persisted across a 24-month follow-up interval, the magnitude of the effect diminished ($P = .02$ at 18 months; $P = .05$ at 24 months).

A 4-site effectiveness study led by Garber and colleagues[62] is being conducted using a variant of the CWS program developed by Clarke and colleagues.[61] Known as the Prevention of Depression in At-Risk Adolescents Study, Garber and colleagues[62] have modified the CWS program to include 8 weekly and 6 monthly continuation sessions and have recruited 316 teenagers (nearly 80 from each site) who have been assigned randomly to the Cognitive Behavioral Prevention Program (CBP) or the UC condition. Results indicate that, through the 8-month follow-up assessment conducted at the completion of the monthly continuation sessions, significantly fewer teenagers in the CBP group had a probable or definite episode of depression, compared with adolescents in the UC condition.[63] Moreover, this main intervention effect was moderated by current parental depression at baseline, such that among adolescents whose parents were not depressed at baseline, CBP was much more effective in preventing the incidence of depressive episodes than UC. Among adolescents in both conditions with a currently depressed parent, rates of incident depression were not significantly different from each other.[63] It should be noted that the studies by Clarke and colleagues and Garber and colleagues are a combination of selective and indicated preventive interventions, that is, the parents have depression (selective prevention) and some of the children are also symptomatic (indicated prevention). A long-term follow-up of this sample is currently underway.

Family-based program

Several intervention programs for the prevention of depression in children and adolescents have incorporated the family system as an integral target of intervention. One such study by Compas and colleagues[64] assessed the efficacy of a family CB preventive intervention aimed at preventing depression in the offspring of parents with a history of depression. The 111 families were randomly assigned to an intervention or control condition. The intervention condition consisted of 8 weekly and 4 monthly sessions with up to 4 families per group, in which both the parents and the children participated. The family CB intervention was designed to educate families about depressive disorders, help families recognize and deal with stress, promote adaptive coping responses to stress, improvement of parenting skills, and increasing family awareness of the effect that stress and depression can have on functioning. The families were also assessed at 2, 6, and 12 months after intervention.

Results indicated that overall, the family CB program produced the strongest effects for positive parent and child outcomes, relative to the control condition. The intervention, relative to the control condition, produced significant benefits in children in terms of depressive symptoms, anxiety symptoms, and internalizing symptoms with marginally significant effects on externalizing symptoms. Depressive symptoms in children were also significantly less in the intervention group as compared with the control group at all 3 assessment points.

Beardslee and colleagues[65] have also developed 2 public health interventions for families when parents are depressed. Their approaches emphasize a cognitive orientation and focus on building strengths and resilience in youth. They also focus on the family as a unit of change and aim to increase parents' understanding of depression and the effects of their depression on their spouses and children. In the Beardslee clinician-facilitated intervention approach, six to eight 45- to 90-minute sessions were conducted with a clinician and individual families, culminating with a family meeting in which the clinician facilitated a family discussion of depression and its effects on the family. The lecture control condition consisted of 2 small group lectures for parents only. Although children did not attend these lecture sessions directly, parents were encouraged to discuss with their children the effects of depression on the family.

Beardslee and colleagues[65–69] have examined the efficacy of the Beardslee prevention approaches. In this research, 100 families with parental depression and a nondepressed child aged 8 to 15 years were assigned randomly to either the clinician-facilitated or the lecture group condition. The families were assessed at baseline, immediately after intervention, and then at approximately 1-year intervals over several years. Both conditions were associated with positive changes in parents' behaviors and attitudes regarding their children, in general family improvements, and in decreased depressive symptoms in children. However, relative to the lecture group condition, the clinician-facilitated condition was associated with greater understanding by children of their parents' depressive illness and improved communication between children and parents. Intervention effects were sustained at 2.5- and 4-year follow-up intervals.[65,66] Moreover, families in which parents reported the most change in behavior and attitude had children who showed the greatest increase in their understanding of their parents' illness, one of the main targets of this preventive intervention.

It is noteworthy that since the development of these intervention approaches, several research groups have adapted the general principles of these programs to new populations and have evaluated these approaches in effectiveness trials. Podorefsky and colleagues[70] adapted the clinician-facilitated intervention approach for use in a low-income urban population and found that families who participated in the intervention reported positive change in family communication, understanding, and focus on the child. They also recently adapted it for use with Latino mothers.[71] Several European countries have developed countrywide programs for children of people with mental illness. Solantaus and Toikka[72] have developed a successful program in Finland and selected the clinician intervention, as one of several interventions, for widespread use. It proved possible both to adapt this program to the Finnish context and to train clinicians in its use.[73]

Unlike other researchers examining the prevention of youth depression in teenagers identified based on their elevated depressive symptoms or family history of depression, Sandler and colleagues[74] focused on preventing negative outcomes in children at risk based on difficult life circumstances, including parental divorce and bereavement. Their research programs rely on correlational studies that identify protective and vulnerability factors that may be addressed through intervention. Both Sandler's parental divorce and bereavement programs have been evaluated experimentally to learn about the effects of these interventions on changing these factors to promote resilience.

Based on research indicating that parental divorce, although common, places children at risk for adjustment difficulties after divorce, Tein and colleagues[75] and Wolchik and colleagues[76] developed and evaluated the New Beginnings Program (NBP), a preventive intervention for divorced families that consists of 2 components: a mother program and a dual-component program that targeted mothers and children in separate but concurrent intervention approaches. These 2 active intervention programs were contrasted to a self-study literature control program in which, during a 6-week period, mothers and children received written materials pertaining to parental divorce.

In a study of 240 recently (within the past 2 years) divorced families with a female primary residential parent and at least one child aged 9 to 12 years, families were assigned randomly to either the mother program, the dual-component (mother and child) intervention, or the self-study control condition.[77] Overall, the mother program was associated with positive change in the mother-child relationship, discipline, and the child's relationship with the father compared with families who were assigned to the self-study control condition, although some of these changes were not sustained during the 6-month follow-up. In addition, the mother program was associated with mother and child reports of children's decreased internalizing and externalizing of problems. At the 6-year follow-up, youths in the dual-component intervention compared with youths in the control condition tended to have fewer diagnosed mental disorders ($P = .007$).[77] Children in the NBP improved more on total psychiatric symptoms, externalizing problems, substance use, grade point average, and had a reduced number of sexual partners.[77]

Sandler and colleagues[78–81] and Tein and colleagues[82] have also developed the Family Bereavement Program (FBP), which aims to prevent mental health problems in bereaved children aged 8 to 16 years and promote resilient outcomes for children and families facing parental loss. The FBP targeted key family-level variables, including the quality of the caregiver-child relationship, mental health problems in the caregiver, the child's exposure to negative life events, and discipline.[79] The FBP is a 2-component program that includes separate groups for parents and/or caregivers and for bereaved children. Sandler and colleagues[81] evaluated the FBP in an RCT of 156 families in which a parent had died between 4 and 30 months before enrollment and in which neither the surviving parent nor the child (aged 8–16 years) were receiving mental health or bereavement services. Families were assigned randomly to either the FBP or to a self-study control program, in which books about grief were distributed to parents and children at monthly intervals.

Overall, the results indicated that, relative to families in the self-study control group, families in the FBP demonstrated improved family and individual risk factors immediately after intervention. However, the FBP was not associated with a change in children's mental health problems after test. At 11-month follow-up, the FBP program was found to improve self-report mental health outcomes for girls, and for children who exhibited more internalizing and externalizing difficulties at baseline. Finally, new main effects of the program emerged at 6-year follow-up for youths' self-esteem and externalizing behaviors.[81] Work by Sandler and colleagues[74] highlights the importance of intervening with families during times of stress. In addition, this work suggests the possibility that intervention effects may emerge gradually over time and that the effects of intervention strategies may vary by sex. At present, Sandler and colleagues are examining longer-term intervention effects and exploring the effects of intervention on clinical diagnoses of depression.

Indicated Prevention Programs

Internet-based programs

In recent years, the Internet has joined the ranks of preventive intervention tools because programs have begun to use the accessibility and cost-effectiveness of Internet-based programs. Van Voorhees and colleagues[83] have implemented a pilot study of a primary care, Internet-based depression prevention intervention for at-risk adolescents, "Project CATCH-IT." The program combines CB therapy, behavioral activation, and interpersonal psychotherapy techniques. A family training program was also included in the intervention to enhance family resiliency by targeting and improving parenting skills. The intervention consisted of a primary care interview, followed by the Internet-based intervention, which was followed by an additional primary care interview and data collection, approximately 4 to 6 weeks postintervention. Preliminary findings indicated that adolescents were willing to engage in the intervention and viewed the program favorably.

Van Voorhees and colleagues[84] further explored the efficacy of Internet-indicated prevention programs by determining the willingness of adolescents to participate based on the type of primary care physician engagement provided. The participants were randomly assigned to one of 2 Internet-based prevention groups: Brief Advice (BA) plus Internet Program, and Motivational Interview (MI) plus Internet Program. Participation and satisfaction were measured over a 12-month period in order to assess the willingness of at-risk adolescents to use an Internet-based prevention of depression program.

Results indicated that the MI group had significantly higher engagement responses to the Internet program than did the BA group in terms of total time on site ($P = .03$), number of sessions ($P = .04$), longer duration of session activity on the Internet ($P = .04$), and more characters typed into the exercises ($P = .01$). Furthermore, the MI group displayed higher trust in their physician ($P = .05$) and greater satisfaction in the Internet component relative to the BA group ($P = .01$). As this study demonstrates, motivational interviews with the primary care physician may encourage adolescent participation in Internet-based prevention programs for depression, allowing for prevention to reach a population that may not be responsive to traditional prevention programs.

Interpersonal

Based on an effective interpersonal psychotherapy treatment program for depressed adolescents,[85,86] the IPT-AST program was developed and evaluated for effectiveness in preventing the onset of depressive disorders in high-risk teenagers. This school-based group intervention focuses on psychoeducation regarding depression and its prevention and skill building that targets interpersonal role disputes, role transitions, and interpersonal deficits. Young and colleagues[87] report a school-based study of IPT-AST in which 41 primarily Hispanic youth aged 11 to 16 years with elevated scores on a measure of depressive symptoms were assigned randomly to either the intervention group or to a school counseling control group. The IPT-AST intervention included 2 initial individual sessions, followed by 8 weekly 90-minute group sessions. Sessions were conducted during the school day and implemented by school guidance counselors and/or psychologists trained by the research team.

Results indicated that, relative to children in the school counseling control condition, adolescents in the IPT-AST group reported fewer symptoms of depression, controlling for baseline depression scores, and better overall functioning and that these differences were sustained across the 6-month follow-up. In addition, across the 6-month follow-up interval, 3.7% of the teenagers in the IPT-AST group met diagnostic criteria for a clinical diagnosis of depression, compared with 28.6% of the teenagers assigned to the control group. This difference was marginally significant ($P = .08$). Although promising, it is concerning that only half of eligible youth elected to participate in this program. Nonetheless, this work suggests that it may be possible to prevent depressive disorders with relatively short interventions, and as the investigators themselves have suggested, it may well make sense to combine this approach with more-traditional CB approaches to depression prevention in youth.[88]

SUMMARY AND DISCUSSION

The specific depression prevention programs reviewed in the previous sections share several meaningful characteristics. In general, the content of these interventions was outlined in manuals and based on evidence-based treatment programs for adolescent depression, those implementing the protocols were carefully trained, and fidelity to the intervention protocols was assessed. The interventions were based on an understanding of risk and protective factors for youth depression, generally targeted an opportune developmental window for depression prevention, and were consistent with universal, selective, and indicated prevention models.

Overall, it seems that there is reason for hope regarding the role of interventions in preventing depressive disorders in youth. Certainly, it seems that such prevention programs decrease children's levels of depressive symptoms, and as symptoms clearly are forerunners of full-blown episodes, they are an important positive outcome in and of themselves. There is evidence that prevention interventions can produce meaningful family change and that this change in family functioning can have long-term positive benefits on children and adolescents.

This review highlights several directions for future research on the prevention of depression in youth.

1. Given the high cost of depression once it occurs and the promise of the initial studies that have been described for selective and indicated prevention, much more attention needs to be focused on depression prevention efforts. Even though none of these programs is ready for widespread dissemination at present, we think that should be the goal over the long-term.
2. We believe that further research will continue to establish an empirical base for the prevention of depression in high-risk youth. Thus, short-term manual-based preventive interventions for youth at high risk for depression should be considered for widespread use and should be considered core parts of the resources available to clinicians and families at high risk for depression. It is important that future interventions both be assessed for and able to contribute to long-term positive outcomes.
3. Selected and indicated prevention approaches appear to be more effective than universal prevention approaches.[46]
4. It is important to attend to moderators of intervention effects. It seems that some intervention programs work better for youth at particularly high risk for depression,

based on individual risk variables and/or family risk. Additional important moderators to consider in future research include sex and exposure to recent stressors.[52,89]

5. It is important to consider approaches that can be widely used and easily taught in addition to more specialized approaches. The family approaches of the Preventive Intervention Project and the development of countrywide programs in Scandinavia emphasize that when good public health interventions are available, they can be widely disseminated.

6. Prevention programs targeting youth depression should include efforts to enhance the family environment. Avenevoli and Merikangas[88] argue that family-based programs are indicated because parental psychopathology is associated with general dysfunction in parental and/or family environment, such that changing the environment of at-risk youth may lower their risk for depression. In fact, family factors may maintain depression in youth[90,91] and have been found to predict outcome and treatment response among depressed children and adolescents. Moreover, adverse family environments are among the most consistent risk factors for adolescent depression.[37] The Preventive Intervention Project, as well as the programs developed by Sandler and colleagues,[74] are examples of effective family-based programs. Similar programs targeting the prevention of youth depression are warranted. More generally, the IOM report on prevention emphasized the value of programs that enhance parenting for families.

7. While not the primary focus of this article, careful study of risk factors for depression emphasizes the importance of both specific and nonspecific risk factors. In terms of the nonspecific risk factors, attention to poverty, exposure to violence, child sexual abuse, and circumstances in which children are exposed to multiple adversities in childhood are needed. Clearly, we would substantially reduce the illness burden for a wide array of childhood and adolescent difficulties including depression if we more fully assessed these nonspecific risk factors.

8. As more is understood about the underlying neuroscience dimensions of depression, effective prevention strategies are likely to be suggested. For example, if it becomes possible to identify those at highest risk earlier in the course of childhood because of genetic vulnerability, it may well be possible to more effectively target specific prevention approaches.

9. More research is needed on the dissemination phase of prevention research. Efforts to demonstrate the effectiveness of prevention programs need to consider the unique needs and experiences of children from different ethnic and cultural groups.[92]

10. There needs to be much greater coordination among efforts for the prevention of depression in children and adolescents. It would be useful if one of the federal agencies took the lead in coordinating this across the National Institute of Health, and also involving other research resources such as those supported by foundations. Through coordinating different research efforts, it is much more likely that broadly disseminated programs could be identified.

REFERENCES

1. Kessler RC, Berglund P, Demler O, et al. The epidemiology of major depressive disorder: results from the National Comorbidity Survey Replication (NCS-R). JAMA 2003;289:3095–105.
2. World Health Organization. The global burden of disease. (CE). Geneva (Switzerland): WHO Press; 1996.

3. Greenberg PE, Kessler R, Birnbaum H. The economic burden of depression in the United States: how did it change between 1990 and 2000? J Clin Psychiatry 2003;64:1465–75.
4. Lynch F, Clarke G. Estimating the economic burden of depression in children and adolescents. Am J Prev Med 2006;31:S143–51.
5. Mueller TI, Leon AC, Keller MB, et al. Recurrence after recovery from major depressive disorder during 15 years of observational follow-up. Am J Psychiatry 1999;156:1000–6.
6. National Research Council and Institute of Medicine. Prevention Committee. Preventing mental, emotional, and behavioral disorders among young people: progress and possibilities. Washington, DC: National Academies Press; 2009.
7. Kovacs M. Next steps for research on child and adolescent depression prevention. Am J Prev Med 2006;31:S184–5.
8. Costello EJ, Pine DS, Hammen C, et al. Development and natural history of mood disorders. Biol Psychiatry 2002;52:529–42.
9. Kessler R, Walters EE. Epidemiology of DSM-III-R major depression and minor depression among adolescents and young adults in the National Comorbidity Survey. Depress Anxiety 1998;7:3–15.
10. Birmaher B, Ryan ND, Brent D, et al. Child and adolescent depression: a review of the past ten years. Part I. J Am Acad Child Adolesc Psychiatry 1996;35:1427–39.
11. Birmaher B, Ryan ND, Williamson DE, et al. Child and adolescent depression: a review of the past ten years. Part II. J Am Acad Child Adolesc Psychiatry 1996;35:1575–83.
12. Lewinsohn PM, Clarke GN, Seeley JR, et al. Major depression in community adolescents: age at onset, episode duration, and time to recurrence. J Am Acad Child Adolesc Psychiatry 1994;33:809–18.
13. Kessler R, Wai CT, Demler O, et al. Prevalence, severity, and comorbidity of 12-month DSM-IV disorders in the National Comorbidity Survey replication. Arch Gen Psychiatry 2005;62:617–27.
14. March JS, Silva S, Petrycki S. Treatment for Adolescents with Depression Study Team. Fluoxetine, cognitive-behavioral therapy, and their combination for adolescents with depression. JAMA 2004;292:807–20.
15. Kovacs M, Feinberg TL, Crouse-Novak MA, et al. Depressive disorders in childhood: I. A longitudinal prospective study of characteristics and recovery. Arch Gen Psychiatry 1984;41:229–37.
16. Kovacs M, Feinberg TL, Crouse-Novak MA, et al. Depressive disorders in childhood: II. A longitudinal prospective study of characteristics and recovery. Arch Gen Psychiatry 1984;41:643–9.
17. Bardone AM, Moffitt T, Caspi A, et al. Adult mental health and social outcomes of adolescent girls with depression and conduct disorder. Dev Psychopathol 1996; 8:811–29.
18. Bardone AM, Moffitt T, Caspi A. Adult physical health outcomes of adolescent girls with conduct disorder, depression and anxiety. J Am Acad Child Adolesc Psychiatry 1998;37:594–601.
19. Lewinsohn PM, Pettit JW, Joiner TE, et al. The symptomatic expression of major depressive disorder in adolescents and young adults. J Abnorm Psychol 2003; 112:244–53.
20. Rao U, Ryan ND, Birmaher B, et al. Unipolar depression in adolescents: clinical outcome in adulthood. J Am Acad Child Adolesc Psychiatry 1995;34:566–78.
21. Weissman MM, Wolk S, Goldstein RB, et al. Depressed adolescents grown up. JAMA 1999;17:7–13.

22. Rubin KH, Both L, Zahn-Waxler C, et al. Dyadic play behaviors of children of well and depressed mothers. Dev Psychopathol 1991;3:243–51.
23. Harnish JD, Dodge KA, Valente E. Mother–child interaction quality as a partial mediator of the roles of maternal depressive symptomatology and socioeconomic status in the development of child behavior problems. Child Dev 1995;66:739–53.
24. Centers for Disease Control and Prevention, National Center for Injury Prevention and Control. In: Web-based Injury Statistics Query and Reporting System (WISQARS). Atlanta (GA): Centers for Disease Control and Prevention; 2010. Available at: http://www.cdc.gov/ncipc/wisqars. Accessed August 23, 2010.
25. Centers for Disease Control and Prevention. Youth risk behavior surveillance-United States 2009. MMWR Surveill Summ 2010;59:1–142, SS–5.
26. Clarke G, Hornbrook M, Lynch F, et al. A randomized trial of a group cognitive intervention for preventing depression in adolescent offspring of depressed parents. Arch Gen Psychiatry 2001;58:1127–34.
27. Garber J, Clarke G, Weersing VR, et al. Prevention of depression in at-risk adolescents: a randomized controlled trial. JAMA 2009;301:2215–24.
28. Kessler RC, McGonagle KA, Zhao S, et al. Lifetime and 12-month prevalence of DSM-III-R psychiatry disorders in the United States. Arch Gen Psychiatry 1994;51: 8–19.
29. Treatment of depression and bipolar disorder. In: Evans DL, Foa EB, Gur RE, et al, editors. Treating and preventing adolescent mental health disorders: what we know and what we don't know. New York: Oxford University Press; 2005. p. 30–54.
30. Kennard BD, Silva SG, Tonev S, et al. Remission and recovery in the Treatment for Adolescents with Depression Study (TADS): acute and long-term outcomes. J Am Acad Child Adolesc Psychiatry 2009;48:186–95.
31. Curry J, Rohde P, Simons A. Predictors and moderators of acute outcome in TADS. J Am Acad Child Adolesc Psychiatry 2006;45:1427–39.
32. Birmaher B, Brent DA, Kolko D, et al. Clinical outcome after short-term psychotherapy for adolescents with major depressive disorder. Arch Gen Psychiatry 2000;57:29–36.
33. Brent DA, Kolko DJ, Birmaher B, et al. Predictors of treatment efficacy in a clinical trial of three psychosocial treatments for adolescent depression. J Am Acad Child Adolesc Psychiatry 1998;37:906–14.
34. Clarke G, Hops H, Lewinsohn PM, et al. Cognitive-behavioral group treatment of adolescent depression: prediction of outcome. Behav Ther 1992;23:341–54.
35. Emslie GJ, Rush AJ, Weiberg WA, et al. Fluoxetine in child and adolescent depression: acute and maintenance treatment. Depress Anxiety 1998;7:32–9.
36. Mrazek PJ, Haggerty RJ. Reducing risks for mental disorders: frontiers for preventive research. Washington, DC: National Academy Press; 1994.
37. Evans DL, Foa EB, Gur RE, et al, editors. Treating and preventing adolescent mental health disorders: what we know and what we don't know. New York: Oxford University Press; 2005.
38. The National Advisory Mental Health Council Workgroup on Child and Adolescent Mental Health Intervention Development and Deployment. Blueprint for change: research on child and adolescent mental health. Washington, DC: The National Institute of Mental Health, Office of Communications and Public Liaison; 2001.
39. National Research Council, Institute of Medicine. The etiology of depression. In: Depression in parents, parenting, and children. Washington, DC: National Academies Press; 2009. p. 73–118.

40. Defining depression and bipolar disorder. In: Evans DL, Foa EB, Gur RE, et al, editors. Treating and preventing adolescent mental health disorders: what we know and what we don't know. New York: Oxford University Press; 2005. p. 4–27.

41. Joorman J, Eugene F, Gotlib IH. Parental depression: impact on offspring and mechanisms underlying transmission of risk. In: Nolen-Hoeksema S, Hilt LM, editors. Handbook of depression in adolescence. New York: Taylor & Francis Group; 2009. p. 441–72.

42. Beardslee WR, Podorefsky D. Resilient adolescents whose parents have serious affective and other psychiatric disorders: importance of self-understanding and relationships. Am J Psychiatry 1988;145:63–9.

43. Gilman SE, Kawachi I, Fitzmaurice GM, et al. Socioeconomic status in childhood and the lifetime risk of major depression. Int J Epidemiol 2002;31:359–67.

44. Widom CS, Dumont K, Czaja SJ. A prospective investigation of major depressive disorder and comorbidity in abused and neglected children grown up. Arch Gen Psychiatry 2007;64:49–56.

45. Horowitz JL, Garber J. The prevention of depressive symptoms in children and adolescents: a meta-analytic review. J Consult Clin Psychol 2006;74:401–15.

46. Gillham JE, Shatte AJ, Freres DR. Preventing depression: a review of cognitive-behavioral and family interventions. Appl Prev Psychol 2000;9:63–88.

47. Kaslow NJ, Thompson MP. Applying the criteria for empirically supported treatments to studies of psychosocial interventions for child and adolescent depression. J Clin Child Psychol 1998;27:146–55.

48. Spence SH, Sheffield JK, Donovan CL. Preventing adolescent depression: an evaluation of the problem solving for life program. J Consult Clin Psychol 2003;71:3–13.

49. Spence SH, Sheffield JK, Donovan CL. Long-term outcome of a school-based, universal approach to prevention of depression in adolescents. J Consult Clin Psychol 2005;73:160–7.

50. Shochet IM, Dadds MR, Holland D, et al. The efficacy of a universal school-based program to prevent adolescent depression. J Clin Child Psychol 2001;30:303–15.

51. Merry S, McDowell H, Wild CJ, et al. A randomized placebo-controlled trial of a school-based depression prevention program. J Am Acad Child Adolesc Psychiatry 2004;43:538–47.

52. Horowitz JL, Garber J, Ciesla JA, et al. Prevention of depressive symptoms in adolescence: a randomized trial of cognitive behavioral and interpersonal prevention programs. J Consult Clin Psychol 2007;75:693–706.

53. Clarke G, Gladstone T, DeBar L, et al. Coping with stress course: prior effectiveness research, revision and improvements. Paper presented at the American Academy of Child and Adolescent Psychiatry. Boston, October 23–28, 2007.

54. Gillham J, Reivich K, Jaycox L, et al. The Penn Resiliency Program. Philadelphia: University of Pennsylvania; 1990.

55. Gillham J, Brunwasser SM, Freres DR. Preventing depression in early adolescence. In: Abela JRZ, Hankin BL, editors. Handbook of depression in children and adolescents. New York: Guilford Press; 2008. p. 309–22.

56. Gillham JE, Hamilton J, Freres DR, et al. Preventing depression among early adolescents in the primary care setting: a randomized controlled study of the Penn Resiliency Program. J Abnorm Child Psychol 2006;34:203–19.

57. Gillham JE, Reivich KJ, Freres DR, et al. School-based prevention of depression and anxiety symptoms in early adolescence: a pilot of a parent intervention component. Sch Psychol Q 2006;21:323–48.

58. Cardemil EV, Reivich KJ, Seligman ME. The prevention of depressive symptoms in low-income minority middle school students. Prev Treat 2002;5(1).

59. Cardemil EV, Reivich KJ, Beevers CG, et al. The prevention of depressive symptoms in low-income minority children: two-year follow-up. Behav Res Ther 2007; 45:313–27.
60. Lewinsohn PM, Roberts R, Seeley J, et al. Adolescent psychopathology: II. Psychosocial risk factors for depression. J Abnorm Psychol 1994;103:302–15.
61. Clarke G, Hawkins W, Murphy M, et al. Targeted prevention of unipolar depressive disorder in an at-risk sample of high school adolescents: a randomized trial of a group cognitive intervention. J Am Acad Child Adolesc Psychiatry 1995;34: 312–21.
62. Garber J, Clarke G, Brent D, et al. Preventing depression in at-risk adolescents: design and sample characteristics. Paper presented at the American Academy of Child and Adolescent Psychiatry. Boston, October 23–28, 2007.
63. Weersing R, Brent D, Garber J, et al. Prevention of depression in at-risk adolescents: outcome at 8 months. Paper presented at the American Academy of Child and Adolescent Psychiatry. Boston, October 23–28, 2007.
64. Compas BE, Champion JE, Reeslund KL, et al. Randomized controlled trial of a family cognitive-behavioral preventive intervention for children of depressed parents. J Consult Clin Psychol 2009;77:1007–20.
65. Beardslee WR, Gladstone TRG, Wright EJ, et al. A family-based approach to the prevention of depressive symptoms in children at risk: evidence of parental and child change. Pediatrics 2003;112:E99–111.
66. Beardslee W, Salt P, Versage E, et al. Sustained change in parents receiving preventive interventions for families with depression. Am J Psychiatry 1997; 154:510–5.
67. Beardslee W, Versage E, Wright E, et al. Examination of preventive interventions for families with depression: evidence of change. Dev Psychopathol 1997;9: 109–30.
68. Beardslee WR, Wright EJ, Salt P, et al. Examination of children's responses to two preventive intervention strategies over time. J Am Acad Child Adolesc Psychiatry 1997;36:196–204.
69. Beardslee W, Wright E, Gladstone T, et al. Long-term effects from a randomized trial of two public health preventive interventions for parental depression. J Fam Psychol 2007;21:703–13.
70. Podorefsky DL, McDonald-Dowdell M, Beardslee WR. Adaptation of preventive interventions for a low-income, culturally diverse community. J Am Acad Child Adolesc Psychiatry 2001;40:879–86.
71. D'Angelo EJ, Llerena-Quinn R, Shapiro R, et al. Adaptation of the preventive intervention program for depression for use with predominantly low-income Latino families. Fam Process 2009;48(2):269–91.
72. Solantaus T, Toikka T. The effective family programme: preventative services for the children of mentally ill parents in Finland. Int J Ment Health Promot 2005;3:37–43.
73. Solantous T, Toikka S, Alasuutari M, et al. Safety, feasibility, and family experiences of preventive interventions for children and families with parental depression. Int J Ment Health Promo 2009;11:15–24.
74. Sandler IN, Wolchik SA, Davis CH, et al. Correlational and experimental study of resilience for children of divorce and parentally-bereaved children. In: Luthar SS, editor. Resilience and vulnerability: adaptation in the context of childhood adversities. New York: Cambridge University Press; 2003. p. 213–40.
75. Tein JY, Sandler IN, MacKinnon DP, et al. How did it work? Who did it work for? Mediation in the context of a moderated prevention effect for children of divorce. J Consult Clin Psychol 2004;72:617–24.

76. Wolchik SA, West SG, Sandler IN, et al. An experimental evaluation of theory-based mother and mother–child programs for children of divorce. J Consult Clin Psychol 2000;68:843–56.
77. Wolchik SA, Sandler IN, Millsap RE, et al. Six-year follow-up of preventive interventions for children of divorce: a randomized controled trial. J Am Acad Child Adolesc Psychiatry 2002;288:1874–81.
78. Sandler IN, Ayers TS, Romer AL. Fostering resilience in families in which a parent has died. J Palliat Med 2002;5:945–56.
79. Sandler IN, Ayers TS, Wolchik SA, et al. The Family Bereavement Program: efficacy evaluation of a theory-based prevention program for parentally bereaved children and adolescents. J Consult Clin Psychol 2003;71:587–600.
80. Sandler IN, Wolchik SA, Ayers TS. Resilience rather than recovery: a contextual framework on adaptation following bereavement. Death Stud 2008;32:59–73.
81. Sandler IN, Wolchik SA, Ayers TS, et al. Linking theory and intervention to promote resilience of children following parental bereavement. In: Stroebe M, Hansson M, Stroebe W, et al, editors. Handbook of bereavement research: consequence, coping and care. Washington, DC: American Psychological Association; 2008.
82. Tein JY, Sandler IN, Ayers TS, et al. Mediation of the effects of the Family Bereavement Program on mental health problems of bereaved children and adolescents. Prev Sci 2006;7:179–95.
83. Van Voorhees BW, Vanderplough-Booth K, Fogel J, et al. Integrative internet-based depression prevention for adolescents: a randomized clinical trial in primary care for vulnerability and protective factors. J Can Acad Child Adolesc Psychiatry 2008;17:184–96.
84. Van Voorhees BW, Fogel J, Pomper BE, et al. Adolescent dose and ratings of an internet-based depression prevention program: a randomized trial of primary care physician brief advice versus a motivational interview. J Cogn Behav Psychother 2009;9:1–19.
85. Mufson L, Dorta KP, Moreau D, et al. Interpersonal psychotherapy for depressed adolescents. 2nd edition. New York: Guilford Press; 2004.
86. Mufson L, Dorta KP, Wickramaratne P, et al. A randomized effectiveness trial of interpersonal psychotherapy for depressed adolescents. Arch Gen Psychiatry 2004;61:577–84.
87. Young JF, Mufson L, Davies M. Efficacy of interpersonal psychotherapy-adolescent skills training: an indicated preventive intervention for depression. J Child Psychol Psychiatry 2006;47:1254–62.
88. Avenevoli S, Merikangas KR. Implications of high-risk family studies for prevention of depression. Am J Prev Med 2006;31:s126–35.
89. Sims B, Nottelmann E, Koretz DS, et al. Prevention of depression in children and adolescents [erratum]. Am J Prev Med 2007;32:451–5.
90. Brent D, Holder D, Kolko D, et al. A clinical psychotherapy trial for adolescent depression comparing cognitive, family and supportive therapy. Arch Gen Psychiatry 1998;54:877–85.
91. Hammen C, Rudolph K, Weisz J, et al. The context of depression in clinic-referred youth: neglected areas in treatment. J Am Acad Child Adolesc Psychiatry 1999;38:64–71.
92. Barrera M. Directions for expanding the prevention of depression in children and adolescents. Am J Prev Med 2006;31:S182–3.

Preventing Postpartum Depression

Laura J. Miller, MD[a],*, Elizabeth M. LaRusso, MD[b]

KEYWORDS

- Postpartum depression • Prevention
- Preconception counseling

Depression is one of the most common illnesses complicating the postpartum period. Its period prevalence has been estimated at 21.9% of women within the first year of giving birth.[1] Over 40% of women experiencing a postpartum depressive episode may experience a recurrent episode after a subsequent pregnancy.[2]

The consequences of postpartum depression can be devastating. Suicide is a major cause of perinatal maternal death.[3] Depressed mothers are less likely to breastfeed, read or sing to their babies, bring their babies to pediatric visits, and implement infant safety practices.[4,5] Adverse effects of maternal postpartum depression on offspring are apparent during infancy and persist through adolescence, including effects on emotion regulation, stress reactivity, and cognition.[6,7]

Although the causes of postpartum depression are not fully understood, certain factors have been found to correlate with increased risk of developing postpartum depression. These include genetic vulnerabilities, hormonal changes, stressors, insufficient social supports, nutritional deficits, sleep and circadian rhythm changes, and reduction in physical activity. It is posited that improvements in one or more of these areas could:

- reduce vulnerability to postpartum depression (primary prevention)
- reduce severity and duration of symptoms when postpartum depression occurs (secondary prevention)
- improve functioning, relationships, and prognosis for women and their offspring (tertiary prevention).

This article summarizes emerging evidence for interventions that may prevent postpartum depression and mitigate its adverse effects. It is worth noting the limitations of this body of knowledge.[8] Most studies to date have been underpowered for detection of prevention effects and have used symptom rating scales rather than diagnostic

a Department of Psychiatry, Brigham and Women's/Faulkner Hospitals, Harvard Medical School, 75 Francis Street, Boston, MA 02115, USA
b Department of Psychiatry, Dartmouth Medical School, Dartmouth Hitchcock Medical Center, One Medical Center Drive, Lebanon, NH 03756-0001, USA
* Corresponding author.
E-mail address: lmiller23@partners.org

Psychiatr Clin N Am 34 (2011) 53–65
doi:10.1016/j.psc.2010.11.010
0193-953X/11/$ – see front matter © 2011 Elsevier Inc. All rights reserved.

psych.theclinics.com

criteria for major depression. There has been no consensual definition of women at risk, thus limiting comparison of findings across studies. Perhaps most important, most studies to date have isolated a single intervention modality—for example, anti-depressant medication or telephone-based social support. However, risk for post-partum depression is multifactorial, with several influences interacting with one another and accounting for a portion of the variance.[9] In individual women, some of these influences may be more salient than others. Conceptual frameworks for preven-tion posit that when vulnerability to distress is multifactorial, mitigating influences are likely to be more powerful when acting cumulatively rather than individually.[10] There-fore, this article begins with a description of assessment of factors that may increase risk of postpartum depression, then summarizes interventions designed to address each modifiable risk factor.

ASSESSMENT OF RISK FOR POSTPARTUM DEPRESSION
Risk Factors for Postpartum Depression

Early identification of women at risk for postpartum depression is crucial to successful prevention. Risk factors associated with developing a postpartum depressive episode have been extensively studied and encompass elements of a woman's genetics, hormonal and reproductive history, and life experiences.[11] Biologic factors that have consistently been found to be associated with increased risk of postpartum depression include experiencing depressed mood or anxiety during pregnancy, a past history of depression or premenstrual dysphoric disorder, and a family history of depression.[11-14] Psychosocial factors, including stressful life events and lack of perceived social support, have also consistently been found to predict postpartum depression.[9,11,12,14] Several other factors, including low socioeconomic status, low self-esteem (particularly in relation to parenting ability), negative birth experience or obstetric complications, difficult infant temperament, and unplanned or unwanted pregnancy, have been less consistently demonstrated to be risk factors for developing postpartum depression.[11,12,14,15]

Formal Risk Assessment Tools

Although several tools have been created to attempt to identify women with known risk factors for postpartum depression, existing tools generally have low sensitivities and poor predictive values. In addition to the lack of a well-validated tool, there is no consensus on the optimal timing of prenatal risk assessment and no evidence on the cumulative impact of having more than one risk factor. Of the available tools, some take into account factors in the immediate postpartum period, decreasing their utility in primary prevention, whereas others can be used during pregnancy. Among the latter, the two that are the most well-studied have significant limitations. The Preg-nancy Risk Questionnaire only considers psychosocial risk and has low predictive value. The Postpartum Depression Predictors Inventory-Revised, a self-report ques-tionnaire developed based on findings from meta-analyses, appears to have good positive predictive value but may miss many true positives.[16,17]

Clinical Risk Assessment for Primary Prevention

In the absence of a widely validated screening tool, clinical assessment is the best strategy for early identification of women at risk for developing postpartum depres-sion. Key elements of a clinical assessment include:

- history of depressive episodes, including postpartum episodes
- history of premenstrual dysphoric symptoms

- family history of depression, including postpartum depression
- current and past stressors
- inventory of available social supports, particularly those in a position to offer practical assistance with the care of a newborn
- the patient's attitudes toward pregnancy and its ensuing role changes, including her expectations of herself as a mother.

For primary prevention, risk assessment optimally occurs during a preconception counseling session, while a woman is considering or planning a pregnancy. Clinicians can increase the likelihood of successful prevention by proactively encouraging preconception risk assessments in patients with depression who are of reproductive age.

Screening and Assessment for Secondary and Tertiary Prevention

A key to secondary and tertiary prevention is early and effective detection and treatment of perinatal depressive symptoms. There is substantial evidence that formal depression screening is significantly superior to routine clinical assessment at detecting perinatal depression.[18] Two frequently used screening tools are the Edinburgh Postnatal Depression Scale, which has been extensively validated in perinatal populations,[19] and the Patient Health Questionnaire-9, which has been extensively validated in primary care settings.[20] Tertiary prevention can also include assessment of mother-infant interaction and caretaking skills[21] to identify whether specific interventions are needed to support parenting and bonding.

PREVENTION STRATEGIES

One approach to designing a postpartum depression prevention strategy is to identify optimal protective factors, and to craft an individual plan to help each patient approximate this ideal. Evidence to date suggests that a woman with optimal resilience:

- is protected from the effects of abrupt hormonal flux on key neurotransmitter systems
- has excellent stress management skills
- knows how to negotiate for social support
- has a healthy eating pattern, including key nutrients
- has at least 30 minutes of aerobic physical activity daily
- gets enough light exposure during the day, and knows how to protect her sleep
- breastfeeds if she desires
- has babies when she wants to.

Depending on which of the above factors need strengthening for a given patient, preventive efforts can include antidepressant medication, cognitive-behavioral psychotherapy, interpersonal psychotherapy, strengthened social support, stress reduction and stress management, dietary improvements, exercise, sleep hygiene, breastfeeding support, and family planning. The applicability of each of these to preventing postpartum depression is summarized below.

Antidepressant Medication

Preventive antidepressant medication may be indicated for women with a history of medication-responsive major depressive episodes, particularly if some or all of the prior episodes were postpartum. Randomized double-blind placebo-controlled trials have shown a significant reduction in postpartum recurrence of major depression with sertraline[22] but not with nortriptyline.[23] It is unclear whether this is because the nortriptyline study was underpowered, or because serotonin-selective reuptake inhibitor agents are more effective than tricyclic antidepressants for preventing postpartum depression.

When considering the preventive use of antidepressant medication in asymptomatic women, a key question is when to begin the medication. In the sertraline study, starting immediately postpartum was effective. However, the risk of recurrence of major depressive episodes during pregnancy may be as high as 68%.[24] Weighing the relative risks of symptom relapse versus antidepressant medication on women and their fetuses in each case helps determine whether to begin antidepressant use during pregnancy.

Duration of preventive treatment is another key question. Studies show high relapse rates if medication is discontinued before 6 months.[25] Epidemiologic data suggest heightened risk of depression throughout the first year postpartum.[1] Although a subset of women only become depressed postpartum, most women at risk for postpartum depression are also at risk for subsequent non-postpartum episodes. For some women, use of an antidepressant for 6 months postpartum allows enough time to learn and implement nonpharmacologic strategies that will be sufficiently protective thereafter. Other women may need ongoing antidepressant use to prevent recurrence.

Psychotherapy

For women who are struggling emotionally and interpersonally with the transition to motherhood, interpersonal psychotherapy can reduce the risk of developing postpartum depression.[26,27] This form of brief psychotherapy, conducted individually or in groups, focuses on navigating social role transitions and negotiating effectively for support.

Cognitive-behavioral therapy (CBT) has not been uniformly found to be effective for preventing postpartum depression. Some data suggest that the most effective CBT strategies for preventing postpartum depression focus on challenging unrealistic "perfect mom" beliefs, and on improving problem-solving skills.[28] Variants of CBT such as behavioral activation and mindfulness-based cognitive therapy show promise in preventing recurrence of depression in general, and are being studied for prevention of postpartum depression.[29]

Social Support

Insufficient social support is a predictor of postpartum depressive symptoms in a variety of cultural contexts.[30–32] Perceived support, availability of support, and a woman's desire for the support are more robust predictors of reduced risk of postpartum depression than is the amount of social support received.[33,34] Social support appears to buffer the effects of stress on postpartum depression, reducing perceived stress and increasing adaptive stress responses.[35,36]

Most studies of natural social supports (ones that are in place within a woman's family, community, or culture) find that they reduce the risk of postpartum depression. Traditional postpartum cultural practices and rituals appear to protect against postpartum depression when they provide desired social support, regardless of the specific nature of the ritual or practice.[37] Conversely, contextual factors that reduce social support postpartum, such as giving birth to a girl in a culture that preferentially values boys, increase the risk of postpartum depression.[30] Reciprocal emotional support with a partner is especially influential.[38] Partners can also play a key role in secondary prevention of risks to offspring; for example, fathers' provision of social support to depressed mothers appears to reduce subsequent behavioral risks in their children.[39]

What is less clear is whether professionally administered social support is effective for preventing postpartum depression and, if so, what kind and with what intensity. Randomized controlled trials of preventive social support interventions have had mixed results, with most showing no short-term preventive effect and none demonstrating a sustained, long-term preventive effect.[40,41] Many of these studies were under powered, so it is not known whether the interventions would show effectiveness in a larger sample.

Examining the interventions with the most demonstrable efficacy to date may highlight promising preventive strategies. One group of effective approaches involves teaching women skills to enhance or activate social support networks, rather than providing social support directly.[42,43] Among interventions that directly provide support, the most effective seems to be outreach by public health nurses or midwives.[40]

Nutrition

Certain nutrients are essential for the biosynthesis and normal functioning of monoamine neurotransmitters. Among these, deficiencies in omega-3 essential fatty acids (n-3 EFA), folate, vitamin B-12, iron, and vitamin D have been associated with increased risk of depressive symptoms.[44] Mean dietary intake of these nutrients is below recommended amounts in pregnant women in the United States.[44]

Particularly important in preventing perinatal depression are n-3 EFAs due to their ability to promote γ-aminobutyric acid receptor binding[45] and reduce inflammation.[46] An analysis of studies from 23 countries showed that high n-3 EFA levels in breast milk, and higher seafood consumption (the food richest in n-3 EFA), predicted lower rates of postpartum depression.[47] Conversely, in another study, lower serum levels of n-3 EFA predicted the occurrence of postpartum depression.[48] However, studies of n-3 EFA supplements for treatment of perinatal depression have had inconsistent results.[49] Some fish rich in n-3 EFA have relatively high mercury content, whereas n-3 EFA supplements from reputable manufacturers are relatively free of this contaminant.[49]

Low serum folate levels are associated with increased occurrence, severity, and duration of symptoms of major depression, and with reduced response to antidepressant medication.[50] Taking prenatal vitamins with folate has not been shown to reduce the prevalence of depression during pregnancy.[51] However, methylfolate has been found to be effective as adjunctive or monotherapy for reducing depressive symptoms in patients with either normal or low serum folate levels.[52]

Iron deficiency anemia increases the risk of developing postpartum depression.[53] To date, no studies have established whether iron repletion prevents postpartum depression.

Overall, direct evidence is lacking that adequate nutrient intake can protect against postpartum depression. However, the evidence that adequate levels of n-3 EFA, folate, and iron protect against depression in general is relatively strong and intake of these nutrients is often insufficient during pregnancy and postpartum.

Physical Activity

Animal studies demonstrate that aerobic exercise protects neurons from the toxic effects of stress, resulting in less depression-like behavior.[54] Although it is not yet clear that a similar protective effect occurs in humans, studies to date suggest that higher levels of physical activity during pregnancy may reduce the risk of postpartum depressive symptoms.[55-58] The American College of Obstetrics and Gynecology recommends at least 30 minutes of moderate exercise on most, if not all, days of the week for pregnant women.[59] Many pregnant women reduce their physical activity to well below this recommended level, citing barriers such as discomfort, pregnancy complications, and insecurity about exercising while pregnant.[60] Among previously sedentary women who try to exercise regularly while pregnant, adherence to their intended exercise plan decreases as pregnancy progresses.[61] Overcoming the barriers to regular perinatal exercise may require considerable support from health care providers. **Box 1** summarizes recommended support strategies.

Sleep and Circadian Rhythm

Sleep disturbance is one of the most potent predictors of postpartum depression. Nearly all mothers of newborns experience frequent nighttime awakenings to care for their babies. By themselves, those awakenings are not associated with increased rates of postpartum depression. Rather, correlates of postpartum depression include a wake time of more than 2 hours between midnight and 6 AM, daytime sleep of less than an hour, and more subjective daytime sleepiness.[63] This suggests that difficulty falling back to sleep after caring for a baby, and insufficient opportunity for daytime naps, may increase the risk of postpartum depression. Environmental factors may contribute to these problems (eg, a noisy environment or the need to care for other children). Perinatal alterations in hormonal circadian rhythms, particularly disturbances of the diurnal rhythm of cortisol[64] and melatonin,[65] may also play a role. In addition, maternal depression and infant sleep disturbances may adversely affect one another. Babies of mothers with depressive symptoms or a history of major depressive disorders have been found to take longer to fall asleep and to have lower sleep efficiency than babies of mothers without depressive symptoms or history.[66]

There are few studies to date directly addressing the role of sleep and circadian rhythm improvement in preventing postpartum depression. One study improved maternal sleep immediately postpartum in women at high risk of postpartum depression through a combination of longer hospital stays, private rooms, infant rooming out overnight, and benzodiazepines as needed. The women receiving this intervention were less likely to develop postpartum depression and had fewer postpartum psychiatric admissions than the control group of women.[67] Another study compared the effects of morning phototherapy (use of a therapeutic light box) versus a control condition (red light) in women with postpartum depressive symptoms and found no difference in symptom improvement.[68] This study (N = 15) was likely underpowered.

By contrast, several studies have demonstrated the efficacy of strategies to improve sleep in general[69] and postpartum.[70] These are summarized in **Box 2**.

Box 1
Strategies for clinicians to engage patients in increasing physical activity

Dispel myths about exercise being dangerous during pregnancy.

Help patients plan realistic ways to increase their physical activity.

Give written prescriptions for the chosen exercise regimens; follow up to identify and overcome barriers to adherence.[62]

Enlist support from significant others in supporting the exercise plan (eg, by participating with them or assuming child care responsibilities to free up patients' time).

Sponsor clinic-based exercise programs or telephone reminders for home-based exercise programs.[58]

Box 2
Strategies to improve sleep postpartum
Breastfeeding and cosleeping with the infant, with safety measures such as a firm bed or attached infant bed
Breastfeeding while lying on one's side
Taking daytime naps
Learning and practicing effective "wind-down" and relaxation techniques
Arranging the physical environment to be conducive to sleep (eg, reduced noise, reduced light, cooler surroundings)
Avoiding stimulants before bedtime (eg, caffeine, nicotine, activating prescription medications)

Breastfeeding Decision Support

It has been posited that breastfeeding could protect against maternal depression by reducing the inflammatory response and attenuating a woman's physiologic response to stress.[46] Indeed, breastfeeding has been shown to reduce cortisol responses to acute stress exposure.[71] However, it has not been demonstrated that this reduces the risk of postpartum depression or that breastfeeding cessation increases the risk of postpartum depression. Evidence suggests that it is more common for postpartum depression to precede weaning rather than to be triggered by weaning.[72] Depression has been found in several studies to influence early cessation of breastfeeding.[5,73,74]

In certain contexts, breastfeeding and the pressure to breastfeed can become a stressor. Factors that increase the stress of breastfeeding include biological variables (insufficient milk supply, infant health problems, physical challenges, sleep deprivation), social variables (lack of support from families or workplaces), and psychological variables (lack of interest, lack of confidence, reactivated memories of sexual trauma).[75,76] Breastfeeding may also become a barrier to a mother's acceptance of antidepressant treatment, due to the mother's concerns about neonatal medication exposure.[77]

Taken together, these findings suggest that psychological reactions to breastfeeding are highly variable. For a given mother-infant pair, breastfeeding can be stressful, relaxing, or both. Preventing or reducing postpartum depressive symptoms may be facilitated by a flexible approach to breastfeeding (eg, providing lactation support for depressed women who want to breastfeed, while also supporting a woman's decision not to breastfeed if its stresses outweigh its benefits in her case).

Family Planning

Nearly half of pregnancies worldwide are unintended.[78] Numerous studies have found that unintended pregnancies, whether unwanted or poorly timed, increase the risk of postpartum depressive symptoms and major depression in a variety of cultural contexts.[79–83] Women with depression may tend to choose less effective contraceptive methods.[84] Depression is the most commonly cited reason for discontinuing contraceptive pills[85] and reduces condom use by adolescent girls.[86]

To date, no studies have directly ascertained whether family planning initiatives reduce the risk of postpartum depression. Clinical guidelines have recommended providing proactive, noncoercive family planning counseling after a woman recovers from a major depressive episode.[87] When feasible, such counseling can involve the

Table 1
Risk factors and preventive interventions for postpartum depression

Risk Factor	Interventions
Biological (genetic, hormonal) vulnerability	Antidepressant medication
Stress	Cognitive-behavioral therapy with a focus on realistic expectations, stress management, relaxation, and problem-solving skills
Insufficient social support	Interpersonal psychotherapy with a focus on negotiating for needed support Outreach (eg, by public health nurses or midwives)
Nutritional deficiencies	Nutritional education and counseling Specific supplements as indicated (eg, n-3 EFA, folate, iron)
Insufficient physical activity	Education about perinatal physical activity Support in helping a woman find and maintain realistic ways to increase physical activity
Sleep deprivation	Education about perinatal sleep hygiene Medication if needed
Breastfeeding decision support	Lactation support if a woman wants to breastfeed but is having difficulties Support for weaning if a woman is finding breastfeeding too stressful
Family planning	Proactive, noncoercive family planning counseling Psychotherapeutic support of assertiveness and effective communication with partner if needed

woman's partner. Psychiatric side effects of specific contraceptive methods can be reviewed and interpersonal considerations (eg, whether a woman could benefit from assertiveness training to negotiate with her partner about condom use) can be identified.

SUMMARY

The prevalence and substantial risks of postpartum depression suggest that finding effective prevention strategies should be a high priority for clinical investigations and public health initiatives. To date, few studies of individual interventions are adequately powered to demonstrate a preventive effect. Since vulnerability to postpartum depression appears to be multifactorial, it is posited that combinations of interventions targeted to a woman's specific vulnerabilities would be a more effective intervention strategy than focusing on a "one-size-fits-all" single intervention modality.

Primary prevention can best be accomplished through a preconception planning session in which a woman is assessed for risk factors for vulnerability to depression; interventions are recommended to target the identified risk factors. If a woman has already developed postpartum depressive symptoms, early detection through systematic screening can promote secondary and tertiary prevention. Specific risk factors and interventions that most directly address them are summarized in **Table 1**.

It should be noted that the factors listed in **Table 1** interact in complex ways. Interventions in one domain may positively influence others (eg, getting more sleep may allow a woman to exercise more and to have enough energy to prepare more nutritious meals). Further, there are marked individual variations in risks and response to interventions that are not well understood. For example, one woman with a strong personal and family history of postpartum depression might successfully prevent further episodes without medication by being careful to manage stress, garner social support, eat a healthy diet, exercise regularly, and maintain adequate sleep. Another woman with a similar personal and family history might need medication to prevent further episodes, no matter how meticulously she applies other strategies.

In conclusion, evidence to date suggests promising interventions that, taken together and targeted to specific risk factors, may help reduce the risks of postpartum depression. Research is underway that may substantially improve efforts to characterize risk for postpartum depression through genetic and neurohormonal biomarkers. Further study may add to the repertoire of interventions that can prevent postpartum depression with modalities such as targeted psychotherapies, pharmacotherapy, neuroprotection, neuromodulation, and neurofeedback.

REFERENCES

1. Gaynes BN, Gavin N, Meltzer-Brody S, et al. Perinatal depression: prevalence, screening accuracy, and screening outcomes. Evidence report/technology assessment 119. Rockville (MD): AHRQ; 2005. p. 36.
2. Wisner KL, Perel JM, Peindl KS, et al. Timing of depression recurrence in the first year after birth. J Affect Disord 2004;78(3):249–52.
3. Shadigian E, Bauer ST. Pregnancy-associated death: a qualitative systematic review of homicide and suicide. Obstet Gynecol Surv 2005;60:183–90.
4. Paulson JF, Dauber S, Leiferman JA. Individual and combined effects of postpartum depression in mothers and fathers on parenting behavior. Pediatrics 2006;118(2):659–68.
5. Field T. Postpartum depression effects on early interactions, parenting, and safety practices: a review. Infant Behav Dev 2010;33(1):1–6.
6. Feldman R, Granat A, Pariente C, et al. Maternal depression and anxiety across the postpartum year and infant social engagement, fear regulation, and stress reactivity. J Am Acad Child Adolesc Psychiatry 2009;48(9):919–27.
7. Hay DF, Pawlby S, Waters CS, et al. Antepartum and postpartum exposure to maternal depression: different effects on different adolescent outcomes. J Child Psychol Psychiatry 2008;49(10):1079–88.
8. Lumley J, Austin MP. What interventions may reduce postpartum depression. Curr Opin Obstet Gynecol 2001;13:605–11.
9. Dennis CL, Janssen PA, Singer J. Identifying women at-risk for postpartum depression in the immediate postpartum period. Acta Psychiatr Scand 2004; 110(5):338–46.
10. Priest SR, Austin MP, Barnett BB, et al. A psychosocial risk assessment model (PRAM) for use with pregnant and postpartum women in primary care settings. Arch Womens Ment Health 2008;11:307–17.
11. Beck CT. Predictors of postpartum depression: an update. Nurs Res 2001;50(5): 275–85.
12. Robertson E, Grace S, Wallington T, et al. Antenatal risk factors for postpartum depression: a synthesis of recent literature. Gen Hosp Psychiatry 2004;26: 289–95.
13. Bloch M, Rotenberg N, Koren D, et al. Risk factors for early postpartum depressive symptoms. Gen Hosp Psychiatry 2006;28:3–8.
14. Matthey S, Phillips J, White T, et al. Routine psychosocial assessment of women in the antenatal period: frequency of risk factors and implications for clinical services. Arch Womens Ment Health 2004;7:223–9.

15. Goyal D, Gay C, Lee KA. How much does low socioeconomic status increase the risk of prenatal and postpartum depressive symptoms in first-time mothers? Womens Health Issues 2010;20:96–104.
16. Austin MP, Hadzi-Pavlovic D, Saint K, et al. Antenatal screening for the prediction of postnatal depression: validation of a psychosocial Pregnancy Risk Questionnaire. Acta Psychiatr Scand 2005;112:310–7.
17. Oppo A, Mauri M, Ramacciotti D, et al. Risk factors for postpartum depression: the role of the Postpartum Depression Predictors Inventory-Revised (PDPI-R). Arch Womens Ment Health 2009;12:239–49.
18. Gjerdingen DK, Yawn BP. Postpartum depression screening: importance, methods, barriers, and recommendations for practice. J Am Board Fam Med 2007;20:280–8.
19. Gibson J, McKenzie-McHarg K, Shakespeare J, et al. A systematic review of studies validating the Edinburg Postnatal Depression Scale in antepartum and postpartum women. Acta Psychiatr Scand 2009;119:350–64.
20. Kroenke K, Spitzer RL, Williams JB. The PHQ-9: validity of a brief depression severity measure. J Gen Intern Med 2001;16:606–13.
21. Fowles ER, Horowitz JA. Clinical assessment of mothering during infancy. J Obstet Gynecol Neonatal Nurs 2006;35:662–70.
22. Wisner KL, Perel JM, Peindl KS, et al. Prevention of postpartum depression: a pilot randomized clinical trial. Am J Psychiatry 2004;161(7):1290–2.
23. Wisner KL, Perel JM, Peindle KS, et al. Prevention of recurrent postpartum depression: a randomized clinical trial. J Clin Psychiatry 2001;62(2):82–6.
24. Cohen LS, Altshuler LL, Harlow BL, et al. Relapse of major depression during pregnancy in women who maintain or discontinue antidepressant treatment. JAMA 2006;295(5):499–507.
25. Sunder KR, Wisner KL, Hanusa BH, et al. Postpartum depression recurrence versus discontinuation syndrome: observations from a randomized controlled trial. J Clin Psychiatry 2004;65(9):1266–8.
26. Spinelli MG, Endicott J. Controlled clinical trial of interpersonal psychotherapy versus parenting education program for depressed pregnant women. Am J Psychiatry 2003;160:555–62.
27. Crockett K, Zlotnick C, Davis M, et al. A depression preventive intervention for rural low-income African-American pregnant women at risk for postpartum depression. Arch Womens Ment Health 2008;11(5–6):319–25.
28. Chabrol H, Teissendre F, Saint-Jean M, et al. Prevention and treatment of postpartum depression: a controlled randomized study on women at risk. Psychol Med 2002;32(6):1039–47.
29. Dimidjian S, Davis KJ. Newer variations of cognitive-behavioral therapy: behavioral activation and mindfulness-based cognitive therapy. Curr Psychiatry Rep 2009;11(8):453–8.
30. Kozinszky Z, Dudas RB, Csatordai S, et al. Social dynamics of postpartum depression: a population-based screening in South-Eastern Hungary. Soc Psychiatry Psychiatr Epidemiol March 19, 2010 [online].
31. Ozbasaran F, Coban A, Kucuk M. Prevalence and risk factors concerning postpartum depression among women within early postnatal periods in Turkey. Arch Gynecol Obstet February 27, 2010 [online].
32. Xie RH, He G, Koczycki D, et al. Fetal sex, social support, and postpartum depression. Can J Psychiatry 2009;54(11):750–6.
33. Sheng X, Le HN, Perry D. Perceived satisfaction with social support and depressive symptoms in perinatal Latinas. J Transcult Nurs 2010;21(1):35–44.

34. Logsdon MC, Birkimer JC, Usni WM. The link of social support and postpartum depressive symptoms in African-American women with low incomes. MCN Am J Matern Child Nurs 2000;25(5):262–6.
35. Cheng CY, Picslar RH. Effects of stress and social support on postpartum health of Chinese mothers in the United States. Res Nurs Health 2009;32(6):582–91.
36. Lau Y, Wong DF. The role of social support in helping Chinese women with postnatal depressive symptoms cope with family conflict. J Obstet Gynecol Neonatal Nurs 2008;37:556–71.
37. Grigoriadis S, Erlick Robinson G, Fung K, et al. Traditional postpartum practices and rituals: clinical implications. Can J Psychiatry 2009;54(12):834–40.
38. Bielinski-Blattman D, Lemola S, Jauss C, et al. Postpartum depressive symptoms in the first 17 months after childbirth: the impact of an emotionally supportive partnership. Int J Public Health 2009;54(5):333–9.
39. Letourneau N, Duffett-Leger L, Salmani M. The role of paternal support in the behavioural development of children exposed to postpartum depression. Can J Nurs Res 2009;41(3):86–106.
40. Dennis CL, Creedy D. Psychosocial and psychological interventions for preventing postpartum depression. Cochrane Database Syst Rev 2004;4:CD001134.
41. Boath E, Bradley E, Henshaw C. The prevention of postnatal depression: a narrative systematic review. J Psychosom Obstet Gynaecol 2005;26:185–92.
42. Elliott SA, Leverton TJ, Sanjack M, et al. Promoting mental health after childbirth: a controlled trial of primary prevention of postnatal depression. Br J Clin Psychol 2006;39:223–41.
43. Zlotnick C, Miller IW, Pearlstein T, et al. A preventive intervention for pregnant women on public assistance at risk for postpartum depression. Am J Psychiatry 2006;163:1443–5.
44. Leung BM, Kaplan BJ. Perinatal depression: prevalence, risks, and the nutrition link—a review of the literature. J Am Diet Assoc 2009;109:1566–75.
45. Sogaard R, Werge TM, Bertelsen C, et al. GABA(A) receptor function is regulated by lipid bilayer elasticity. Biochemistry 2006;45:13118–29.
46. Kendall-Tackett K. A new paradigm for depression in new mothers: the central role of inflammation and how breastfeeding and anti-inflammatory treatments protect mental health. Int Breastfeed J 2007;30:2–6.
47. Hibbeln JR. Seafood consumption, the DHA content of mothers' milk and prevalence rates of postpartum depression: a cross-national, ecological analysis. J Affect Disord 2003;69:15–29.
48. DeVriese SR, Christophe AB, Maes M. Lowered serum n-3 polyunsaturated fatty acid (PUFA) levels predict the occurrence of postpartum depression: further evidence that lowered n-PUFAs are related to major depression. Life Sci 2003; 73:3181–7.
49. Freeman MP. Complementary and alternative medicine for perinatal depression. J Affect Disord 2009;112:1–10.
50. Bodnar LM, Wisner KL. Nutrition and depression: implications for improving mental health among childbearing-age women. Biol Psychiatry 2005;58:679–85.
51. Cho YJ, Han JY, Choi JS, et al. Prenatal multivitamins containing folic acid do not decrease prevalence of depression among pregnant women. J Obstet Gynaecol 2008;28(5):482–4.
52. Fava M, Mischoulon D. Folate in depression: efficacy, safety, differences in formulations, and clinical issues. J Clin Psychiatry 2009;70(Suppl 5):12–7.
53. Corwin EJ, Murray-Kolb LE, Beard JL. Low hemoglobin level is a risk factor for postpartum depression. J Nutr 2003;133(12):4139–42.

54. Marais L, Stein DJ, Daniels WM. Exercise increases BDNF levels in the striatum and decreases depressive-like behavior in chronically stressed rats. Metab Brain Dis 2009;24(4):587–97.
55. Strom M, Mortensen EL, Halldorson TI, et al. Leisure-time physical activity in pregnancy and risk of postpartum depression: a prospective study in a large national birth cohort. J Clin Psychiatry 2009;70:1707–14.
56. Armstrong K, Edwards H. The effectiveness of a pram-walking exercise programme in reducing depressive symptomatology for postnatal women. Int J Nurs Pract 2004;10:177–94.
57. Norman E, Sherburn M, Osborne RH, et al. An exercise and education program improves well-being of new mothers: a randomized controlled trial. Phys Ther 2010;90(3):348–55.
58. Heh S, Huang L, Ho S, et al. Effectiveness of an exercise support program in reducing the severity of postnatal depression in Taiwanese women. Birth 2008; 35:60–5.
59. ACOG Committee Obstetric Practice. ACOG Committee opinion, number 267, January 2002: exercise during pregnancy and the postpartum period. Obstet Gynecol 2002;99(1):171–3.
60. Hegaard HK, Kjaergaard H, Damm P, et al. Experience of physical activity during pregnancy in Danish nulliparous women with a physically active life before pregnancy: a qualitative study. BMC Pregnancy Childbirth 2010;10(1):33.
61. Yeo S, Cisewski J, Lock EF, et al. Exploratory analysis of exercise adherence patterns with sedentary pregnant women. Nurs Res 2010;59(4):280–7.
62. Sorensen J, Sorensen JB, Skovgaard T, et al. Exercise on prescription: changes in physical activity and health-related quality of life in five Danish programmes. Eur J Public Health April 5, 2010 [online].
63. Goyal D, Gay C, Lee K. Fragmented maternal sleep is more strongly correlated with depressive symptoms than infant temperament at three months postpartum. Arch Womens Ment Health 2009;12:229–37.
64. Taylor A, Glover V, Marks M, et al. Diurnal pattern of cortisol output in postnatal depression. Psychoneuroendocrinology 2009;34(8):1184–8.
65. Parry BL, Meliska CJ, Sorenson DL, et al. Plasma melatonin circadian rhythm disturbances during pregnancy and postpartum in depressed women and women with personal or family histories of depression. Am J Psychiatry 2008; 165(12):1551–8.
66. Armitage R, Flynn H, Hoffmann R, et al. Early developmental changes in sleep in infants: the impact of maternal depression. Sleep 2009;32(5):693–6.
67. Steiner M, Fairman M, Jansen K, et al. Can postpartum depression be prevented [Abstract]? Presented at Marce Soceity International Biennial Scientific Meeting. Sidney (Australia), September 10–13, 2002.
68. Corrall M, Wardrop AA, Zhang H, et al. Morning light therapy for postpartum depression. Arch Womens Ment Health 2007;10(5):321–4.
69. Berk M. Sleep and depression: theory and practice. Aust Fam Physician 2009; 38(5):302–4.
70. Hunter LP, Rychnovsky JD, Yount SM. A selective review of maternal sleep characteristics in the postpartum period. J Obstet Gynecol Neonatal Nurs 2009;38:60–8.
71. Heinrichs M, Meinlschmidt S, Neumann I, et al. Effects of suckling on hypothalamic-pituitary-adrenal axis responses to psychosocial stress in postpartum lactating women. J Clin Endocrinol Metab 2001;86(10):4798–804.
72. Misri S, Sinclair DA, Kuan AJ. Breastfeeding and postpartum depression: is there a relationship? Can J Psychiatry 1997;42(10):1081–5.

73. Kehler HL, Chaput KH, Tough SC. Risk factors for cessation of breastfeeding prior to six months postpartum among a community sample of women in Calgary, Alberta. Can J Public Health 2009;100(5):376–80.
74. Lau Y, Chan KS. Perinatal depressive symptoms, sociodemographic correlates, and breastfeeding among Chinese women. J Perinat Neonatal Nurs 2009; 23(4):335–45.
75. Thuller D, Mercer J. Variables associated with breastfeeding duration. J Obstet Gynecol Neonatal Nurs 2009;38(3):259–68.
76. Kendall-Tackett K. Breastfeeding and the sexual abuse survivor. J Hum Lact 1998;14(2):125–30.
77. Misri S, Kostaras X. Benefits and risks to mother and infant of drug treatment for perinatal depression. Drug Saf 2002;25(13):903–11.
78. Cleland J. Contraception in historical and global perspective. Best Pract Res Clin Obstet Gynaecol 2009;23(2):165–76.
79. Chang D, Schwartz EB, Douglas E, et al. Unintended pregnancy and associated maternal preconception, prenatal and postpartum behaviors. Contraception 2009;79(3):194–8.
80. Nakku JE, Nakasi G, Mirembe F. Postpartum major depression and six weeks in primary healthcare: prevalence and associated factors. Afr Health Sci 2006;6(4): 207–14.
81. Csatordai S, Kozinszky Z, Devosa I, et al. Obstetric and sociodemographic risk of vulnerability to postnatal depression. Patient Educ Couns 2007;67(1–2):84–92.
82. Iranfar S, Shareri J, Ranjbar M, et al. Is unintended pregnancy a risk factor for depression in Iranian women? East Mediterr Health J 2005;11(4):618–24.
83. Owoeye AO, Aina OF, Marakinyo O. Risk factors of postpartum depression and EPDS scores in a group of Nigerian women. Trop Doct 2006;36(2):100–3.
84. Garbers S, Correa N, Tobier N, et al. Association between symptoms of depression and contraceptive methods choices among low-income women at urban reproductive health centers. Matern Child Health J 2010;14(1):102–9.
85. Kulkarni J. Depression as a side effect of the contraceptive pill. Expert Opin Drug Saf 2007;6(4):371–4.
86. Smith PB, Buzi RS, Weinman ML. Mental health screening in family-planning clinics: a sexual risk-reduction opportunity. J Sex Marital Ther 2010;36(3):181–92.
87. David HP, Morgall JM. Family planning for the mentally disordered and retarded. J Nerv Ment Dis 1990;178(6):385–91.

Preventing Depression in Later Life: State of the Art and Science Circa 2011

Fawzi Hindi, BA[a], Mary Amanda Dew, PhD[b],
Steven M. Albert, PhD, MSPH[c], Francis E. Lotrich, MD, PhD[d],
Charles F. Reynolds III, MD[c,e],*

KEYWORDS

- Prevention - Selective/Indicated - Depression - Later life

That our ability to understand, treat, and even cure disease has reached its current state and improves still further every year is remarkable. Nonetheless, the ultimate goal of medicine and health care is prevention of illness: the reduction of incidence through preempting new cases of illness, in addition to protection from downstream consequences of already established illness. The 2008 National Institute of Mental Health (NIMH) Strategic Plan (http://www.nimh.nih.gov/about/strategic%2Dplanning%2Dreports/) includes prevention as one of its key objectives with respect to mental disorders such as depression. By preventing depression, one hopes ultimately to enhance health span and life span.

Supported in part by P30 MH71944, P60 MD00107, T32 MH019986, the UPMC Endowment in Geriatric Psychiatry the John A. Hartford Center of Excellence in Geriatric Psychiatry Department of Psychiatry, University of Pittsburgh School of Medicine.
The authors have nothing to disclose.
[a] Department of Psychiatry, Western Psychiatric Institute and Clinic, University of Pittsburgh, School of Medicine, 3811 O'Hara Street, Pittsburgh, PA 15213, USA
[b] Department of Psychiatry, Western Psychiatric Institute and Clinic, University of Pittsburgh, School of Medicine, 3811 O'Hara Street, Suite 502, Iroquois Building, Pittsburgh, PA 15213, USA
[c] Department of Behavioral and Community Health Sciences, Graduate School of Public Health, University of Pittsburgh, A211 Crabtree Hall, Pittsburgh, PA 15261, USA
[d] Department of Psychiatry, Western Psychiatric Institute and Clinic, University of Pittsburgh, School of Medicine, 3811 O'Hara Street, TDH 1408, Pittsburgh, PA 15213, USA
[e] Department of Psychiatry, Western Psychiatric Institute and Clinic, University of Pittsburgh, School of Medicine, 3811 O'Hara Street, 758 Bellefield Towers, Pittsburgh, PA 15213, USA
* Corresponding author. Department of Psychiatry, Western Psychiatric Institute and Clinic, University of Pittsburgh, School of Medicine, 3811 O'Hara Street, 758 Bellefield Towers, Pittsburgh, PA 15213.
E-mail address: reynoldscf@upmc.edu

Because unipolar major depression is among the leading contributors to the global burden of illness-related disability,[1] and is predicted to be the greatest contributor to illness burden by 2030,[2] it is a matter of public health significance to identify people at high risk for depression and/or who are already mildly symptomatic, and to discover ways of implementing timely and rational risk reduction strategies to preempt major depression.[3] In this article, the published literature is reviewed to summarize what is known about depression prevention in older adults, and, ultimately, to inform future research.

PUBLIC HEALTH CONTEXT AND RATIONALE FOR DEPRESSION PREVENTION IN LATER LIFE

Two questions provide the organizing framework for depression prevention research and practice in older adults: (1) Can early intervention targeted to older individuals at increased risk or already living with subthreshold symptoms of depression reduce incidence, severity, or duration of incident major depression to a clinically significant degree? and (2) How are interventions to prevent major depression in a community-dwelling elderly population best organized and implemented?

The goals of research in this area are to improve accuracy in predicting major depression in older adults and their caregivers, to guide the timely introduction of risk reduction strategies, and to determine whether there are additional health and economic benefits to prevention of major depression in older adults. These could include slower progression of cognitive decline, better control of pain, better indicators of cardiovascular and cerebrovascular health, less caregiver burden, and less cost to the health care delivery system. All of these are significant downstream burdens that could be mitigated through depression prevention in later life.

From a public health perspective, prevention of major depression in later life is important for the following reasons[3]: (1) depressive episodes in older adults are prevalent and disabling (6%–10% in primary care settings), 30% in medical and long-term care settings; it is estimated that incidence rates of new episodes are about half of prevalence; (2) depression is associated with significant excess mortality after myocardial infarction, stroke, and cancer, and it is the major risk factor for suicide in old age; (3) available treatments are only partially satisfactory in reducing symptom burden, sustaining remission and health-related quality of life, and in averting years lived with disability; (4) milder or subthreshold states increase the risk of developing the full clinical disorder but may be more reversible than the advanced clinical state and may be associated with neurobiological changes at an earlier and more modifiable stage of development; (5) the geriatric mental health workforce issues confronting the nation drive the imperative for devising effective, scalable, depression prevention models that can be implemented by general medical rather than mental health specialty clinicians[4]; and (6) preventing depression in older adults may be cost-effective.[5]

By preventing depression in older adults, the aim is to prevent the downward spiral of depression to disability and death and thereby enhance and prolong older adults' capacity for independence. Because depression diminishes both health span and life span, the ultimate goal of depression prevention is to protect and enhance both.[3]

The doubling of the number of older adults living with a mental disorder by 2030 is only part of the public health challenge of, and rationale for, preventing clinically significant depressive syndromes in old age. Specifically, older adults of lower socioeconomic status have increased risk for chronic illnesses and for depression. The social worlds that put older adults at risk for depression, especially poverty and living in dangerous neighborhoods, also act to reduce the effectiveness of antidepressant treatment.[6] Thus, studies of depression prevention must also involve adults on low income (who are often racial minorities). For example, a randomized controlled prevention trial evaluating problem-solving therapy (PST) to prevent episodes of major depression, diminish disability, and improve health-related quality of life in adults on lower income who have risk factors for depression and are already living with mild symptoms of depression is currently under way.[7] The control condition is health education in dietary practices, chosen because of the high rate of obesity among participants and the need to provide an attentional control. Relative to white participants in the trial, black participants have (1) lower household income and less formal years of education, (2) higher rates of health hazards (obesity, diabetes, hypertension), (3) higher rates of physical disability, and (4) more frequent histories of alcohol or substance abuse.[8] About one-third of both blacks and whites report a remote prior history of major depressive episodes. Subjects are being followed for 2 years, with booster sessions of PST or health education every 6 months. As reviewed later, successful depression prevention research requires an infrastructure of community partnerships with primary care and social service agencies that reach the vulnerable populations most in need of preventive interventions.

RATIONALE FOR SELECTIVE AND INDICATED PREVENTION

The literature suggests that depression prevention in later life may be most efficiently accomplished by targeting the elderly who experience risk factors, particularly functional limitations as a result of illnesses such as stroke or macular degeneration, have a small social network, and/or have subthreshold symptoms.[9,10] Efficiency of interventions to prevent depression encompasses both the effect of the intervention and the effort required to implement it. The effect is reflected in the proportion of cases that would be prevented if the adverse effects of the targeted risk factor were completely blocked (attributable fraction). Effort is reflected by the number of persons who would need to receive a depression prevention intervention to avoid 1 new case of late-life depression (number needed to treat [NNT]). Schoevers and colleagues[11] have estimated that the risk factor for which preventive interventions would have the greatest effect and least effort is subthreshold depressive symptoms (NNT of 3–4 vs NNT of 7–9 in selective prevention).[11] That is, preventive interventions may have a greater effect in older adults with subthreshold symptoms (indicated prevention) than in patients without such symptoms who may have other risk factors such as disabilities from medical illness (selective prevention). For example, a recent, randomized, controlled prevention trial from Amsterdam has shown the effectiveness of stepped-care prevention of anxiety disorders and major depressive disorders in 170 primary care patients aged 75 years and older with subthreshold symptoms not meeting the full diagnostic criteria for syndromal disorders.[12] This intervention was implemented by mental health nurses for 1 year and encompassed a stepped-care algorithm of 3 months of watchful waiting, 3 months of bibliotherapy, 3 months of PST, and referral to a general practitioner if symptoms persisted. It thus allowed the parsimonious use of resources as needed for older patients with persistent symptoms of depression or anxiety. The intervention reduced the incidence of anxiety disorders and major depressive episodes by 50% in 1 year, relative to care as usual (24% vs 12%).

Clinically, depression merits considerable effort in prevention because of its contributions to disability, morbidity, and mortality. In patients suffering terminal illnesses, such as cancer, depression is a major source of suffering coexistent with all the discomforts and burdens of cancer therapy. For such individuals already undergoing distressing treatment, the prevention of a major source of suffering is a worthwhile clinical objective. Depression has also been linked with increased risk of mortality in congestive heart failure,[13] stroke,[14] various forms of cancer,[15] suicide during treatment of cancer,[16] and reduced quality of life for terminally ill patients such as those suffering from brain tumors.[17] It is apparent, therefore, that whether as the patient's presenting illness or a comorbidity significantly altering the treatment and outcome of another disease, the effect of depression is worth preempting by preventive measures.

Before discussing depression prevention further, however, the limitations of current depression treatment need to be discussed. Assume that, in a given primary care setting, evidence-based interventions are practiced with 100% insurance coverage providing for all types of interventions, both mainstream and experimental. Even in this idealized scenario, however, one study shows that the burden of depression, which is measured in years lived with disability, would be averted only by 34%.[18] Such a success rate in ideal circumstances is clearly inadequate. Now, however, assume a more realistic situation in which insurance coverage is only 70%. In such a situation, years averted with disability decreases to around 25%.[18] This finding is even more concerning, in that it underscores the limited access to, and effectiveness of, existing treatments and the need for better preventive interventions.

There are additional important shortcomings of current depression treatment that underscore the need for prevention. These are the findings that full remission occurs only in one-third of those treated with a newer antidepressant and that each subsequent drug intervention is associated with progressively poorer response rates.[19] Compounding this already troubling dilemma, there is the problem of dissemination of treatment: the limited access that certain populations, especially older, racial, and ethnic minorities, have to evidence-based mental health care.

In summary, currently available treatment, even if it were to be administered in an ideal evidence-based way and available to all populations, remains only partially satisfactory in assuaging depression-related disability. From a public health perspective, depression prevention is needed to reduce incidence rates, that is, to preempt episodes of major depression in those with known risk factors (and perhaps already mildly symptomatic), and thereby to mitigate the global burden of depression's illness-related disability.

OBJECTIVES OF DEPRESSION PREVENTION

Implicit in the discussion of depression prevention in older adults are 3 underlying objectives: the preemption of incident episodes of depression, the prevention of recurrent episodes of depression, and, protection from depression's medical and psychosocial complications.[3]

Several types of depression prevention were outlined by the Institute of Medicine in both its 1994[20] and 2009[21] reports: universal, selective, and indicated prevention. In universal prevention, the entire population base, regardless of whether they are at risk for depression, is targeted. An example would be outreach through media to educate the general population about the early warning signs of depression, to dispel stigma about depression, and to encourage help seeking; or educational outreach to primary care physicians to educate them about the risk factors (such as depression) for suicide in older adults.

As opposed to this wide-scale intervention, selective prevention focuses on those patients presenting with established susceptibility, based on a set of risk factors. For example, in the case of late-life depression, such well-known risk factors include disability, social isolation, bereavement, and chronic insomnia.[9,11] Moving toward greater severity of risk are preventive measures directed to patients already living with some symptoms of depression, although remaining subsyndromal; so-called indicated prevention. To date, most of the limited data in the literature are derived from studies of selective and indicated prevention. The sample size requirements for studies of universal prevention are substantially greater than the samples of 150 to 300 generally seen in studies of selective and indicated prevention.

THE FEASIBILITY OF DEPRESSION PREVENTION

Using PubMed (searching for "depression prevention" and using limits such as "randomized controlled trials") and cross-referencing with published papers, we were able to identify 30 randomized controlled trials of depression prevention, of which only 4 were conducted in older adults.[8,10,12,22]

Capturing the state of the field, 1 meta-analytic review of 19 trials using mixed-aged samples reported a pooled incidence rate ratio of 0.78 (95% confidence interval [CI] 0.65–0.93), indicating a reduction in incidence of diagnosable major depression of nearly 20% in 1 year.[23] Several published papers support the efficacy of selective and indicated prevention of depression in either at-risk or already mildly symptomatic older individuals. Some of the studies have used as their primary outcome variable the occurrence of major depressive episodes (typically studies of indicated prevention), whereas other studies have encompassed both major and minor depressive episodes as their primary outcome (typically studies of selective prevention).

A study exemplifying selective prevention enrolled patients with recent stroke.[10] Depression occurs in 30% to 40% of stroke victims, and poststroke depression has been implicated as a contributing factor to impaired recovery of stroke victims, along with increased mortality. In the study, nondepressed patients receiving placebo were significantly more likely to suffer a major or minor depressive episode in a 12-month period than those patients administered either a selective serotonin reuptake inhibitor (SSRI) alone (low-dose escitalopram, 5 mg/d), or receiving a course of PST.[10] This study found an NNT of approximately 8.

A recent report from Amsterdam[12] evaluated indicated prevention in Dutch primary care patients older than of 75 years of age. With the objective of determining the efficacy of an indicated stepped-care prevention program, 170 individuals with subthreshold symptom levels of depression or anxiety were followed. Although these individuals did not yet meet the diagnostic criteria for their respective disorders, they were offered either a preventive stepped-care program or usual care. The intervention program comprised 4 sequential steps, each of 3 months' duration: watchful waiting, cognitive-behavioral therapy–based bibliotherapy, PST, and referrals to primary care if the patient so needed. The incidence of major depressive and anxiety disorders was reduced by more than 50% at a 1-year follow-up. Thus, about 24% of patients randomly assigned to treatment as usual experienced the onset of major depressive episodes or of anxiety disorders, compared with 11% of participants receiving the stepped-care for depression prevention.

Despite evidence of efficacy, the question may arise as to whether the benefits of such a preemptive strategy come at an affordable cost. To address this issue, the cost-effectiveness of the stepped-care depression prevention program reported from Amsterdam versus routine primary care was estimated at $700 per recipient and $5431 per disorder-free year gained.[5]

Beyond just reducing the incidence of depression, however, prevention also entails protecting older adults from the downstream consequences of depression.[3] One such downstream consequence is suicide. The PROSPECT (Prevention of Suicide in

Primary Care Elderly: Collaborative Trial) study[24,25] portrays the efficacy of prevention strategies of suicide. PROSPECT showed that by exporting depression care management strategies to urban and rural primary care practices in New York, Philadelphia, and Pittsburgh, a 2.2-fold decrease in suicidal ideation was observed within 2 years. The available data, although still limited, suggest the feasibility, efficacy, and affordability of selective and indicated depression prevention in older adults.

FROM RESEARCH TO PRACTICE

Although current evidence supports the feasibility, efficacy, and affordability of depression prevention, there are many issues that need to be addressed before such interventions can become reality in the modern health care system.

The first is the need for more efficacy trials with a longer duration of study than 12 months. The reason for recommending longer trials derives from the goal of preventing depression, not just delaying it. Moreover, long-term efficacy trials in at-risk patients such as the elderly, low socioeconomic groups, ethnic minorities, and family caregivers are needed to establish the broader clinical usefulness and effect of depression prevention. Moreover, such efforts could assist health care professionals in understanding the specific needs of these groups to better tailor preventive measures to particular patients.

The second issue is the need for better pathophysiological models of depression. A better understanding of the causes of depression should facilitate identifying risk factors for depression. Subsequently, with a better comprehension of risk factors, physicians can better focus their efforts on those with established vulnerabilities, enabling depression prevention, in the long-term, to become more personalized, efficient, and affordable. Examples of this strategy are illustrated by the work of Lenze and colleagues[26] and Lotrich and colleagues.[27] Even more fundamental than individualizing depression prevention, is the need for pathophysiological models to identify how to prevent depression. To date, most depression prevention strategies have been based on depression treatment strategies (eg, PST and use of SSRIs). What are the causal mechanisms leading to depression that need to be interrupted?

The third issue is that, if depression prevention was practiced throughout all primary care facilities, there still remains the issue of improving the rate of patient participation in such programs. The availability of programs does not mean that patients will choose to take advantage of them. Greater use of strategies aimed at potential participants in depression prevention services, such as media campaigns to reduce stigma (promotion and universal prevention, to borrow from the Institute of Medicine's 2009 lexicon[21]) is needed.

The fourth issue is the opportunity afforded by the Internet.[3] With the Internet revolutionizing most aspects of daily life, it is imperative that the mental health community learn to use this powerful tool for the benefit of older adults at risk for depression. Doing so may enable the field to move beyond selective and indicated prevention to universal prevention, by disseminating depression prevention interventions globally to reduce health disparities, especially when the local health care system cannot provide care to those who need it.[3] This will entail confirming important ethical issues, such as the need to inform users that Internet-based dissemination is not intended as a vehicle for emergency mental health services.

RECOMMENDATION FOR FUTURE DEPRESSION PREVENTION RESEARCH IN OLDER ADULTS

To move the field forward and to maximize clinical and policy changes, several strategies are recommended: (1) use of fewer exclusion criteria to recruit clinically representative participants with medical, neurologic, and/or psychosocial risk factors/ comorbidities; (2) partnerships with primary care practices and community-based agencies reaching low-income adults where public health need is greatest; (3) use of lean assessment batteries with low respondent burden and appropriate for people with less formal education; (4) specification of prevention-relevant outcomes beyond symptom ratings, such as burden of coexisting medical illness (especially cardiovascular and cerebrovascular illness), cognitive and functional impairment, and caregiver burden; (5) follow-up periods of at least 12 months and, preferably, 24 months to derive more accurate and clinically meaningful estimates of true incidence reduction; and (6) use of a structured but flexible menu of approaches to be carried out by general medical clinicians (rather than mental health specialists). Research projects need to be powered to detect moderately large effect sizes of interventions on the cumulative incidence of major depression for 1- and 2-year follow-up periods. Based on the limited published data, this means sample sizes of 150 to 300 participants (or 75–150 in each of the experimental and control arms).

General Approach

Because of the diversity of challenges inherent in risk for depression in later life, interventions need to allow for some degree of tailoring to meet the specific needs of the individual and his/her caregiver. Thus, a structured but at the same time tailored approach to delivering the interventions responsive to individual needs is appropriate. There are important synergies, for example, to be attained by simultaneously intervening with the caregiver and the care recipient. That is, dyadic intervention may have greater potential because of effects on factors such as effective support seeking and support provision within the dyad.[28]

Interventions that have already been shown to promote self-efficacy and resilience in prior studies of depression treatment seem to be promising candidates. The focus should be on assessing the value of such strategies before older adults become ill, in the face of the most pervasive risk factors for depression in old age: disabilities related to medical and cognitive impairments, social isolation, caregiving burden, bereavement, and poor sleep.[9,11]

Promising Interventions

Simple, brief, learning-based approaches, already shown to have efficacy in the treatment of depressive disorders, pain, or insomnia disorders, seem promising to address the mandate of the NIMH Strategic Plan (2.3) "to develop and test innovative interventions to reduce risk and positively alter trajectories of illness." Although antidepressant medications are the most widely used modality for treating prevalent cases of major depression, their use in subthreshold depression may be ill-advised because of a lack of evidence for efficacy in mild depression, as well as adverse effects in older adults such as hyponatremia, risk for falls, bone demineralization, and cataracts.[29] Psychological interventions may be preferable for reasons of safety and patient preference. PST has been used successfully in depression prevention studies,[10,12,22,30] is more easily learned than interpersonal psychotherapy or CBT, and can be embedded within a clear service model.[31] Teaching coping skills may diminish the sense of loss of control (helplessness) at the core of depression. Similarly, teaching strategies for better sleep (because poor sleep is a known and well-established risk factor for depression) may diminish affective reactivity and enhance cognitive flexibility on the part of both care recipients and caregivers.[32] In this context, brief behavioral treatment of insomnia (BBTI) is particularly promising, because it has been shown to improve sleep quality and reduce symptoms of depression and anxiety.[32] Moreover, learning-based interventions are effective for prevalent cases of depression and insomnia. Interventions such as PST and BBTI are also practicable, that is, safe, cheap, deliverable by general medical clinicians (including nurses and social workers), and more likely to be acceptable to older adults than the use of antidepressant medication before major depression is diagnosable. An important caveat in this discussion, however, are data that SSRI pharmacotherapy is effective in the prevention of recurrent episodes depression, an enormously important clinical issue in the care of older adults.[33]

Important Measurement Domains

The literature suggests a core of shared measurement domains in keeping with the general logic model articulated here: depression and anxiety (both categorical measures and dimensional measures of severity), comorbid medical burden, social and physical disability, insomnia, pain, cognitive status, social isolation/support, caregiver burden, self-efficacy, problem-solving skills, and promising biopredictors of depression (eg, proinflammatory cytokines).[7,8,27] Biopredictors of depression may enable depression prevention to focus on individuals at highest risk and offer guidance as to when and where in the pathway to depression one might best intervene.

Need to Personalize Depression Prevention Strategies

Because most older adults do not get depressed after a disabling medical event or negative life event such as bereavement, the efficiency of depression prevention efforts need to be further enhanced. To address the question of which patients are most likely to benefit from depression prevention, it seems important to investigate biosignatures of depression risk and of response to prophylactic interventions (eg, cytokine activity, sleep). That is, the field should seek to understand biological correlates of (1) the likelihood of depression, (2) time period of risk, and (3) risk reduction using psychosocial or biological strategies. This is in keeping with the general goal of research, to develop models for estimating depression risk (using sociodemographic, clinical, and biological variables easily obtained in community settings), to guide the rationale, and timely and clinically appropriate introduction of risk reduction strategies in persons who need them most.

As suggested earlier, an important dimension of risk for depression and anxiety is poor sleep.[34] Insomnia is known to be a potent risk factor for depression and anxiety, not simply a prodrome. What is not yet known is whether protecting sleep or improving sleep quality prevents depression in older adults. Poor sleep is also highly prevalent in later life, especially among those living with social and financial strain, in those living with chronic pain and related medical disabilities, and in those with mild cognitive impairment and progressive cognitive disability. Poor sleep also affects caregivers, often leading to a decision to place a family member in long-term care. Furthermore, there seems to be a bidirectional relationship between poor sleep and increase in proinflammatory cytokine activity. Both seem to be depressogenic.[27] Thus, improving sleep fits well into the conceptual framework of depression prevention articulated here.[32] Good sleep is important for affective regulation, decreasing stress reactivity, and helping to mitigate chronic pain. It is also essential to information processing, cognitive flexibility, and problem solving. Insomnia is a modifiable precursor and risk factor for depression occurrence and reoccurrence. Teaching people healthy sleep habits, getting them to understand and experience first hand how changing behavior affects health, is a unique entry to sustainable, health-promoting life styles. In this context, the authors have recently published clinical trial data showing that curtailing time in bed and allowing less sleep is associated with poorer health outcomes in

Table 1
Methodologic challenges confronting depression prevention research in older adults

Components of the Mission	What is Needed to Address the Mission	Related Methodologic Challenges
Prevention of episodes of depression	Better understanding of the nature of and interrelationships among risk factors to target when and how to intervene	Identification, modification, validation of efficient (low burden, feasible, strong psychometrics) assessments for multiple domains of factors Development of statistical methods to better characterize complex sets of risk factors and their trajectories over time Development of classification techniques that allow care providers to efficiently gauge risk for depression in their clients
	Wider range of strategies to deliver prevention interventions	Migration of traditional face-to-face intervention delivery to telemedicine-based formats without loss of fidelity and effectiveness
	Appropriate timing/sequencing of interventions	Development/adaptation of research designs and analytic strategies – to incorporate multiple durations and sequences of treatments – to accommodate care provider/patient preferences
	Accurate identification of change in clinical status	Development of efficient, low cost measures acceptable to patients/providers and sensitive to change Determination of whether depression outcome and risk factor assessments are feasible, acceptable, and valid
Depression prevention in the community, particularly in underserved, low-income populations	Better engagement/retention of underserved older adults in interventions; facilitation of their response to intervention	Development/adaptation of research designs and analytic strategies to accommodate patient preferences for preventive care Determination of acceptability of depression and risk factor assessments to community-based assessors/care providers
	Engagement of community-based health care and services providers as prevention partners	
Sustainability of depression prevention efforts	Strategies to facilitate transportability of prevention interventions into the community for sustained use	Refinement/application of a standardized approach to characterize intervention delivery and content Evaluation of costs and reimbursability of prevention interventions Development of assessments for depression outcomes and risk factors that can be easily used by community-based care providers Development/adaptation of research designs and analytic strategies to accommodate patient/care provider preferences for preventive care Dissemination of approaches to increase intervention transportability to new settings, populations, and care providers Dissemination of new assessment tools, research design strategies, and analytic tools for prevention effectiveness trials
	Training of the next generation of researchers conducting effectiveness and dissemination studies	

adults aged 75 years and older, during a 30-month period of observation.[35] There seem to be close relationships between sleep duration/quality, health span and lifespan.

SUMMARY OF METHODOLOGICAL CHALLENGES FOR THE FUTURE

Implicit in this review are important methodological challenges to progress in depression prevention research in older adults. The missions and related methodological challenges of late-life depression prevention are summarized in **Table 1**.

Paramount among these challenges is the need for a better understanding of the nature and interrelationships among risk factors to target when and how to intervene. Also needed is a wider range of strategies to deliver prevention interventions (eg, using the Internet), together with evidence bearing on the appropriate timing and sequencing of interventions. Methods for better engagement of underserved older adults in interventions and improved engagement of health care and services providers in prevention programs need to be developed and tested. Strategies to facilitate the transportability of prevention interventions into the community for sustained use are much needed.

SUMMARY

Depression is a disorder with a significant public health burden that not only reduces the duration and quality of life of those with depression but also negatively affects the course of comorbid illnesses. Current modalities of depression prevention, although efficacious, fall short of the ideal, especially regarding the need to personalize intervention. In the future, a better understanding of the pathophysiological risk factors for depression that help to identify when and how to intervene in at-risk patients, along with a mastery of the Internet as a powerful dissemination tool, may pave the way to making depression prevention a widely practiced and effective intervention. What is now still revolutionary may become mainstream practice.

REFERENCES

1. World Health Organization. Global health statistics: a compendium on incidence, prevalence and mortality estimates for over 200 conditions, in the global burden of disease. Cambridge (MA): Harvard University Press; 1996.
2. Mathers CD, Loncar D. Projections of global mortality and burden of disease from 2002 to 2030. PLoS Med 2006;3:e442.
3. Reynolds CF. The cutting edge: prevention of depressive disorders. Depress Anxiety 2009;26:1062–5.
4. Institute of Medicine of the National Academies. Retooling for an aging America: building the health care workforce. 2008. Available at: http://www.iom.edu/?ID=53452. Accessed August 1, 2010.
5. Van't Veer-Tazelaar P, Smit F, van Hout HP, et al. Cost-effectiveness of a stepped care intervention to prevent depression and anxiety in late life: randomised trial. Br J Psychiatry 2010;196:319–25.
6. Cohen A, Houck PR, Szanto K, et al. Social inequalities in response to antidepressant treatment in older adults. Arch Gen Psychiatry 2006;63:50–6.
7. Sriwattanakomen R, Ford AF, Thomas SB, et al. Preventing depression in later life: translation from concept to experimental design and implementation. Am J Geriatr Psychiatry 2008;16:460–8.

8. Sriwattanakomen R, McPherron J, Chatman J, et al. A comparison of the frequencies of risk factors for depression in older black and white participants in a study of indicated prevention. Int Psychogeriatr 2010;22:1240–7.

9. Smit F, Ederveen A, Cuijpers P, et al. Opportunities for cost-effective prevention of late-life depression: an epidemiological approach. Arch Gen Psychiatry 2006;63: 290–6.

10. Robinson RG, Jorge RE, Moser DJ, et al. Escitalopram and problem-solving therapy for prevention of poststroke depression: randomized controlled trial. JAMA 2008;299:2391–400.

11. Schoevers RA, Smit F, Deeg DJ, et al. Prevention of late-life depression in primary care: do we know where to begin? Am J Psychiatry 2006;163:1611–21.

12. van't Veer-Tazelaar PJ, van Marwijk HW, van OP, et al. Stepped-care prevention of anxiety and depression in late life: a randomized controlled trial. Arch Gen Psychiatry 2009;66:297–304.

13. Jiang W, Alexander J, Christopher E, et al. Relationship of depression to increased risk of mortality and rehospitalization in patients with congestive heart failure. Arch Intern Med 2001;161:1849–56.

14. Robinson RG. Poststroke depression: prevalence, diagnosis, treatment, and disease progression. Biol Psychiatry 2003;54:376–87.

15. Pinquart M, Duberstein PR. Depression and cancer mortality: a meta-analysis. Psychol Med 2010;40:1797–810.

16. Breitbart W. Suicide in cancer patients. Oncology (Williston Park) 1987;1:49–55.

17. Pelletier G, Verhoef MJ, Khatri N, et al. Quality of life in brain tumor patients: the relative contributions of depression, fatigue, emotional distress, and existential issues. J Neurooncol 2002;57:41–9.

18. Andrews G, Issakidis C, Sanderson K, et al. Utilising survey data to inform public policy: comparison of the cost-effectiveness of treatment of ten mental disorders. Br J Psychiatry 2004;184:526–33.

19. Rush AJ. Limitations in efficacy of antidepressant monotherapy. J Clin Psychiatry 2007;68(Suppl 10):8–10.

20. Institute of Medicine, Committee on Prevention of Mental Disorders, Division of Biobehavorial Science and Mental Disorders. Reducing risks for mental disorders: frontiers for preventive intervention research. Washington, DC: The National Academies Press; 1994.

21. Institute of Medicine. Preventing mental, emotional, and behavioral disorders among young people: progress and possibilities. Washington, DC: The National Academies Press; 2009.

22. Rovner BW, Casten RJ, Hegel MT, et al. Preventing depression in age-related macular degeneration. Arch Gen Psychiatry 2007;64:886–92.

23. Cuijpers P, van Straten A, Smit F, et al. Preventing the onset of depressive disorders: a meta-analytic review of psychological interventions. Am J Psychiatry 2008;165:1272–80.

24. Alexopoulos GS, Reynolds CF, Bruce ML, et al. Reducing suicidal ideation and depression in older primary care patients: 24-month outcomes of the PROSPECT study. Am J Psychiatry 2009;166:882–90.

25. Bruce ML, Ten Have TR, Reynolds CF, et al. Reducing suicidal ideation and depressive symptoms in depressed older primary care patients: a randomized controlled trial. JAMA 2004;291:1081–91.

26. Lenze EJ, Munin MC, Skidmore ER, et al. Onset of depression in elderly persons after hip fracture: implications for prevention and early intervention of late-life depression. J Am Geriatr Soc 2007;55:81–6.

27. Lotrich FE, Ferrell RE, Rabinovitz M, et al. Risk for depression during interferon-alpha treatment is affected by the serotonin transporter polymorphism. Biol Psychiatry 2009;65:344–8.

28. Schulz R, Czaja SJ, Lustig A, et al. Improving the quality of life of caregivers of persons with spinal cord injury: a randomized controlled trial. Rehabil Psychol 2009;54:1–15.

29. Fournier JC, DeRubeis RJ, Hollon SD, et al. Antidepressant drug effects and depression severity: a patient-level meta-analysis. JAMA 2010;303:47–53.

30. Ciechanowski P, Wagner E, Schmaling K, et al. Community-integrated home-based depression treatment in older adults: a randomized controlled trial. JAMA 2004;291:1569–77.

31. Baldwin C. Preventing late-life depression: a clinical update. Int Psychogeriatr 2010;22(8):1216–24.

32. Germain A, Moul DE, Franzen PL, et al. Effects of a brief behavioral treatment for late-life insomnia: preliminary findings. J Clin Sleep Med 2006;2:403–6.

33. Reynolds CF, Dew MA, Pollock BG, et al. Maintenance treatment of major depression in old age. N Engl J Med 2006;354:1130–8.

34. Ford DE, Kamerow DB. Epidemiologic study of sleep disturbances and psychiatric disorders. An opportunity for prevention? JAMA 1989;262:1479–84.

35. Reynolds CF, Serody L, Okun ML, et al. Protecting sleep, promoting health in later life: a randomized clinical trial. Psychosom Med 2010;72:178–86.

Prevention of Posttraumatic Stress Disorder

Heather M. Sones, BS[a], Steven R. Thorp, PhD[b,c,*],
Murray Raskind, PhD[d,e]

KEYWORDS

- Posttraumatic stress disorder • Prevention • Mental health
- Psychological distress

Most men and women in the United States report experiencing a severe traumatic event at some point, but the psychological distress that often follows naturally subsides for most people.[1] For some individuals, distress persists and develops into posttraumatic stress disorder (PTSD). PTSD is a highly prevalent anxiety disorder, affecting nearly 7% of the general population.[2] The hallmarks of PTSD are reexperiencing symptoms (such as flashbacks and nightmares), avoidance of thoughts and stimuli related to the traumatic event, emotional numbing, and hyperarousal symptoms (such as hypervigilance and difficulty sleeping).[3] PTSD is characterized by subjective distress and functional deficits (Thorp and Stein, 2005),[4] and it is associated with poorer physical health,[5] increased risk of additional mental health disorders,[1] and more frequent suicide attempts.[6] Individuals with PTSD miss an average of 4 days of work per month, resulting in a loss of almost $3 billion per year in productivity within the United States alone.[7]

Because PTSD results from a specific, identifiable event, the disorder lends itself to the application of prevention strategies for at-risk individuals. For example, combat personnel can be targeted before deployment, and attempts can be made to inoculate emergency personnel to potentially traumatic events they may witness or experience. Similarly, although natural disasters can rarely be predicted, those individuals

[a] San Diego State University/University of California, San Diego Joint Doctoral Program in Clinical Psychology, 6363 Alvarado Court, Suite 103, San Diego, CA 92120-4913, USA
[b] Center of Excellence in Stress and Mental Health, VA San Diego Healthcare System, 8810 Rio San Diego Drive, Mail Code 116A4Z, San Diego, CA 92108, USA
[c] Department of Psychiatry, The University of California, San Diego, 9500 Gilman Drive, Mail Code 0603, La Jolla, CA 92093-0603, USA
[d] Education and Clinical Center, VA Puget Sound Health Care System, Seattle Division, 1660 South Columbian Way, Box 358280, Seattle, WA 98108, USA
[e] Department of Psychiatry and Behavioral Sciences, University of Washington, Box 356560, Seattle, WA 98195, USA
* Corresponding author. Center of Excellence in Stress and Mental Health, VA San Diego Healthcare System, 8810 Rio San Diego Drive, Mail Code 116A4Z, San Diego, CA 92108.
E-mail address: sthorp@ucsd.edu

Psychiatr Clin N Am 34 (2011) 79–94
doi:10.1016/j.psc.2010.11.001
0193-953X/11/$ – see front matter. Published by Elsevier Inc.

psych.theclinics.com

exposed to the disaster can be identified quickly as candidates for preventive treatment. The identification of a causal event may make prevention efforts for PTSD more feasible and effective than for other psychological disorders.

Three levels of prevention to reduce the risk of mental health disorders have been identified: universal, selected, and indicated.[8] Universal, or primary, preventions are applied to everyone in a population, regardless of individual risk factors. For PTSD, universal prevention efforts aim to reduce the exposure to traumatic events for everyone in a given population. An example is educational programs for women to decrease rates of sexual assault. Selective, or secondary, prevention targets individuals who are at particular risk for developing a disorder, although they have not yet exhibited symptoms. For PTSD, selective prevention efforts could target individuals who have been exposed to a traumatic stressor or life event, and are therefore at greater risk for developing the disorder. Examples include brief psychotherapy for traumatized persons. Selective prevention efforts can be further refined to target traumatized individuals who have additional risk factors that increase the likelihood of PTSD development. Indicated, or tertiary, prevention targets individuals who are exhibiting subclinical symptoms of the disorder, although full criteria have not been met. For PTSD, these efforts target those traumatized persons who are beginning to exhibit symptoms of PTSD such as sleep disturbance. These interventions could also target individuals meeting criteria for acute stress disorder (ASD) with the goal of preventing chronic PTSD.

THEORETICAL PERSPECTIVES AND RISK FACTORS

Examining theories of PTSD development as well as risk factors associated with PTSD can provide the rationale for prevention measures. Theories of PTSD etiology and risk factors for PTSD development have been reviewed elsewhere.[9–11] Many PTSD theories have attributed the development of the disorder to an interruption in the proper consolidation of the traumatic memory. Brewin and colleagues,[12] through their dual representation theory, suggested that trauma memories are represented in both verbally accessible memories (VAMs) and situationally accessible memories (SAMs). VAMs contain information about the event that the victim had consciously and fully processed. VAMs are committed to long-term memory and are able to be verbally retrieved when desired. SAMs consist of the lower-level perceptual information from the event, including sights, sounds, smells, emotions, and bodily reactions. These memories are often vague and difficult to recall verbally, but may be involuntarily triggered by reminders of the event. Because these memories are not properly integrated in the victim's memory, they may result in the reexperiencing of symptoms of PTSD.

A theory proposed by Pitman[13] states that traumatic events can result in the release of stress hormones that cause an overconsolidation of the traumatic memory. Pitman notes that, in mammals, exposure to stressful events causes the release of hormones that enhance the consolidation of the traumatic memory and the formation of extinction-resistant conditioned responses to trauma-related triggers. Although this process is often adaptive (ie, it may protect the mammal from future dangerous situations), extreme stress can result in disorders such as PTSD. Individuals who experience extreme trauma can become superconditioned via a deeply embedded trauma memory that causes intrusive symptoms.[13]

Several factors have been identified that can interfere with the consolidation of traumatic memories. Peritraumatic emotional responses and the release of stress hormones such as cortisol and adrenaline have been shown to disrupt the normal formation of memories.[14] Intense affect during a traumatic event, including intense feelings of fear, helplessness, and horror, have also been associated with physiological arousal[15] and the development of PTSD.[10] Peritraumatic dissociation, or detachment of awareness during the traumatic experience, has been found to be one of the most significant predictors of PTSD.[10] Dissociation can result in incomplete and less-accessible information that prevents the proper consolidation of the trauma memory.[14]

Another common theme in theories explaining PTSD development is fear conditioning. Many theories have drawn on Mowrer's[16] 2-factor theory, which states that previously neutral stimuli become associated with fear responses through the process of classical conditioning. Although repeated exposure to these stimuli and memories would extinguish this learned association, continual avoidance of these triggers maintains this conditioned fear response.[17] Foa and Kozak[18] and Foa and Rothbaum[19] suggested that stimuli and responses conditioned during a traumatic event form a fear network. When this network is activated via a trauma-related trigger, it causes an escape response in the individual. These networks become pathological when they contain an inaccurate representation of the event, when they are resistant to modification, or when the escape response is activated by safe stimuli. Given this component of PTSD theory, it follows that attention bias for trauma-related information and post-trauma experiential avoidance can serve as risk factors for the development of PTSD.

Another theme common in PTSD theories is that of cognitive dissonance. The information learned during a traumatic event does not easily integrate into the victim's prior belief system, which can be problematic and lead to illness. Several theories have highlighted commonly held beliefs that are contradicted by the experiencing of a traumatic event. Janoff-Bulman[20] argued that such an event can disrupt a victim's assumptions about self, others, and the world (including the belief that bad things happen only to bad people). Bolton and Hill[21] postulated that, in the absence of trauma, people believe in their own competence and that the world is predictable. An unpredictable traumatic event, especially one in which the individual questions his response, may contradict these beliefs and cause distress. Horowitz[22] stated that individuals have a need for new events to be integrated into their prior belief system. When information about a traumatic event is not easily incorporated, it may remain an active memory, and result in the intrusive symptoms of PTSD. Individuals who develop PTSD may incorporate the traumatic event into their belief system by either changing their interpretation of the event (ie, assimilation) or making extreme, maladaptive changes to their prior beliefs (ie, overaccommodation).[23] Maladaptive beliefs related to the traumatic event have been found to be a risk factor for the development of PTSD.[24]

PSYCHOSOCIAL INTERVENTIONS FOR PTSD

Female gender, younger age, minority status, low socioeconomic status, and less education may increase an individual's risk for developing PTSD.[11] Although these variables are fixed (or, in the case of socioeconomic status and education, challenging to modify), they can serve as indicators for at-risk populations that could be targeted by prevention programs. Other measures have focused on factors that are more malleable.

Several different psychotherapeutic approaches have been applied in an effort to prevent the development of PTSD. Although psychosocial methods have proved effective at reducing PTSD symptoms once the disorder has developed, intervention efforts that attempt to prevent the development of PTSD have had mixed results. This article reviews the literature in 2 categories: (1) psychological debriefing programs (immediate, single-session approaches), and (2) brief-delay, multiple-session psycho-logical interventions.

PSYCHOLOGICAL DEBRIEFING (IMMEDIATE, SINGLE-SESSION APPROACHES)

Psychological debriefing interventions typically occur within hours or days after a trau-matic event.[25] Debriefing is often administered to everyone exposed to the event in a single meeting. During these sessions, victims are encouraged to share their experi-ences and emotional reactions to the event. Victims are also offered psychoeducation regarding normal reactions to trauma. Although several variations of these single-session interventions have been tested, the most common form of psychological debriefing is critical incident stress debriefing (CISD).[26]

CISD is a secondary prevention effort that invites all victims of a traumatic event to a single 3- to 4-hour session. The CISD team helps to normalize stress responses and provide education on typical reactions to stressful events. The team teaches coping skills, encourages participants to share their experiences and emotional reactions, and offers additional resources for those who may need it.[25] CISD teams often comprise individuals familiar with the organization (eg, nurses in an emergency depart-ment) and mental health professionals.[27] The CISD approach is designed to be flexible and so it is loosely structured. CISD was originally developed for use with individuals indirectly exposed to traumatic events because of their occupation, such as fire-fighters or emergency medical personnel, and was not designed to prevent PTSD. However, CISD has been applied to direct victims of trauma in an effort to prevent PTSD[28] despite evidence that it may be ineffective for that purpose.[29,30] CISD has resulted in more severe psychopathology, including PTSD symptoms, compared with a control condition.[31] Thus, CISD may be ineffective for PTSD prevention and may have harmful effects.[32]

Several possible reasons exist as to why single-session debriefings such as CISD are generally ineffective at decreasing PTSD symptoms. First, all trauma victims are invited to the debriefing, regardless of their risk for developing PTSD. Risk for PTSD varies based on environmental and personal variables.[11] Therefore, individuals attending CISD meetings may range from virtually unaffected by the event to severely traumatized. Those who have more severe symptoms may decline the invitation to attend because avoidance of trauma-related stimuli is a hallmark of psychological trauma, or, if they participate, they may have more difficulty seeing their response as normal when others report a less intense reaction. Conversely, there is the potential for those who are severely traumatized to cause distress in otherwise asymptomatic individuals when everyone in the group is sharing detailed personal accounts of the traumatic experience. As originally designed, CISD would gather people who know one another, such as firefighter units. However, sharing traumatic experiences with strangers, such as in mass-disaster sites, could be maladaptive. In single-session approaches there is little time to become familiar with others. There are potential ethical implications if all trauma victims are mandated to attend the session and disclose to others, as may happen in work-related incidents. In addition, single-session approaches may not provide sufficient opportunities to practice new skills.

BRIEF DELAY, MULTIPLE-SESSION PSYCHOLOGICAL INTERVENTIONS

Brief delay, multiple-session programs typically occur within the first weeks to months following the traumatic event, and tend to be more structured than debriefing programs like CISD. In contrast to letting participants freely discuss an event and their reactions in the presence of a facilitator, these approaches are more didactic and follow a more detailed protocol. These interventions typically target individuals considered to be at greater risk for the development of PTSD. Although several variations of these interventions exist, the most studied is trauma-focused cognitive behavioral therapy (TFCBT).

TFCBT has received the greatest amount of empirical support for the prevention of PTSD. Several randomized controlled trials have found TFCBT to be more effective than supportive counseling for reducing ASD symptoms and PTSD diagnosis at 3 to 6 months after treatment in individuals diagnosed with ASD.[33] The exact protocol for TFCBT varies across studies, but most studies that have found TFCBT to be effective have included some element of psychoeducation, cognitive restructuring, and/or exposure therapy.

Given the variable components of TFCBT across studies, researchers have begun to question which component(s) of the intervention are most effective at reducing PTSD. Exposure components have been included to reduce traumatic stress symptoms via extinction of trauma-related fear conditioning. Cognitive restructuring is designed to help correct maladaptive thoughts about the event and to help victims integrate the informational and emotional components of the memory.[34] One study sought to compare non–exposure-based early interventions with prolonged exposure (PE) therapy for individuals diagnosed with ASD.[35] At 6-month follow-up, the participants who had received exposure therapy were less likely to meet criteria for PTSD and more likely to have fully remitted. To date, most effective exposure models have been conducted in individual (one-on-one) psychotherapy format, whereas cognitive restructuring is done in both individual and group formats. Thus, available resources and the number of victims may help determine which components are chosen.

Another multiple-session exposure intervention that has been implemented is memory structuring.[36] This 2-session intervention is based on the premise that memories of traumatic events are typically fragmented and rely heavily on somatosensory and emotional information. In the first session, the therapist helps the victim to compose a detailed narrative of the trauma that includes emotional reactions, sensory experiences, and factual information from the event. Both the therapist and patient read this aloud, and the patient is asked to read the account to others before the second session. In the second session, the account is reviewed again, and the therapist discusses sources of social support for the patient. Although similar to PE, this intervention differs in that the trauma account is read only once during the first session (compared with many times in PE), the narrative is shared with others outside of therapy, and there are only 2 sessions (compared with about 10 sessions in PE). A pilot study found memory structuring to be more effective at reducing PTSD symptoms, compared with the supportive listening control condition, for motor vehicle accident victims at risk for developing PTSD.[36] However, a second trial did not find a significant difference between the memory structuring intervention and a control condition.[37]

Prevention efforts could apply well-established psychotherapy protocols from chronic PTSD in response to early signs of the disorder. Shalev and colleagues[38] conducted a study comparing PE, cognitive therapy, and selective serotonin reuptake inhibitors (SSRIs) for early PTSD intervention and found that both psychotherapies were effective at reducing PTSD symptoms. SSRIs were not found to be significantly effective at reducing PTSD prevalence. Participants began treatments within a month of the traumatic event, and the psychotherapies decreased PTSD diagnoses to approximately 20% (compared with almost 60% on the waitlist). This research suggests that some of the gold standard treatments for PTSD may also be effective as preventative measures.

Many effective, multiple-session interventions target individuals considered to be at risk for PTSD as opposed to applying the intervention to all victims. Shalev examined a subsample of participants within his study that had exhibited subthreshold symptoms.[39] These individuals, whether on the waitlist or a treatment condition, appeared to recover naturally. It may therefore be more cost-effective to implement these interventions only for individuals who are exhibiting the full disorder. Although TFCBT is effective for trauma victims considered to be at risk for PTSD, it may be ineffective when applied to all individuals irrespective of risk.[33]

Zatzick and colleagues[40] developed an innovative stepped collaborative care (CC) intervention that may hold promise for future PTSD prevention efforts. It is a stepped program in that the amount of care delivered is dependent on the patient's symptoms. In the study, trauma victims who presented to the emergency room were paired with a case manager who helped to coordinate their medical and mental health care, as well as any additional needs expressed by the individual (eg, occupational concerns, finances). The case manager was available 24 hours a day, 7 days a week. All patients who presented with possible alcohol abuse received a motivational interviewing intervention, and those who were exhibiting sustained posttraumatic distress (as indicated by either extreme distress for 24 hours or repeated requests for more intense treatments) were offered a psychiatric evaluation. At 3 months after the trauma, those patients meeting criteria for PTSD were offered their choice of cognitive behavioral therapy, pharmacotherapy, or both. Based on the individual needs of the patient, these treatments were offered throughout the 12-month follow-up. In the control group receiving usual care, standard emergency room and hospital procedures were followed, and participants were given a list of community referrals before leaving the hospital. Overall, the group that received the CC intervention showed significantly better mental health outcomes, less-severe PTSD symptoms, and fewer symptoms of alcohol abuse/dependence than the control group that received usual care. They also showed no overall change in rates of PTSD diagnosis and a decrease in alcohol dependence diagnosis, whereas the control group increased in both PTSD and alcohol dependence diagnoses.[40]

As a whole, although psychosocial programs for PTSD prevention have promise, it is not yet clear which programs work best. The programs vary across studies, making it difficult to interpret results. Nonetheless, there seem to be several themes that run through this body of literature that may help in designing future effective prevention efforts.[25] It seems that the least effective interventions are those implemented within the first few days following the event. Psychosocial programs should instead target the period of several weeks or months following the trauma, with active monitoring of symptoms during that period. Individuals considered at risk should be targeted by prevention efforts, and therefore effective screening tools for PTSD symptoms and other risk factors should be developed and used. Risk factors could include proximity to the traumatic event, peritraumatic physiological symptoms,[36] acute psychological distress immediately following the trauma,[41] or diagnosis of ASD.[34] Effective treatments for chronic PTSD, such as exposure therapy and cognitive reprocessing therapy, may serve as models for prevention programs. Cost-effectiveness is an additional consideration; future discussions should consider cost and feasibility when determining the duration and intensity of prevention programs. As discussed earlier, PTSD costs our society in terms of treatment, physical ailments associated with PTSD, and loss of productivity. Targeting individuals considered to be at risk may maximize cost-effectiveness, but even targeted programs could be costly. For example, if an intensive program like stepped CC were implemented, for how long could individuals be followed after trauma given the resources required (eg, fully accessible case management)?

POTENTIAL PHARMACOLOGIC APPROACHES TO PTSD PREVENTION

When the body encounters a severe stressor, such as a traumatic event, various neurobiological pathways are activated. For example, these stressors stimulate release of the adrenergic catecholamines epinephrine (EPI) and norepinephrine (NE) and the hormone cortisol as important components of the classic fight-or-flight response. In addition to their prominent effects on cardiovascular function, metabolism, and immunity, catecholamines and cortisol have important effects on memory and on fear conditioning, memory retrieval, and consolidation of emotionally distressing memories.[42,43]

Given the various neurobiological pathways implicated in the development of PTSD, the use of pharmacological interventions is a plausible means for reducing the incidence of PTSD following a traumatic event. This area has received increasing attention in the literature. The development of effective prophylactic medications could have many advantages, including efficiency (ie, the ability to treat many people in a fraction of the time therapeutic interventions may take), ease of administration, and less of a demand on mental health professionals. Several drugs have been studied for PTSD prevention, including propranolol, morphine, glucocorticoids, and SSRIs.

PROPRANOLOL: CAN PHARMACOLOGIC BLOCKADE OF THE BRAIN β ADRENORECEPTOR PREVENT PTSD?

The medication that has received the most attention for PTSD prophylaxis is propranolol, a β-adrenergic antagonist (ie, β-blocker) originally used to treat hypertension. Pitman[13] postulated that high adrenergic activity (ie, EPI and NE) during a traumatic event would produce excessively strong emotional memories and fear conditioning in susceptible individuals. The traumatic memories become overconsolidated, or so deeply engraved in the traumatized individual's mind that extinction of the memory is inhibited and the memory continually surfaces through reexperiencing symptoms such as intrusive memories and nightmares. Subsequent animal and human studies specifically implicated stimulation of brain postsynaptic β adrenoreceptors in the consolidation of emotionally aversive memories.[42,44] These findings led to the hypothesis that pharmacologic blockade of brain β adrenoreceptors following a traumatic stress might prevent subsequent PTSD by reducing fear conditioning and preventing overconsolidation of distressing memories. Increased heart rate following trauma, likely caused by cardiac β-adrenergic stimulation, is a predictor of subsequent PTSD following trauma.[45] This finding provides further support for the posited model of PTSD prevention via β-adrenergic blockage. Because propranolol is a clinically available β adrenoreceptor that easily crosses from blood into brain after oral administration, this drug was a good candidate for studies testing this hypothesis.

Several pilot studies have examined the effectiveness of propranolol for preventing PTSD. In the first clinical trial, Pitman and colleagues[46] administered propranolol or a placebo to patients in the emergency department, most of whom experienced a motor vehicle accident, within 6 hours of experiencing the trauma. Participants were given 10 days of either 40 mg propranolol (n = 18) given 4 times per day or an equivalent placebo (n = 23).[41] PTSD symptoms were rated at 1 month and 3 months following trauma, and psychophysiologic response to script-driven trauma imagery was also measured at 3 months. There were no significant differences in PTSD symptoms between the propranolol and placebo groups at either follow-up assessment. However, at the 3-month follow-up, the propranolol group experienced significantly less physiological arousal during the imagery task compared with the placebo group. The significant reduction of fear conditioning in the propranolol group despite no relative difference in PTSD reduction between groups suggests that the excessive fear conditioning model of PTSD pathogenesis may be overly simplistic.

One other randomized controlled trial examined the use of propranolol for PTSD prevention. Patients admitted to a surgical trauma center were randomized to either 14 days of propranolol (n = 17), the anticonvulsant gabapentin (n = 14), or an equivalent placebo regimen (n = 17).[47] Although PTSD symptoms assessed by the PTSD checklist declined in all 3 groups with time, there were no differences between treatment at 1-, 4-, or 8-month follow-up. At 4-month follow-up, rates of PTSD were 25% in both the propranolol and placebo groups. Only 10% of eligible potential subjects agreed to participate, which reveals the difficulty of recruiting acutely traumatized persons into randomized PTSD prevention trials. Taken together, the findings of these 2 placebo-controlled studies do not support efficacy for propranolol administration after trauma to prevent PTSD.

There is significant controversy about the use of propranolol for PTSD prevention. Because the β-blocker can attenuate the emotional response and memory of a traumatic event, several professionals have argued against its use. An entire issue of the Journal of Bioethics was dedicated to this topic.[48] Studies have shown that propranolol not only decreases emotional memory but also episodic memory for the traumatic event.[49] This leads to various ethical concerns, considering that the long-term implications of emotional and episodic memories are not yet well understood. For example, although aspects of these memories may contribute to PTSD, other aspects may be adaptive (eg, helping survivors to avoid certain people or situations associated with the traumatic event). There may also be legal implications of forgetting (eg, a survivor testifying against a perpetrator may lose details or emotions that were tied to the memory).

OTHER ANTIADRENERGIC APPROACHES TO PREVENTION OF PTSD

Although blocking the β adrenoreceptor with propranolol is the only antiadrenergic approach to PTSD prevention that has been tested in controlled trials, there are rationales for other approaches. If brain release of NE during traumatic stress contributes to PTSD pathogenesis, then inhibiting NE release with an α-1 adrenoreceptor agonist, such as clonidine or guanfacine, might reduce the incidence or severity of PTSD. That opiates reduce brain NE release and have been associated with reduced PTSD incidence in naturalistic studies (see later discussion) provides further rationale. Although open-label studies in southeast Asian refugees suggest that clonidine may reduce symptoms of established PTSD,[50] the only placebo-controlled trial of an α-2 adrenoreceptor agonist for established PTSD was negative.[51] That this multisite study in a large sample of American veterans with chronic PTSD showed no effect of guanfacine versus placebo reduces enthusiasm for, but does not eliminate, the possibility of α-2 adrenoreceptor agonist usefulness in PTSD prevention.

OPIATE ADMINISTRATION FOLLOWING TRAUMA

An emerging line of research has begun to study the effects of acute administration of morphine on the development of PTSD. As previously discussed, it has been proposed that a more severe noradrenergic response can lead to the overconsolidation of the traumatic memory, which is believed to result in many of the reexperiencing symptoms associated with PTSD.[14] Morphine and other opiates are potent analgesics and antianxiety drugs widely prescribed to persons who have suffered painful, life-threatening, traumatic physical injury. Peritraumatic pain seems to predict the development of PTSD,[52] so the pain reduction offered by opiates may help prevent PTSD.

Moreover, opiates reduce the potentially PTSD-inducing outflow of NE from the locus ceruleus,[53] so morphine administration following trauma could be expected to reduce the risk of PTSD.

Naturalistic studies have consistently shown inverse relationships between the dose of morphine administered and PTSD incidence and symptom severity in physically injured samples. In children hospitalized following acute burns, those receiving higher doses of morphine had greater reductions in PTSD symptoms in 6 months.[54,55] In 155 adults hospitalized following traumatic injury, those prescribed higher doses of morphine had lower incidence of PTSD at 3-month follow-up.[56] In 696 combat-injured US military personnel serving in Iraq, the use of morphine during early trauma care was significantly associated with lower risk of a subsequent PTSD diagnosis.[57] These studies confirm the importance of pain control in physically injured persons, but the potential role of opiates in prevention of PTSD following severe psychological trauma in the absence of painful physical injury remains unclear.

Although promising, several factors should be taken into consideration when evaluating these findings. All the studies discussed earlier were conducted naturalistically, and therefore causal relationships cannot be drawn. Additional factors could be moderating this relationship between morphine use and PTSD, such as pain severity. Pain has been positively associated with PTSD severity across several studies,[52] such that more pain is predictive of more severe PTSD symptoms. Morphine administration may be correlated with the self-reported pain of victims, making self-reported pain the moderating variable in the relationship between morphine and PTSD. In future studies, drugs that reduce nonadrenergic responses without pain reduction could be used to control for the effects of pain reduction. Because morphine has a range of effects on various neurotransmitter systems, it is unclear whether its effect on the noradrenergic system, specifically, is related to a decrease in PTSD symptoms.

CORTISOL ADMINISTRATION FOLLOWING TRAUMA

Given the key role of cortisol in the fear response and development of PTSD, researchers have theorized that the use of glucocorticoids in the aftermath of trauma may prevent the development of PTSD. Several previous studies have found cortisol levels to be lower in individuals with PTSD compared with those without the disorder. For example, low cortisol concentrations have been found in chronic PTSD,[58] and low posttrauma cortisol levels have been identified as a risk factor for PTSD in motor vehicle accident victims,[59] which provides a rationale for evaluating exogenous cortisol administration following trauma as a possible PTSD prevention strategy. Although the cognitive effects of cortisol are complex,[60] the ability of cortisol to impair retrieval of long-term memory[61] in humans could be a mechanism by which cortisol reduces PTSD incidence or intensity.

Although randomized placebo-controlled trials of cortisol have not been performed, several naturalistic studies have been conducted examining the usefulness of cortisol to prevent PTSD in trauma victims. Overall, the researchers have found that patients who had been administered glucocorticoids either during or immediately following the trauma were significantly less likely to develop PTSD than those who were not.[62,63] In long-term survivors of septic shock, patients receiving stress doses of cortisol had significantly lower incidence of PTSD.[64,65] Similar beneficial effects of cortisol on PTSD symptoms were suggested in a study of patients undergoing cardiac surgery.[62] These studies were also conducted naturalistically, and often in hospital settings, and therefore other medications and treatment procedures could not be controlled. In addition, the effect of potentially life threatening physical injury could not be controlled in these studies. However, these findings offer promise and should be investigated further in future studies. The findings from observational studies provide support for future rigorous, randomized, placebo-controlled trials of cortisol specifically to prevent PTSD.

SSRIs

The SSRI antidepressants are the most widely used drugs to treat PTSD. They have been shown to be modestly effective for civilian trauma PTSD studies, but no better than placebo for PTSD in American military veterans.[66,67] In the PTSD prevention psychotherapy trial by Shalev and colleagues,[38] discussed earlier, the SSRI escitalopram was also evaluated compared with placebo. The SSRI was no better than placebo in reducing the incidence of PTSD.

ISSUES TO CONSIDER ABOUT PHARMACOLOGICAL INTERVENTIONS

Although the ease of medication is appealing, there are several issues that should be considered when exploring the use of medications to prevent PTSD. First, mass administration of medications in the aftermath of traumatic events could lead to so-called overpathologizing of what may be a normal stress response for most individuals. There are no exact methods of predicting who will develop PTSD. Not everyone who may receive the drug would have developed PTSD. Second, as noted by several studies, the ideal dosage and timing of medication administration after an event (24 hours? One week? One month?) are not yet established. Third, many of the aforementioned studies involved administration of the medications while in the emergency room or other crisis setting. However, victims of crisis events may not be considered competent to consent in the acute phase of recovery. Fourth, patients may be taking other medications that may interact with PTSD prevention drugs, they may be predisposed to addiction to certain drugs (eg, morphine), or they may face unpleasant or dangerous side-effects from the prophylactic drug. These risks must be weighed against potential benefits. Fifth, cost to the victim should be considered. Generic, cheaper medications that require only a few administrations are more affordable and that may improve medication adherence. Sixth, the enduring psychological, legal, and social effects of potential memory loss or alteration must also be taken into consideration. The literature that describes the costs and benefits of electroconvulsive therapy for depression may serve as a guide in this area. In sum, although pharmacological prevention efforts are promising, there are several issues that must be examined before the systematic adoption of preventative medications for people at risk for PTSD.

FUTURE DIRECTIONS

It is evident that PTSD prevention research is only in its infancy. Most studies to date have focused on CISD, and these have found little support for its use as a preventative intervention. Researchers have only recently begun to develop alternative programs, such as the stepped CC intervention, that hold promise for the future of PTSD prevention. However, these studies need to be replicated across various populations before they can be recommended for widespread use. In addition, various other prevention efforts have been developed and implemented despite their lack of empirical support to date. These programs deserve recognition and should be a focus of future research efforts to determine whether they are truly effective at preventing PTSD. Two of these programs are psychological first aid (PFA) and pretrauma stress management.

Psychological first aid is a form of single-session psychological debriefing. This intervention was developed by both the National Child Traumatic Stress Network and the National Center for PTSD, with the most recent edition of the manual published in 2006.[68] PFA is based on past empirical research of early interventions for trauma, and an expert panel was involved throughout its development.[69] PFA consists of 8 core components: contact and engagement, safety and comfort, stabilization, information gathering, practical assistance, connection with social supports, information on coping support, and linkage with collaborative services.[68] Although this prevention program seems promising, particularly because it was designed to work across settings, ages, and cultures, no empirical studies have been done to determine its effectiveness.[69]

Pretrauma interventions vary greatly in their content, but typically target individuals at higher risk for exposure to trauma, such as police officers, firefighters, and military personnel. Individuals in these higher risk groups are often provided with training to enhance skills, such as is done in training facilities to prepare troops for combat (eg, www.strategic-operations.com). Virtual reality simulators have also been used to prepare soldiers and police officers for situations that are likely to arise. In addition to instilling occupational skills (eg, protocols to follow and weapons use during firefights), these training programs could teach stress management. Moreover, they could explicitly and systematically be harnessed to inoculate individuals through exposure to situations similar to traumatic situations that they could experience.

Although the main goal of these training programs is to help participants execute their responsibilities under stress, it is likely that these interventions could also decrease rates of PTSD. This prediction is consistent with the classic idea of latent inhibition. Within learning theory, latent inhibition refers to the delayed learning that occurs as a result of preexposure to a stimulus without a consequence.[34,70] Exposing an individual to a stimulus for which there are no consequences (eg, simulated combat situation) decreases the likelihood of fear conditioning during the actual event. Related research indicates that individuals who experience events that are perceived as uncontrollable and/or unpredictable are, in general, at greater risk of developing PTSD.[71] Exposure to stressful simulations could help to reduce the peritraumatic arousal that is often associated with a greater risk of PTSD. Despite all of these factors that indicate the potential usefulness of these types of stress management trainings to reduce PTSD, we know of no empirical study of the effectiveness of such programs.

Sleep disruption, and particularly disruption of rapid eye movement (REM) sleep, are increasingly implicated in the pathophysiology of PTSD.[72,73] Recurrent nightmares of the traumatic event are one of the most debilitating symptoms of PTSD. Trauma-related nightmares may arise from abnormal REM sleep, and fragmentation of REM sleep is associated with subsequent development of PTSD.[74] Because trauma nightmares vividly reenact the traumatic stressor and are accompanied by adrenergic arousal, they are possibly retraumatizing stimuli that lower the threshold for PTSD development. Studies have found that the presence of trauma-related nightmares immediately following the event can predict the development and severity of PTSD symptoms 6 to 12 months after the trauma.[34] Nightmare prevention may thus help prevent the development of PTSD after a traumatic event.

Several treatments have effectively reduced PTSD-related nightmares,[75] and this article discusses 1 promising psychosocial approach and 1 medication. Imagery rehearsal therapy involves the rescripting of the nightmare and rehearsing the modified version every day, and has been shown to effectively reduce sleep disturbance, nightmares, and PTSD symptoms in general.[76] Prazosin is a brain active α-1 adrenoreceptor antagonist that was originally used to treat hypertension. Prazosin has been shown to significantly decrease the number of distressing nightmares in those with PTSD.[77] The hypothesis about nightmares acting as retraumatizing stimuli could be tested by reducing or eliminating posttrauma nightmares and normalizing REM sleep with prazosin. In animal studies, prazosin normalized REM sleep following its disruption by α-1 adrenoreceptor agonists.[78,79] In placebo-controlled studies in chronic PTSD, prazosin markedly reduced trauma nightmares and sleep disturbance, increased total sleep time, and increased sense of well-being and ability to function in military veterans[77,80] and civilians.[81] However, the ability of prazosin to prevent PTSD following acute trauma remains to be tested.

In addition to testing currently used treatments for PTSD as intervention methods, research should focus on the development of new PTSD prevention techniques. These efforts should focus on targeting the mechanisms discussed in the various theories of PTSD development. Although there are many efforts to make the world safer, people will always be confronted with traumatic events. Those who experience such events are at risk for the development of PTSD and the individual and societal costs that entails. PTSD presents a formidable challenge and a clear opportunity. If PTSD can be prevented, it could benefit millions worldwide and it could inform our prevention efforts for other psychological disorders.

REFERENCES

1. Kessler RC, Sonnega A, Bromet E, et al. Posttraumatic stress disorder on the National Comorbidity Survey. Arch Gen Psychiatry 1995;52:1048–60.
2. Kessler RC, Berglund P, Demler O, et al. Lifetime prevalence and age-of-onset distributions of DSM-IV disorders in the National Comorbidity Survey Replication. Arch Gen Psychiatry 2000;62:593–602.
3. American Psychiatric Association. Diagnostic and statistical manual of mental disorders. text revision. 4th edition. Washington, DC: American Psychiatric Association; 2000.
4. Thorp SR, Stein MB. Posttraumatic stress disorder and functioning. PTSD Research Quarterly 2005;16:1–7.
5. Jitender S, Cox BJ, Stein MB, et al. Physical and mental comorbidity, disability, and suicidal behavior associated with posttraumatic stress disorder in a large community sample. Psychosom Med 2007;69:242–8.
6. Krysinska K, Lester D. Post-traumatic stress disorder and suicide risk: a systematic review. Arch Suicide Res 2010;14:1–23.
7. Kessler RC. Posttraumatic stress disorder: the burden to the individual and to society. J Clin Psychiatry 2000;61:4–12.
8. Mrazek PG, Haggerty RJ. Reducing risk for mental disorders: frontiers for preventative intervention research. Washington, DC: The National Academies Press; 1994.
9. Brewin CR, Holmes EA. Psychological theories of posttraumatic stress disorder. Clin Psychol Rev 2003;23:339–76.
10. Ozer EJ, Best SR, Lipsey TL, et al. Predictors of posttraumatic stress disorder and symptoms in adults: a meta-analysis. Psychol Bull 2003;129:52–73.
11. Brewin CR, Andrews B, Valentine JD. Meta-analysis of risk factors for posttraumatic stress disorder in trauma-exposed adults. J Consult Clin Psychol 2000; 68:748–66.
12. Brewin CR, Dalgleish T, Joseph S. A dual representation theory of post traumatic stress disorder. Psychol Rev 1996;103:670–86.
13. Pitman RK. Post-traumatic stress disorder, hormones, and memory. Biol Psychiatry 1989;26:221–3.

14. McCleery JM, Harvey AG. Integration of psychological and biological approaches to trauma memory: Implications for pharmacological prevention of PTSD. J Trauma Stress 2004;17:485–96.
15. Bryant RA, Harvey AG, Guthrie RM, et al. A prospective study of psychophysiological arousal, acute stress disorder, and posttraumatic stress disorder. J Abnorm Psychol 2000;109:341–4.
16. Mowrer OH. Learning theory and behavior. New York: Wiley; 1960.
17. Keane TM, Zimering RT, Caddell RT. A behavioral formulation of PTSD in Vietnam veterans. Behav Therapist 1985;8:9–12.
18. Foa EB, Kozak MJ. Emotional processing of fear: exposure to corrective information. Psychol Bull 1986;99:20–35.
19. Foa EB, Rothbaum BO. Treating the trauma of rape: cognitive behavioral therapy for PTSD. New York: Guilford Press; 1998.
20. Janoff-Bulman R. Shattered assumptions: towards a new psychology of trauma. New York: Free Press; 1992.
21. Bolton D, Hill J. Mind, meaning, and mental disorder. Oxford: Oxford University Press; 1996.
22. Horowitz MJ. Stress response syndromes. 2nd edition. Northvale (NJ): Jason Aronson; 1986.
23. Resick PA, Schnicke MK. Cognitive processing therapy for sexual assault victims. J Consult Clin Psychol 1992;60:748–56.
24. Bryant RA. Early predictors of posttraumatic stress disorder. Biol Psychiatry 2003; 53:789–95.
25. Gray MJ, Maguen S, Litz BT. Acute psychological impact of disaster and large-scale trauma: limitations of traditional interventions and future practice recommendations. Prehosp Disaster Med 2004;19:64–72.
26. Mitchell JT. When disaster strikes…the critical incident stress debriefing. JEMS 1983;8:36–9.
27. McCabe B, Boudreaux ED. Emergency psychiatry: critical incident stress management: II. Developing a team. Psychiatr Serv 2000;51:1499–500.
28. Everly GS Jr, Mitchell JT. Critical incident stress management (CISM): a new era and standard of care in crisis intervention. 2nd edition. Elliot City (MD): Chevron; 1999.
29. van Emmerik AA, Kamphuis JH, Hulsbosch AM, et al. Single session debriefing after psychological trauma: a meta-analysis. Lancet 2002;360:766–71.
30. Litz BT, Gray MJ, Bryant RA, et al. Early intervention for trauma: current status and future direction. Clin Psychol Sci Pract 2002;9:112–34.
31. Bisson JI, Jenkins PL, Alexander J, et al. Randomised controlled trial of psychological debriefing for victims of acute burn trauma. Br J Psychiatry 1997;171: 78–81.
32. Bledsoe BE. Critical incident stress management (CISM): benefit or risk for emergency services? Prehosp Emerg Care 2002;7:272–9.
33. Kornor H, Winje D, Ekeberg O, et al. Early trauma-focused cognitive-behavioural therapy to prevent chronic post-traumatic stress disorder and related symptoms: a systematic review and meta-analysis. BMC Psychiatry 2008;8:81.
34. Feldner MT, Monson CM, Friedman MJ. A critical analysis of approaches to targeted PTSD prevention: current status and theoretically derived future directions. Behav Modif 2007;31:80–116.
35. Bryant RA, Moulds ML, Guthrie RM, et al. A randomized controlled trial of exposure therapy and cognitive restructuring for posttraumatic stress disorder. J Consult Clin Psychol 2008;76:695–703.

36. Gidron Y, Reuven G, Freedman S, et al. Translating research findings to PTSD prevention: results of a randomized-controlled pilot study. J Trauma Stress 2001;14:773–80.
37. Gidron Y, Gal R, Givati G, et al. Interactive effects of memory structuring and gender in preventing posttraumatic stress symptoms. J Nerv Ment Dis 2007; 195:179–82.
38. Shalev AY, Freedman S, Adessky R, et al. Prevention of PTSD by early treatment: a randomized controlled study. Preliminary results from the Jerusalem Trauma Outreach and Prevention Study (J-TOP). In: Program Book for the American College of Neuropsychopharmacology 46th Annual Meeting. Boca Raton (FL); 2007. p. 63. Available at: http://www.acnp.org/annualmeeting/programbooks. aspx. Accessed November 11, 2010.
39. Busko M. Early psychotherapy, not SSRI therapy, prevents chronic PTSD in large trial. Available at: http://www.medscape.com/viewarticle/567859. Updated December 21, 2007. Accessed July 9, 2010.
40. Zatzick D, Roy-Byrne P, Russo J, et al. A randomized effectiveness trial of step-ped collaborative care for acutely injured trauma survivors. Arch Gen Psychiatry 2004;61:498–506.
41. Bisson JI, Shepherd JP, Joy D, et al. Early cognitive-behavioural therapy for post-traumatic stress symptoms after physical injury. Br J Psychiatry 2004;184:63–9.
42. Cahill L, Prins B, Weber M, et al. Beta-adrenergic activation and memory for emotional events. Nature 1994;371:702–4.
43. Schelling G, Kilger E, Roozendaal B, et al. Stress doses of hydrocortisone, trau-matic memories and post-traumatic stress disorder in patients after cardiac surgery: a randomized study. Biol Psychiatry 2004;55:627–33.
44. Van Stegeren AH, Everaerd W, Cahill L, et al. Memory for emotional events: differ-ential effects of centrally versus peripherally acting beta-blocking agents. Psychopharmacology (Berl) 1998;138:305–10.
45. Shalev AY, Sahar T, Freedman S, et al. A prospective study of heart rate responses following trauma and the subsequent development of PTSD. Arch Gen Psychiatry 1998;55:553–9.
46. Pitman RK, Sanders KM, Zusman RM, et al. Pilot study of secondary prevention of posttraumatic stress disorder with propranolol. Biol Psychiatry 2002;51:189–92.
47. Stein MB, Kerridge C, Dimsdale JE, et al. Pharmacotherapy to prevent PTSD: results from a randomized controlled proof-of-concept trial in physically injured patients. J Trauma Stress 2007;20:923–32.
48. Henry M, Fishman JR, Youngner SJ. Propranolol and the prevention of post-trau-matic stress disorder: is it wrong to erase the 'sting' of bad memories? Am J Bio-eth 2007;7:12–20.
49. Reist C, Duffy JG, Cahill L, et al. Beta-adrenergic blockade and emotional memory in PTSD. Int J Neuropsychopharmacol 2001;4:377–83.
50. Kinzie JD, Sacks RL, Riley CM. The polysomnographic effects of clonidine on sleep disorders in posttraumatic stress disorders: a pilot study with Cambodian patients. J Nerv Ment Dis 1994;182:585–7.
51. Neylan TC, Lenoci M, Samuelson KW, et al. No improvement of posttraumatic stress disorder symptoms with guanfacine treatment. Am J Psychiatry 2006;163:2186–8.
52. Norman SB, Stein MB, Dimsdale JE, et al. Pain in the aftermath of trauma is a risk factor for post-traumatic stress disorder. Psychol Med 2008;38:533–42.
53. Shiekhattar R, Aston-Jones G. Modulation of opiate responses in brain noradren-ergic neurons by the cyclic AMP cascade: changes with chronic morphine. Neuroscience 1993;57:879–85.

54. Saxe G, Stoddard F, Courtney D, et al. Relationship between acute morphine and the course of PTSD in children with burns. J Am Acad Child Adolesc Psychiatry 2001;40:915–21.
55. Stoddard FJ, Sorrentino EA, Ceranoglu TA, et al. Preliminary evidence for the effects of morphine on posttraumatic stress disorder symptoms in one- to four-year-olds with burns. J Burn Care Res 2009;30:836–43.
56. Bryant RA, Creamer MC, O'Donnell ML, et al. A study of the protective function of acute morphine administration on subsequent posttraumatic stress disorder. Biol Psychiatry 2009;65:438–40.
57. Holbrook TL, Galarneau MR, Dye JL, et al. Morphine use after combat injury in Iraq and post-traumatic stress disorder. N Engl J Med 2010;362:110–7.
58. Yehuda R, Halligan SL, Grossman R, et al. The cortisol and glucocorticoid receptor response to low dose dexamethasone administration in aging combat veterans and holocaust survivors with and without posttraumatic stress disorder. Biol Psychiatry 2002;52:393–403.
59. Delahanty DL, Raimonde AJ, Spoonster E, et al. Injury severity, prior trauma history, urinary cortisol levels, and acute PTSD in motor vehicle accident victims. J Anxiety Disord 2003;17:149–64.
60. Roozendaal B. Stress and memory: opposing effects of glucocorticoids on memory consolidation and memory retrieval. Neurobiol Learn Mem 2002;78:578–95.
61. De Quervain DF, Roozendaal B, McGaugh JL. Stress and glucocorticoids impair retrieval of long-term spatial memory. Nature 1998;394:787–90.
62. Schelling G, Roozendaal B, DeQuervain DJ. Can posttraumatic stress disorder be prevented with glucocorticoids? Ann N Y Acad Sci 2004;1032:158–66.
63. Schelling G, Briegel B, Roozendaal B, et al. The effect of stress doses of hydrocortisone during septic shock on posttraumatic stress disorder in survivors. Biol Psychiatry 2001;50:978–85.
64. Schelling G, Stoll C, Kapfhammer HP, et al. The effect of stress doses of hydrocortisone during septic shock on posttraumatic stress disorder and health-related quality of life in survivors. Crit Care Med 1999;27:2678–83.
65. Briegel J, Forst F, Haller M, et al. Stress doses of hydrocortisone reverse hyperdynamic septic shock: a prospective, randomized, double-blind, single center study. Crit Care Med 1999;27:723–32.
66. Raskind MA. Pharmacologic treatment of PTSD. In: Shiromani PJ, Keane TM, LeDoux JE, editors. Post-traumatic stress disorder: basic science and clinical practice. New York: Humana Press; 2009. p. 337–61.
67. Friedman MJ, Marmar CR, Baker DG, et al. Randomized, double-blind comparison of sertraline and placebo for posttraumatic stress disorder in a Department of Veterans Affairs setting. J Clin Psychiatry 2007;68:711–20.
68. Brymer M, Jacobs A, Layne C, et al. National Child Traumatic Stress Network and National Center for PTSD. Psychological first aid: field operations guide. 2nd edition, July, 2006. Available at: http://www.nctsn.org/nctsn_assets/pdfs/pfa/2/PsyFirstAid.pdf. Accessed August 1, 2010.
69. Ruzek JI, Brymer MJ, Jacobs AK, et al. Psychological first aid. J Ment Health Counsel 2007;29:17–49.
70. Lubow RE, Moore AU. Latent inhibition: The effect of non-reinforced exposure to the conditioned stimulus. J Comp Physiol Psychol 1959;52:415–9.
71. Foa EB, Zinberg R, Rothbaum BO. Uncontrollability and unpredictability in post-traumatic stress disorder: an animal model. Psychol Bull 1992;112:218–38.
72. Pace-Schott EF, Millad MR, Orr SP, et al. Sleep promotes generalization of extinction of conditioned fear. Sleep 2009;32:19–26.

73. Stickgold R. Of sleep, memories and trauma. Nat Neurosci 2007;10:540–2.
74. Mellman T, Bustamante V, Fins A, et al. Rapid eye movement sleep and the early development of posttraumatic stress disorder. Am J Psychiatry 2002;159: 1696–701.
75. Maher MJ, Rego SA, Asnis GM. Sleep disturbances in patients with post-traumatic stress disorder: Epidemiology, impact and approaches to management. CNS Drugs 2006;20:567–90.
76. Krakow B, Hollifield M, Johnston L, et al. Imagery rehearsal therapy for chronic nightmares in sexual assault survivors with posttraumatic stress disorder: a randomized controlled trial. JAMA 2001;286:537–45.
77. Raskind MA, Peskind ER, Hoff DJ, et al. A parallel group placebo controlled study of prazosin for trauma nightmares and sleep disturbance in combat veterans with post-traumatic stress disorder. Biol Psychiatry 2007;61:928–34.
78. Hilakivi I, Leppavuori A. Effects of methoxamine, an alpha-1 adrenoreceptor agonist, and prazosin, an alpha-1 antagonist, on the stages of the sleep-waking cycle in the rat. Acta Physiol Scand 1984;120:363–72.
79. Pellejero T, Monti JM, Baglietto J, et al. Effects of methoxamine and alpha-1 adrenoreceptor antagonists, prazosin and yohimbine, on the sleep-waking cycle of the rat. Sleep 1984;7:365–72.
80. Raskind MA, Peskind ER, Kanter ED, et al. Reduction of nightmares and other PTSD symptoms in combat veterans by prazosin: a placebo-controlled study. Am J Psychiatry 2003;160:371–3.
81. Taylor FB, Martin P, Thompson C, et al. Prazosin effects on objective sleep measures and clinical symptoms in civilian trauma PTSD: a placebo-controlled study. Biol Psychiatry 2008;63:629–32.

Prevention of the First Episode of Psychosis

William R. McFarlane, MD[a,b],*

KEYWORDS

- Psychosis • Schizophrenia • Prevention • Mood disorder
- Prodromal • High-risk

Among all medical disorders, schizophrenia is one of the most disabling and costly. It is the most severe mental disorder, creating nearly continuous disability for a lifetime in the majority of cases. Somewhat less than 1% (between 0.27% and 0.83%) of the population suffers from this disorder, even though the yearly incidence is low, approximately 0.2 per 1000.[1] In market economies, it is the fifth leading cause of disability and premature mortality among all medical disorders. It is a devastating disorder for families and communities, whose members often assume major caretaking burdens because of the profound functional deficits that this disorder imposes. It has been estimated that the total lifetime cost for a single case of schizophrenia is greater than $10 million.[2] Twenty-five percent of all hospital admissions and disability payments in the United States are accounted for by patients with severe mental illness, most of which is schizophrenia and other psychotic disorders. It is a major drain on the economy: recent estimates put direct and indirect costs to the nation for schizophrenia at more than $62 billion per year.[3] Recent meta-analyses have found that schizophrenia exacts a 25-year reduction in life expectancy, principally secondary to heart disease, cancer, and suicide.[4]

The functional disability that is particularly devastating seems due to biologic and psychosocial deficit processes that usually begin before the psychotic symptoms. These often persist in spite of treatment and usually get worse with time and each subsequent episode. Although improved treatment has ameliorated some of this disability, long-term outcomes in general remain poor. Nationally, substantial reductions in the availability of community-based services have led to a decline in prognosis. At the same time, clinical trials have demonstrated that overall treatment and rehabilitation efficacy has improved substantially; thus, prognosis, in theory,

[a] Department of Psychiatry, Tufts University Medical School, 136 Harrison Avenue, Boston, MA 02111, USA
[b] Center for Psychiatric Research, Maine Medical Center Research Institute, Maine Medical Center, 22 Bramhall Street, Portland, ME 04102, USA
* Maine Medical Center, 22 Bramhall Street, Portland, ME 04102.
E-mail address: mcfarw@mmc.org

Psychiatr Clin N Am 34 (2011) 95–107
doi:10.1016/j.psc.2010.11.012
0193-953X/11/$ – see front matter © 2011 Elsevier Inc. All rights reserved.

should be improving. Given these realities, schizophrenia is not just an interesting and clinically challenging psychiatric disorder but also a significant public health burden.

The most significant empirical influence on the emergence of deliberate efforts to prevent psychotic disorders has been the evidence that the duration of untreated first episode of psychosis has some of the most enduring impacts on the course of illness of any known treatment. Recent studies of first-episode psychosis document that the average time between onset of psychotic symptoms and the initiation of treatment is from 1 to 2 years, depending on the study.[5] These findings are troubling when considering other studies that have shown a deteriorating course and reduced response to treatment as the duration of untreated psychosis (DUP) lengthens and with each episode of psychosis.[6,7]

These and other studies suggest that the earliest signs of development of psychosis arise during adolescence as a consequence of neurodegenerative processes, psychosocial stress, and hormonal changes. The current approach asserts that those processes can be altered and even reversed by earlier treatment.[8–10] In essence, current data support the conclusion that symptomatic and functional outcomes are determined by the number of days that a person has spent in a psychotic state and perhaps by the duration of the untreated prodromal state. The prodromal period, alternatively, can last for months to years, making its identification a feasible means of achieving the goal of indicated prevention. In addition, psychosis is inherently heterogeneous as to ultimate diagnosis. In particular, a substantial proportion of those at high risk for psychosis actually experience the onset of a severe mood disorder, not schizophrenia. The symptomatic phenomena observed during the onset of bipolar disorder with psychosis are similar to those for schizophrenia, with a poor prognosis.[11]

Supporting prevention research is the vast amount of new knowledge that demonstrates the fundamental biologic underpinnings of the disorder combined with a wealth of data showing that this biologic vulnerability is heavily influenced by family, social, and other environmental influences.[12,13] The combined influence of these two strands of scientific and clinical progress has prompted several groups, especially in Europe and Australia, to develop treatment programs explicitly designed to intervene early in the first episode. More recently, they have gone on to intervene in the period between onset of attenuated psychotic symptoms and the onset of frank psychosis, a period termed the *prodrome* or *prodromal phase*, borrowing a term from epilepsy. Thus, at present, prevention of schizophrenia and other psychotic disorders constitutes secondary prevention, or in current terminology, indicated prevention. The cohort to be identified and treated preventively is, in the most technical terms, already experiencing the onset of psychotic symptoms and is often partially disabled cognitively and functionally. The extent of illness does not rise to the level needed to meet current criteria for a schizophrenic or psychotic mood disorder. For the moment, the question of whether or not intervention delays or prevents altogether onset is left to longer-term research. The same is true for the etiologic basis of early phase psychosis, given the current lack of a genetic marker or even clear diagnostic or prognostic implications. Even delaying onset is seen as valuable in itself, because achieving developmental milestones and cognitive maturation seems to be a defense against the neurologic consequences of long-term psychotic disorders. At the least, those persons experiencing such symptoms are vulnerable and at elevated risk for a psychotic disorder, even if they do not experience imminent onset. From a lay perspective, most persons during the prodromal phase are not seen as mentally ill. The focus of this article is on those preventive efforts and the relevant science on which they are based.

INDICATORS AND IDENTIFIERS

In response to the evidence for longer DUP predicting poor outcome, research has increasingly focused on the opposite tendency—to reduce DUP to the minimum possible. Most of this article is devoted to the latter alternative, but these investigations began with this basic observation—that being psychotic for long periods leaves patients vulnerable to increasing severity, more disability, and diminished response to treatment. The practical effect was to spur development of indicators that could predict likelihood of imminent onset of psychosis. Those indicators are based on symptoms that are primarily characteristic of schizophrenia, even though psychosis itself is not limited to a single diagnostic entity. Beginning with well-known risk factors—schizoid tendencies and a family history of psychosis—the effort to develop predicting instruments to select participants at high risk for psychosis has centered mainly on attenuated psychotic symptoms. Thus, 4 well-described criteria sets have arisen, of which 2 are variations on the older *Diagnostic and Statistical Manual of Mental Disorders* (Third Edition Revised) criteria for prodromal schizophrenia. The Comprehensive Assessment of At-Risk Mental States (CAARMS)[14] and the Structured Interview for Prodromal Syndromes (SIPS)[15] define risk for psychosis under 3 categories: (1) attenuated psychotic symptoms, (2) brief intermittent psychotic episodes (1 week to 1 month), or (3) recent marked functional deterioration while having a first-degree relative with a psychotic disorder or schizotypal personality disorder (SPD). The Bonn Scale for the Assessment of Basic Symptoms,[16] based on Huber's[17] original concept of core or basic symptoms of schizophrenia, adds criteria consisting of elements of thought disorder (interference, perseveration, pressure, blockage, derealization, and so forth). It achieves 78% accuracy; nearly 70% of those meeting prodromal criteria experienced conversion to schizophrenia over 9 years.[16] Cornblatt and colleagues[18] added a measure of negative symptoms, theorizing that almost all persons with schizophrenia manifest subtle versions of this deficit-related syndrome even before onset of attenuated psychotic symptoms. In a recent review of 16 follow-up studies,[19] the overall average for conversion to psychosis using the various existing criteria sets is 30% to 35% per year. Also, serial measures in the same location, in particular Melbourne, Australia, have found a decreasing rate of conversion in untreated samples.[20] That observation suggests a longer-term effect of early intervention within a specific population or a natural decrease in incidence generally.[20]

A frequent criticism of indicated prevention for psychosis is that those who do not convert must be false positive for psychosis, reflecting concern that ethical practice dictates watchful waiting to determine diagnosis.[19] There is an emerging consensus, however, that the great majority of such persons are often functionally and neurocognitively impaired, regardless of their near-term likelihood of developing frank psychosis. Nearly all studies of cognitive function in prodromal samples have found substantial impairment, particularly in verbal memory, processing speed, executive function, and olfaction.[21] Other studies have shown lesser degrees of the same type of cortical volume reduction that has been documented in schizophrenia, especially in those patients who do convert.[22] Also, such cases may become psychotic (true positives) later, reflecting the long risk period for onset of psychosis.[23] As discussed previously, one study with a much longer follow-up period found a steadily increasing rate of true positives over time: approximately 70%.[16] As results for indicated prevention improve, intervention is less and less controversial, particularly for those interventions with lower risks and general benefits for mental and physical health.

EFFICACY TRIALS OF INDICATED PREVENTION

The evidence for the long-term negative impact of untreated psychosis has led to early treatment being increasingly considered as the necessary step to preventing deterioration and resistance to treatment. Given the long prodromal period (often up to a year) within which it is possible to identify individuals at risk, early identification and intervention have made possible a substantial improvement in functioning, symptomatology, and prognosis. Recent clinical research has shown that early application of existing and only slightly modified evidence-based treatments for schizophrenia and mood disorders can markedly improve outcome and prognosis. Six clinical trials have consistently found that conversion to psychosis can be limited to approximately half or less of the expected (control) rate with medication and/or psychosocial treatment.[24–29] The international evidence that psychosocial and/or psychopharmacologic treatment may be preventive if applied before onset of frank psychosis is discussed (**Table 1**).

Buckingham

Falloon described a small public health program designed to detect and treat psychotic and prodromal states as early as possible.[30] It was located in Buckingham and an adjoining county in England. Treatment was continued until "all evidence of prodromal features" had remitted. Sixteen patients were identified by this system, after assessing more than 1000 referrals over the 4 years of the project. Thirteen patients with prodromal symptoms "experienced full and usually rapid recovery after brief integrated intervention." One patient with a full psychotic onset of schizophrenia was treated to remission over 4 weeks; another developed bipolar disorder, also treated effectively with antimanic medication; a third went on to experience multiple recurrences of prodromal symptoms but not psychosis. This led to a 10-fold reduction of the incidence rate in the catchment area. The integrated treatment model included family psychoeducation, thiordiazine in low doses, and follow-up via the patients' general practitioners.

Manchester Cognitive Therapy Trial

Morrison and his colleagues[31] mounted a comparative clinical trial, Early Detection and Intervention Evaluation (EDIE), of cognitive therapy for young adults at risk of

Table 1
Psychosis prevention studies

	One-Year Rates for Conversion to Psychosis			
	Control		Experimental	
	n	Converted	n	Converted
PACE	28	10 (35.7%)	31	6 (19.4%)
PRIME	29	11 (37.9%)	31	5 (16.1%)
OPUS	30	10 (33.3%)	37	3 (5.7%)
EDIE	23	6 (26.1%)	35	2 (5.7%)
O-3 FAs	40	11 (27.5%)	41	2 (4.9%)
PIER	0	0	148	13 (8.8%)
Total	150	48	323	31
Mean conversion rate		32.0%	—	9.6%
Without PIER				
Total	150	48	175	18
Mean conversion rate		32.0%	—	10.3%

psychosis to evaluate its efficacy for the prevention of transition to psychosis. They randomized 58 patients at high risk of developing a first episode of psychosis to either cognitive therapy or treatment as usual. Therapy was provided over 6 months, and all patients were monitored on a monthly basis for 12 months. Logistic regression demonstrated that cognitive therapy significantly reduced the likelihood of progressing to psychosis over 12 months. In addition, it significantly reduced the likelihood of being prescribed antipsychotic medication and of meeting criteria for a *Diagnostic and Statistical Manual of Mental Disorders* (Fourth Edition) diagnosis of a psychotic disorder and improved positive symptoms. At 3 years, cognitive therapy significantly reduced likelihood of being prescribed antipsychotic medication, but it did not affect transition to psychosis.[31] Controlling for baseline cognitive factors did yield a significant result for conversion to psychosis. The follow-up rate at 3 years, however, was only 47%; assessments were not blind to treatment condition; and the effect would not have been significant if 2 cases had not been reassigned post hoc. Also, the mean age was 23, substantially older than samples in North America. With those caveats, cognitive therapy seems an acceptable and modestly efficacious intervention for the older range of those young adults whose cognitive development has been largely completed.

German Research Network on Schizophrenia

A second trial of cognitive therapy in the prodromal phase was recently reported from the German Research Network on Schizophrenia.[28] In a multisite study involving centers in Cologne, Bonn, Düsseldorf, and Munich, the protocol involved participants who were in the earliest phase, manifesting basic symptoms (eg, thought disorder and alterations of perception), which were used, along with full psychosis, as outcome indicators. The cognitive therapy addressed thought and perception deficits, negative symptoms, general anxiety and depression, and family and occupational problems. The experimental condition was compared with supportive counseling, which comprised assessment, patient education, and empathic, but unstructured, support. No medication was used. The treatment goal was to improve psychosocial and occupational functioning, which had not been shown to change in previous clinical trials in the prodromal phase; 113 participants were assessed, randomized, and treated. Of some importance was the mean age, 25.8, which was similar to the Manchester sample in being substantially older than the mean ages in North American studies. Although there were significant improvements over time for the sample in both conditions, there were no significant improvements for cognitive behavioral therapy over the comparison treatment. Alternatively, deterioration did not occur and the mean level of functioning did improve in both study treatment conditions. The main methodologic drawback was a large number of participants (40.7%) with missing psychosocial outcome data, reflecting a high dropout rate. This sample was not readily comparable in that it was older and less severe in symptomatology.

Danish National Schizophrenia Project

One large-scale effort that proved preventive in nature was originally focused on early intervention in the initial psychosis. The Danish National Schizophrenia Project (OPUS, in Danish) compared outcomes in three treatments at six sites across a prospective intervention and follow-up period of 2 years, with plans for a 5-year assessment.[32] After being identified as having an initial psychosis, participants, ages 16 to 35, were assigned to (1) supportive psychodynamic psychotherapy (n = 119), (2) integrated treatment (n = 139), or (3) treatment as usual (n = 304). Integrated treatment consisted of multifamily psychoeducational groups,[33] assertive community treatment, and antipsychotic medication, an approach termed *Family-aided Assertive Community Treatment (FACT)* in the United States. It is an evidence-based approach for established schizophrenia.[34] In these first-episode patients, integrated treatment achieved the best results for measures of functioning and negative symptoms. Odds ratios ranged from 3 to 7 for improvements compared with treatment as usual.

A fortuitous result of the OPUS study was that a subsample was recruited with SPD but not psychosis or schizophrenia.[26] Seventy-nine such participants were assigned to the respective treatments, with the targeted outcome being initial conversion to, rather than relapse of, psychosis. At the end of 2 years of treatment, 48.3% of the participants in the treatment-as-usual group had a psychotic episode, compared with 25% of those in the integrated treatment arm, which was a large and significant difference. This study further supported the efficacy of family-based treatment as a preventive intervention but also suggested another avenue for early identification—finding youth and young adults with SPD and offering treatment with evidence-based treatments for schizophrenia.

Personal Assessment and Crisis Evaluation

Personal Assessment and Crisis Evaluation (PACE) is a large-scale version of the Falloon effort, headed by McGorry and colleagues, over the past 12 years in Melbourne, Australia.[24] The PACE program intervened with young people who were seen to be at risk for imminent onset of psychosis. The PACE service relied on referral from a general practitioner, similarly to Falloon's project in the United Kingdom. They also targeted individuals who encounter young people frequently, including school counselors, teachers, and youth workers. The intervention included stress management, social skills training, problem solving, family education and crisis support, symptom monitoring, and targeted medication at low doses (primarily risperidone).

The PACE program has been evaluated in an experimental design. Those participants who met criteria for high risk for psychosis (CAARMS) were randomly assigned to (1) a comparison group consisting of assessment and supportive treatment, an approach termed *needs-based intervention (NBI)*, or (2) an experimental group, specific-preventive intervention (SPI) cognitive therapy and medication (low-dose [1–2 mg] risperidone), given by symptom indication for 6 months, after which they received NBI.[24] Of 522 referrals, 92 met the criteria and of those, 59 were randomly assigned and 33 refused. After 6 months, the NBI cohort had a relapse/conversion rate of 36%; the experimental group receiving and adhering to intensive psychosocial treatment showed a rate of 7% ($P = .03$); those offered but not adhering to medication treatment manifested a rate of 12% (not significant). Measures of functioning were unchanged from baseline. The SPI group had better outcomes for conversion, but more than half did not accept medication, and among that group, there was a higher conversion rate during the second 6-month follow-up period. The SPI group, even without medication or cognitive therapy after 6 months, had no additional conversions. Those results held true at 3 years. The number needed to treat was 4.

Prevention Through Risk Identification, Management, and Education

McGlashan and colleagues,[25] at 4 sites in North America, used olanzapine in an industry-sponsored controlled trial, Prevention through Risk Identification, Management, and Education (PRIME), to treat prodromal schizophrenia and other psychotic disorders. Although their experience has shown that it is difficult to recruit participants using traditional drug trial methodology, the study served as a rigorous test of a pharmacologic strategy to prodromal intervention. This study used an adaptation of the Australian (CAARMS) criteria and the SIPS and its associated Scale of Prodromal

Symptoms. Sixty participants were randomly assigned to olanzapine or placebo and treated for 1 year, followed by observation without treatment for 1 year. The sample averaged 17.7 years of age. The rate of conversion was 38% for the control group and 16% for the treated group ($P = .09$), and the dropout rate was 35% for the placebo and 55% for the treated group. During the second year, 25% (placebo) and 33% (olanzapine), respectively, of the initially nonconverting cases converted. The differences for conversion were at a trend level, but conversion in the placebo group occurred throughout the year, in contrast to the treated group, in which they occurred early in the first year. The treated group had a significantly superior effect for positive symptoms but also experienced marked weight gain (mean 8.8 kg). The number needed to treat was 4.5. During the second year, without medication, symptoms worsened for both groups, but some of the weight gained was lost. A measure of functioning showed a slight, although significant, improvement over time (mean Global Assessment of Functioning improved from 42 to 48). This study, relying almost solely on medication for prevention effect, found that at 2 years, with no treatment in the second year, 79% and 80%, respectively, had converted or dropped out. That was a somewhat discouraging outcome from a public health standpoint.

Prevention of Psychosis by Omega-3 Fatty Acids

A supernutritional strategy was tested by Amminger and colleagues,[29] who conducted a randomized clinical trial in which omega-3 fatty acids (O-3 FAs) (without concomitant second-generation antipsychotics [SGAs]) were tested against placebo for 12 weeks, with psychosocial intervention held constant. At 1 year, the O-3 FAs condition had a conversion rate of 4.9% versus 27.5% in the placebo condition. Effects were correlated with blood level of O-3 FAs at baseline. The preventive effect persisted at 1 year, after the O-3 FAs were discontinued at 12 weeks. Positive and negative symptoms and functioning all improved significantly. The number needed to treat was, again, 4.

Portland Identification and Early Referral

The Portland Identification and Early Referral (PIER) program was developed in 2000, to undertake systematic early detection, intervention, and prevention of psychosis throughout an entire urban area, by providing treatment during the prodromal period. The intent was to reduce incidence of psychotic disorders and schizophrenia specifically for a defined population while also testing the efficacy of family psychoeducation as a preventive treatment. To achieve effectiveness, the PIER program (1) developed a widespread referral network, (2) mounted a major public education campaign, and (3) operated a special multidisciplinary team to treat those young people at the highest risk of onset of psychosis. The initial focus of the PIER team's effort was on educating and training for all school and college counseling professionals, primary health care and pediatric physicians, and mental health clinicians serving youth and young adults. The focus was on a defined catchment area of approximately 340,000.[35] The clinical approach used was FACT, as in OPUS. Specifically, families were engaged systematically in all cases. The model was based on the fact that family intervention was highly effective in established psychotic disorders and that adolescents in particular would be difficult to engage and maintain in treatment without family involvement.[36]

Preliminary outcome data are available for 1 year of treatment over the first 6 years of intake. Between May 7, 2001, and September 30, 2007, of 148 prodromal participants averaging 16.5 years of age, 8.8% developed a full psychosis. The identification and referrals yielded a referral rate of 46% of the expected rate for all psychotic disorders. The mean scores for the Global Assessment of Functioning went from 38 at entry to 55 at the 12-month assessment (functioning in role as expected, but with moderate or intermittent symptoms). The PIER treatment model is currently being tested in a National Institutes of Health–sponsored randomized clinical trial.

SUMMARY OF STUDIES OF INDICATED PREVENTION

Systems of early detection, intervention, and secondary or indicated prevention have been developed and tested in the United Kingdom, Australia, Scandinavia, Germany, Austria, and North America. Most involve specialized treatment with existing, empirically validated methods. These published studies of preventive intervention have achieved a substantial reduction in rates of first frank psychosis and in reducing prodromal and psychotic symptoms. A simple compilation across studies (see **Table 1**) demonstrates that the mean conversion rate across studies is 9.6% of treated participants versus 32% of untreated or treatment-as-usual control participants. In 3 studies, the number needed to treat was 4, comparable or superior to other medical preventive interventions.

To date, some studies have found high dropout rates, and one medication was found to have major side effects. Those studies that have used evidence-based and longer-term family and rehabilitative interventions (Buckingham, OPUS and PIER) have had better retention rates, persistence of effects, patient social and role functioning, and family well being. Psychosocial functioning is emerging as the area requiring the greatest clinical and rehabilitative effort and in which the value of psychosocial intervention is likely to be paramount. The evidence for long-term treatment effects and changes in prognosis is currently modest, much of it extrapolations of long-term outcomes of treatment of typical cases of schizophrenia. Further, some studies found that progression of disorder occurred after discontinuing a 6-month course of treatment. Experience demonstrates that arrest of deterioration, reduction of untreated psychosis, and short-term prevention of onset of psychosis, however, are consistent across studies and sites. The results also confirm that early detection is feasible. The major caveat is that no intervention strategy has yet emerged as superior to others. Rather, several previously efficacious treatments of psychotic disorders have shown at least marginal efficacy in the clinical high-risk population. The most unambiguous results have followed psychosocial and supernutritional treatment, less so after antipsychotic drug therapy.

CURRENT NORTH AMERICAN STUDIES

The principal barrier facing indicator and prevention intervention studies has been sample size. Although schizophrenia and psychotic mood disorders have a relatively high prevalence, they have a low incidence rate. That reality makes demonstration of effects difficult at any one site, at least to the degree that would be necessary for credibility regarding policy or public health initiatives. Two studies are now under way in North America that are attempting to overcome this barrier. Both are multisite studies, and one is recruiting a large proportion of the incident at-risk population within the sites' geographic and/or service areas.

Early Detection and Intervention for the Prevention of Psychosis Project

The Robert Wood Johnson Foundation has funded a 4-year national research demonstration (Early Detection and Intervention for the Prevention of Psychosis [EDIPP]) project to produce the clinical evidence necessary to justify widespread use of the PIER early detection and preventive treatment approach. Five replication sites have been selected and are currently recruiting participants: Zucker Hillside Hospital, Glen Oaks, New York; Washtenaw County Health Organization, Ypsilanti, Michigan;

University of California at Davis, Sacramento, California; University of New Mexico, Albuquerque, New Mexico; and Mid-Valley Behavioral Health Care Network, Salem, Oregon. The sites were selected to create a national sample with representatives of the major geographic, ethnic, and racial subgroups within the United States. Portland's PIER program is the model site and the study coordinating center while also recruiting participants. After initial training, each site has developed the 3 key components of the PIER model: (1) a community outreach and education program to train a large number of professionals from many disciplines outside the traditional mental health system; (2) targeted dissemination of information for the key affected populations regarding severe mental illness, promoting rapid consultation and treatment; and (3) a specialized FACT clinical team, whose multidisciplinary members quickly assess and treat young persons during the earliest phases of psychosis. Each site provides family psychoeducation, supported education and employment, assertive community treatment, and a psychotropic medication protocol for the prodromal population.

Each site has identified and entered into treatment 40 to 80 youth, ages 12 to 25, over the course of the 4-year study, identified from population bases of 300,000 to 500,000. The total sample is more than 335. EDIPP includes an effectiveness study with 3 components: (1) cutpoint assignment to treatment condition, using regression discontinuity methodology (in lieu of a random assignment design); (2) an epidemiologic catchment area comparison design with an historical control period; and (3) a simultaneous assessment of outcomes and cost-effectiveness for hospitalized (ie, not prevented or early) first-episode patients in experimental and control catchment areas.

North American Prodromal Longitudinal Study

This multisite study, the North American Prodromal Longitudinal Study, integrates basic measures and naturalistic outcome assessment over 8 sites in the United States and Canada.[37] Based on participant selection using the same identification system (SIPS) as in the PIER, EDIPP, and PRIME studies, individual sites have been coordinated to achieve a total sample of 888 participants with a high degree of agreement across sites on the Scale of Prodromal Syndromes diagnostic criteria; currently, 651 participants have sufficient data for planned outcome analyses. Approximately 10% have been recruited into medication trials, while the rest are being followed naturalistically. Most (n = 370) were admitted on the basis of heightened clinical risk manifested by current prodromal psychotic symptoms; the remainder consists of individuals with a first-degree relative with a psychotic illness, a *Diagnostic and Statistical Manual of Mental Disorders* (Fourth Edition) SPD diagnosis or a recent, very brief psychotic episode. There are two comparison groups: help-seeking individuals who do not meet any of the high-risk criteria (n = 174) and nonpsychiatric controls (n = 195). A set of common outcome measures will be used to estimate the conversion rate, endpoint diagnosis, and psychosocial outcomes. The first report on an initial subsample demonstrated an overall rate of conversion of 34% by 30 months, but subgroups (eg, those with suspiciousness, a family history, and current substance abuse) converted at up to 81% of those with that clinical profile.[38] A second report details neurocognitive deficits compared with controls.[21]

ALTERNATIVE INTERVENTIONS

One possible treatment alternative has been suggested by a naturalistic treatment study in which psychiatrists treated patients with psychotropic medications but without a randomized or specific drug protocol.[39] Forty-eight adolescents meeting clinical high-risk criteria were treated either with SGA or selective serotonin reuptake inhibitor (SSRI) drugs. No SSRI-treated patients converted. In sharp contrast, 43% of the SGA-treated patients converted, 92% of them after being nonadherent with their SGA medication. This study suggested that there is a major trade-off between efficacy and adherence, favoring a nonantipsychotic drug treatment approach. If confirmed in a randomized clinical trial, the SSRI approach is one that would improve the safety and reduce the negative image of a drug treatment prevention strategy. Another group, Woods and colleagues at Yale, is testing the use of glycine, a precursor of the components of the glutamine neurotransmitter system, to enhance cortical functioning in prodromal participants (unpublished data, 2009).

A small body of evidence and experience is suggesting that direct practice of the neural substrate of cognition, often using sophisticated video games, may substantially improve occupational and social functioning as well as post-treatment scores on neurocognitive testing. Currently, all results in the prodrome are preliminary but promising. The results from an earlier trial are intriguing: schizophrenia participants experienced a larger effect on employment than on changes in the cognitive test scores.[40] The more it becomes clear that positive symptoms and conversion to psychosis are preventable, the more important it will be to intervene to prevent the march of negative symptoms, cognitive deterioration, and functional deficits. Those are the treatment targets that are increasingly apparent as an integral, although more subtle, and probably primary aspect of the prodrome of psychosis.

SUMMARY

As with early identification and intervention in cancer and cardiovascular disease, there are inherent challenges to indicated prevention in psychotic disorders: expanding the accuracy and evidence for the indicators, applying those indicators to earlier stages of illness, and refining and testing the interventions themselves. Both a challenge and an opportunity, the next stage of development will be integrating advanced imaging techniques, neurocognitive assessments, molecular genetic strategies, and knowledge of neurotransmitter functioning with improved psychosocial and psychopharmacologic preventive intervention strategies to achieve enhanced accuracy and efficacy. Meanwhile, the current record of several prevention trials has raised the estimate of prevention efficacy from promising to likely, although earlier studies had substantial shortcomings. As with treatment of established schizophrenia and mood disorders, there is no currently superior single treatment modality. One interpretation of the lack of a clearly superior treatment approach is that much less intensive and risky methods are effective when severity and chronicity are still minimal. This parallels approaches in cancer and heart disease. The efficacy of low-intensity/low-risk family psychoeducational intervention and O-3 FAs illustrates this point.

The complications of antipsychotic drugs argue for staged intervention approaches that begin with psychosocial therapies, such as family and cognitive methods, and supernutritional and general health and wellness methods. Antipsychotic drugs and methods, such as supported employment, would be reserved for the late-stage prodrome, in which positive and negative symptoms are all but at psychotic or diagnostic levels. Given the increasing accuracy of identification methods and the evidence for the preventive efficacy of several intervention models, it seems likely that clinicians will add prevention and early intervention to their treatment approaches. The public health implications of that eventual outcome cannot be underestimated.

REFERENCES

1. Eaton WW. Evidence for universality and uniformity of schizophrenia around the world: assessment and implications. In: Gattaz WF, Hafner H, editors, Search for the causes of schizophrenia, vol. IV. Darmstadt (Germany): Steinkopf; 1999. p. 21–33.
2. Rupp A, Keith SJ. The costs of schizophrenia. Psychiatr Clin North Am 1993; 16(2):413–23.
3. Wu EQ, Birnbaum HG, Shi L, et al. The economic burden of schizophrenia in the United States. J Clin Psychiatry 2005;66:1122–9.
4. Parks J, Svendsen D, Singer P, et al. Morbidity and mortality in people with serious mental illness. Alexandria (VA): National Association of State Mental Health Program Directors, Medical Directors Council; 2006.
5. Perkins DO, Gu H, Boteva K, et al. Relationship between duration of untreated psychosis and outcome in first-episode schizophrenia: a critical review and meta-analysis. Am J Psychiatry 2005;162(10):1785–804.
6. Lieberman JA, Perkins D, Belger A, et al. The early stages of schizophrenia: speculations on pathogenesis, pathophysiology, and therapeutic approaches. Biol Psychiatry 2001;50(11):884–97.
7. Haas GL, Garratt LS, Sweeney JA. Delay to first antipsychotic medication in schizophrenia: impact on symptomatology and clinical course of illness. J Psychiatr Res 1998;32(3–4):151–9.
8. Verdoux H, Liraud F, Bergey C, et al. Is the association between duration of untreated psychosis and outcome confounded ? A two-year follow-up study of first-admitted patients. Schizophr Res 2001;49(3):231–41.
9. Larsen T, More L, Vibe-Hansen L, et al. Premorbid functioning versus duration of untreated psychosis in 1 year outcome in first-episode psychosis. Schizophr Res 2000;45(1–2):1–9.
10. Norman R, Townsend L, Malla A. Duration of untreated psychosis and cognitive functioning in first-episode patients. Br J Psychiatry 2001;179(4):340–5.
11. Correll CU, Penzner JB, Frederickson AM, et al. Differentiation in the preonset phases of schizophrenia and mood disorders: evidence in support of a bipolar mania prodrome. Schizophr Bull 2007;33(3):703–14.
12. Bebbington P, Kuipers L. The predictive utility of expressed emotion in schizophrenia: an aggregate analysis. Psychol Med 1994;24(3):707–18.
13. Tienari PA, Wynne LC, Sorri A, et al. Genotype-environment interaction in schizophrenia-spectrum disorder. Br J Psychiatry 2004;184:216–22.
14. Yung AR, Phillips LJ, Yuen HP, et al. Psychosis prediction: 12-month follow-up of a high-risk ("prodromal") group. Schizophr Res 2003;60:21–32.
15. Miller TJ, McGlashan TH, Rosen JL, et al. Prodromal assessment with the structured interview for prodromal syndromes and the scale of prodromal symptoms: predictive validity, inter-rater reliability and training to reliability. Schizophr Bull 2003;29(4):703–15.
16. Klosterkotter J, Hellmich M, Steinmeyer EM, et al. Diagnosing schizophrenia in the initial prodromal phase. Arch Gen Psychiatry 2001;58(2):158–64.
17. Huber G, Gross G, Schuttler R, et al. Longitudinal studies of schizophrenic patients. Schizophr Bull 1980;6(4):592–605.
18. Cornblatt B, Obuchowski M, Roberts S, et al. Cognitive and behavioral precursors of schizophrenia. Dev Psychopathol 1999;11(3):487–508.
19. Haroun N, Dunn L, Haroun A, et al. Risk and protection in prodromal schizophrenia: ethical implications for clinical practice and future research. Schizophr Bull 2005;32(1):166–78.

20. Yung AR, Yuen HP, Berger GE, et al. Declining transition rates in ultra high risk (prodromal) services: dilution of reduction of risk? Schizophr Bull 2007;33(3):673–81.
21. Seidman LJ, Giuliano AJ, Meyer EC, et al. Neuropsychology of the prodrome to psychosis in the NAPLS consortium: relationship to family history and conversion to psychosis. Arch Gen Psychiatry 2010;67(6):578–88.
22. Sun D, Phillips L, Velakoulis D, et al. Progressive brain structural changes mapped as psychosis develops in 'at risk' individuals. Schizophr Res 2009;108(1–3): 85–92.
23. Kirkbride JB, Fearon P, Morgan C, et al. Heterogeneity in incidence rates of schizophrenia and other psychotic syndromes: findings from the 3-center AeSOP study. Arch Gen Psychiatry 2006;63(3):250–8.
24. McGorry P, Yung A, Phillips L, et al. Randomized controlled trial of interventions designed to reduce the risk of progression to first-episode psychosis in a clinical sample with subthreshold symptoms. Arch Gen Psychiatry 2002; 59(10):921–8.
25. McGlashan TH, Zipursky RB, Perkins D, et al. Randomized, double-blind trial of olanzapine versus placebo in patients prodromally symptomatic for psychosis. Am J Psychiatry 2006;163(5):790–9.
26. Nordentoft M, Thorup A, Petersen L, et al. Transition rates from schizotypal disorder to psychotic disorder for first-contact patients included in the OPUS trial. A randomized clinical trial of integrated treatment and standard treatment. Schizophr Res 2006;83(1):29–40.
27. Morrison AP, French P, Walford L, et al. Cognitive therapy for the prevention of psychosis in people at ultra-high risk: randomised controlled trial. Br J Psychiatry 2004;185(4):291–7.
28. Bechdolf A, Wagner M, Veith V, et al. Randomized controlled multicentre trial of cognitive behaviour therapy in the early initial prodromal state: effects on social adjustment post treatment. Early Interv Psychiatry 2007;1(1):71–8.
29. Amminger GP, Schafer MR, Papageorgiou K, et al. Long-chain omega-3 fatty acids for indicated prevention of psychotic disorders: a randomized, placebo-controlled trial. Arch Gen Psychiatry 2010;67(2):146–54.
30. Falloon IRH. Early intervention for first episodes of schizophrenia: a preliminary exploration. Psychiatry 1992;55(1):4–15.
31. Morrison AP, French P, Parker S, et al. Three-year follow-up of a randomized controlled trial of cognitive therapy for the prevention of psychosis in people at ultrahigh risk. Schizophr Bull 2007;33(3):682–7.
32. Rosenbaum B, Valbak K, Harder S, et al. Treatment of patients with first-episode psychosis: two year outcome data from the Danish National Schizophrenia Project. World Psychiatry 2006;5(2):100–3.
33. McFarlane WR. Multifamily groups in the treatment of severe psychiatric disorders. New York: Guilford Press; 2002.
34. McFarlane W, Stastny P, Deakins S. Family-aided assertive community treatment: a comprehensive rehabilitation and intensive case management approach for persons with schizophrenic disorders. New Dir Ment Health Serv 1992;53:43–54.
35. McFarlane WR, Cook WL, Downing D, et al. Portland identification and early referral: a community-based system for identifying and treating youths at high risk of psychosis. Psychiatr Serv 2010;61(5):512–5.
36. McFarlane WR. Family-based treatment in prodromal and first-episode psychosis. In: Miller T, editor. Early intervention in psychotic disorders. Amsterdam: Kluwer Academic Publishers; 2001. p. 197–230.

37. Addington J, Cadenhead K, Cannon TD, et al. North American Prodrome Longitudinal Study: a collaborative multisite approach to prodromal schizophrenia research. Schizophr Bull 2007;33(3):665–72.

38. Cannon TD, Cadenhead K, Cornblatt B, et al. Prediction of psychosis in youth at high clinical risk. Arch Gen Psychiatry 2008;65(1):28–37.

39. Cornblatt BA, Lencz T, Smith CW, et al. Can antidepressants be used to treat the schizophrenia prodrome. Results of a prospective, naturalistic treatment study of adolescents. J Clin Psychiatry 2007;68:546–57.

40. McGurk SR, Mueser KT, Pascaris A. Cognitive training and supported employment for persons with severe mental illness: one-year results from a randomized controlled trial. Schizophr Bull 2005;31(4):898–909.

Prevention of Metabolic Syndrome in Serious Mental Illness

Rohan Ganguli, MD, FRCP[a,b],*, Martin Strassnig, MD[a]

KEYWORDS

- Metabolic syndrome • Mental illness • Lifestyle management
- Antipsychotic medication

In the past decade, increasing attention has been focused on the nonpsychiatric morbidity and mortality associated with psychiatric disorders. There is evidence from as far back as 1919[1] that individuals with serious mental illnesses had a shortened life span. Nevertheless, many were shocked by recent data showing that, even in the modern era, a person with schizophrenia or bipolar disorder has a 20% to 25% shortening of life expectancy.[2] The most frequent causes of premature mortality in persons with mental illness are heart disease, cerebrovascular disease, and pulmonary disease.[2] A systematic review of cohort studies examining total and all-cause mortality in persons with schizophrenia has shown that life expectancy is 20% lower among those with schizophrenia than in the general population,[3] with cardiovascular disease (CVD) as the most frequent natural cause of death. These data are in close accord with numerous large epidemiologic investigations that have consistently found higher standardized mortality ratios (SMR) and higher rates of CVD for persons with schizophrenia compared with contemporary cohorts in the general population.[4–8] The data for bipolar disorder and other severe mood disorders are similar for persons with schizophrenia with higher SMR and rates of CVD compared with the general population.[9,10] The rates of metabolic syndrome are also higher in persons with schizophrenia[11,12] and those with bipolar disorder.[13,14] Patients with severe mood disorders, including depression, have also been found to be at higher risk for heart

This work was partially supported by a Canadian Institutes of Health Research (CIHR) Tier 1 Canada Research Chair grant to Dr Ganguli, and a 2008 Young Investigator Award to Dr Martin Strassnig, from the National Alliance for Research in Schizophrenia and Depression (NARSAD).

[a] Center for Addiction and Mental Health, University of Toronto, 901 King Street West, Suite 500, Box 13, Toronto, ON M5V 3HS, Canada
[b] Western Psychiatric Institute and Clinic, University of Pittsburgh, 3811 O'Hara Street, Pittsburgh, PA 15213-2593, USA
* Corresponding author. Center for Addiction and Mental Health, University of Toronto, 901 King Street West, Suite 500, Box 13, Toronto, ON M5V 3HS, Canada.
E-mail address: Rohan_Ganguli@camh.net

Psychiatr Clin N Am 34 (2011) 109–125
doi:10.1016/j.psc.2010.11.004
0193-953X/11/$ – see front matter © 2011 Elsevier Inc. All rights reserved.

disease after 2 years of treatment, even though they were not different from the general population at baseline.[15] Thus, in the effort to restore years of life lost by persons with serious mental illness, preventing or postponing the development and progression of heart disease is the natural target of these efforts.

WHAT IS THE METABOLIC SYNDROME?

The term metabolic syndrome was coined to describe a constellation of risk factors (central obesity, insulin resistance, raised blood pressure, and abnormal lipid profile) that were thought to be highly predictive of increased risk for heart disease, especially coronary heart disease.[16] Current criteria for metabolic syndrome are summarized in **Table 1**. Recent meta-analyses confirm that persons with metabolic syndrome have almost double the risk of incident heart disease and coronary artery disease than those without the syndrome.[17,18] Because insulin resistance is a core component of metabolic syndrome, individuals with the syndrome are also at greater risk for developing diabetes, and diabetes is by itself a risk factor for heart disease.[19]

In recent years, questions have been asked about whether the component abnormalities included in the metabolic syndrome are simply additive in their effect on risk, or whether meeting criteria for the syndrome provides any additional predictive power with respect to risk for heart disease.[20] Despite these unresolved questions, the term metabolic syndrome is retained in this article, as it is so well known in the field of risk reduction. However, risk reduction is discussed in terms of the various individual risk factors, because there is no treatment for metabolic syndrome per se. Interventions most likely to reduce the risk of CVD include reduction in weight, treatment of hypertension, treatment of dyslipidemia, treatment of insulin resistance and diabetes, and cessation of smoking. Smoking is not discussed in this article, but the importance of smoking as a risk factor for heart disease needs to be mentioned because of the high rates of smoking among persons with serious mental illness.[21]

Table 1 Metabolic syndrome: screening tools and National Cholesterol Education Program (NCEP) and International Diabetes Federation criteria	
Hypertriglyceridemic waist phenotype: simultaneous presence of	
Fasting triglycerides >2.0 mmol/L	
Waist circumference >90 cm	
Metabolic syndrome criteria met if any 3 of the following are present	
NCEP/ATP-III criteria	International Diabetes Federation
Presence of at least 3 of 5 parameters:	
Blood pressure >130/85 mm Hg	Same, or specific treatment
Fasting glucose ≥6.1 mmol/L (110 mg/dL)	Fasting plasma glucose >100 mg/dL (5.6 mmol/L) or type 2 diabetes diagnosis
Fasting triglycerides ≥1.7 mmol/L (150 mg/dL)	>150 mg/dL (1.7 mmol/L) or active treatment
HDL-C	
Men <1.0 mmol/L 40 mg/dL Women <1.3 mmol/L 50 mg/dL	<40 mg/dL (1.03 mmol/L) for men, <50 mg/dL (1.29 mmol/L) for women
Waist circumference	
Men >102 cm Women >88 cm	Ethnicity specific, in whites, men >94 cm, women >80 cm

METABOLIC SYNDROME AND OBESITY IN SERIOUS MENTAL ILLNESS

There has been a marked increase in overweight and obesity in the past 25 years, with the prevalence of obesity among all adults rising from 13% to 32% for both genders, and among all racial/ethnic and age groups.[22] Obese individuals have an increased risk of several adverse health outcomes, notably hypertension, diabetes, CVD, arthritis, disability, and mortality.[23] Obesity is an independent risk factor for CVD[24] and the degree of obesity correlates with CVD risk.[25]

Exceptionally high rates of obesity have been reported for patients with schizophrenia.[11,26] A survey by Dickerson and colleagues[27] found rates of obesity as high as 50% in women and 42% in men in a random sample of outpatients with schizophrenia compared with US population data and much higher rates of severe obesity (body mass index [BMI], calculated as weight in kilograms divided by the square of height in meters) >40 kg/m^2. The mean baseline BMI in the CATIE study was 29.7 kg/m^2, with 36.6% of men and 73.4% of women classified as having central obesity, defined by a waist circumference in excess of 102 and 88 cm, respectively.[28]

LIFESTYLE MANAGEMENT TO PREVENT WEIGH GAIN AND REDUCE WEIGHT

The foundation of risk reduction in both heart disease and diabetes lies in changing lifestyle, specifically eating and exercise, with the purpose of maintaining a healthy weight (preventing or treating obesity) and increasing physical activity and fitness. Guidelines for weight management were proposed by the National Heart, Lung and Blood Institute (NHLBI) in 1998, as an aid to reduce and postpone the incidence of heart disease. The Canadian Cardiovascular Society and Guidelines[29] and the American Diabetes Association also state that "You can prevent or delay the onset of type 2 diabetes through a healthy lifestyle."[30] These recommendations are supported by several large clinical trials demonstrating that weight loss does delay or prevent the onset of type 2 diabetes in at-risk individuals[31,32] and reduce the risk of heart disease.[33]

Preventing weight gain can, in turn, prevent many of the obesity-related risk factors for CVD (ie, insulin resistance and type 2 diabetes mellitus, dyslipidemia, hypertension, and vascular inflammation).[34] In terms of weight loss, evidence supports that even small reductions in body weight can lead to substantial improvements in a metabolic risk profile predictive of CVD and type 2 diabetes mellitus.[35–37] Weight loss of as little as 5% of initial body weight, if the decrease is predominantly adipose tissue volume, can postpone the onset or prevent CVD, type 2 diabetes, hypertension; hyperlipidemia, cardiorespiratory failure and other chronic degenerative diseases.[38,39]

With regard to glucose metabolism, insulin sensitivity improves rapidly before much weight loss occurs and continues to improve with continued weight loss.[40] In patients who are already obese, for example, and have a risk profile predictive of type 2 diabetes mellitus, a 5% weight loss at the end of 1 year of dietary therapy can decrease fasting blood glucose, insulin, hemoglobin A_{1c} concentration, and the dose of oral hypoglycemic therapy.[41] Modest (5%) weight loss can also have preventative effects, decreasing the 4- to 6-year cumulative incidence of diabetes by more than 50% in obese persons with already impaired glucose tolerance.[32]

In terms of lipid abnormalities, weight loss decreases serum levels of low-density lipoprotein-cholesterol (LDL-C) and triglycerides, whereas increases in serum levels of high-density lipoprotein-C (HDL-C) are typically seen only after weight loss is sustained.[42] The greatest relative improvements in serum triglycerides and LDL-C usually occur within the first 2 months of weight loss versus weight gain.[43,44] A sustained weight loss of 5% is needed to maintain a decrease in serum triglyceride concentrations; serum total cholesterol and LDL-C revert toward baseline if weight loss is not maintained.[45]

Changes in body weight changes can correlate with systolic and diastolic blood pressure in a dose-dependent manner; therefore, greater weight loss is generally associated with decrease in blood pressure, and weight gain with increase in blood pressure.[46] Weight loss and subsequent regaining of weight results in a steady increase in blood pressure toward baseline and beyond.

Unfortunately all large clinical trials of prevention of heart disease and diabetes have systematically excluded patients with severe mental illnesses. Studies on weight reduction in patients with schizophrenia have been taking place only in the last few years.[47] Studies on prevention of weight gain are much fewer. In this article, the evidence on efficacy of weight loss studies and on prevention of weight gain are reviewed, focusing on studies using a randomized controlled design.

There are now several good randomized, controlled, clinical trials of standard behavioral strategies for weight reduction as listed in **Table 2**, and reviewed in detail elsewhere.[47] Almost all of the studies have reported either greater weight loss or less weight gain in subjects who were assigned to the behavioral treatment as opposed to standard care or similar alternative.

In terms of true prevention studies, the evidence base is much smaller, not because of negative studies, but because of the small number of efforts undertaken up to the present time. One recently published study[51] evaluated a dietician-delivered nutritional counseling program to prevent weight gain in patients starting treatment with olanzapine. Fifty-one individuals were randomized to either 6 one-on-one nutrition education sessions, provided by a registered dietician, or to usual care. The primary outcomes were changes in weight and BMI at 3 and 6 months after baseline assessments. Subjects in the intervention group had gained less weight than the controls at both 3 and 6 months (2.0 kg vs 6.0 kg at 3 months [$P <.002$] and 2.0 kg vs 9.9 kg at 6 months [$P <.013$]). At 6 months the BMI of the intervention group had increased by 0.8 kg/m^2 versus an increase of 3.2 kg/m^2 in the controls ($P <.017$). However, the proportion of patients in whom weight gain could be completely prevented was not reported. In a pilot randomized controlled trial, Brar and colleagues[52] applied the standard weight loss strategies in a stepped manner to prevent weight gain in 51 subjects who were starting on a variety of novel antipsychotics. They found that 63% of subjects randomized to the intervention did not gain weight compared with only 22% of those randomized to usual care ($P = .02$).

There have also been attempts to explore the potential for preventing antipsychotic-induced weight gain by pharmacologic means. On a theoretical basis, it was proposed that histamine H2 blockers might interfere with antipsychotic-induced weight gain. However, it was found that nizatidine had only a transient effect of ameliorating olanzapine-induced weight gain.[57] Poyurovsky and colleagues[58] investigated another H2 blocker, famotidine, in a double-blind placebo-controlled trial on patients starting treatment with olanzapine. They found no difference in weight gain between subjects who were randomized to receive famotidine and the controls.

Metformin, an insulin-sensitizing biguanide, is indicated for lowering blood sugar in type 2 diabetics, and is often associated with weight loss. The possibility that it might prevent weight gain associated with olanzapine has been investigated. Early small pilot studies suggested some benefit for weight loss.[59,60] However, a randomized double-blind placebo-controlled trial failed to show any evidence that metformin attenuated olanzapine-induced weight gain.[61] However, a recent trial did find that metformin was more effective in producing weight loss than behavior therapy alone, but that the combination of behavior therapy and metformin was more effective than either of them alone.[62]

Table 2
Randomized controlled clinical trials of lifestyle interventions for weight loss in schizophrenia

Authors	Intervention	N	Duration	Results
Harmatz & Lapuc,[48] 1968	Diet only Diet + group therapy Diet + negative reinforcement	21	10 wk	0% −2% −7%
Rotatori et al,[49] 1980	Behavior therapy adapted from Down syndrome intervention	14	14 wk	Intervention −7.3 lb Controls +0.4 lb
Littrell et al,[50] 2003	Weekly groups on diet and exercise versus usual care	70	16 wk	Intervention −0.3 kg Controls +4.3 kg
Evans et al,[51] 2005	Six 1-hour nutrition education sessions within 3 months in patients started on olanzapine versus usual care	51	6 mo	Intervention +2 kg Controls +9.9 kg (increase of ≥7% bodyweight: 13% of intervention group, and 64% of controls)
Brar et al,[52] 2005	Behavior therapy; nutrition, exercise and behavioral interventions versus usual care	72	14 wk	Intervention −2 kg Controls −1.1 kg (5% weight loss in 32.1% of intervention subjects vs 10.8% in controls)
Weber and Wyne,[53] 2006	Cognitive/behavioral group intervention in outpatients with schizophrenia on novel antipsychotics versus usual care	17	16 wk	Cognitive/behavioral group −5.4 lb Controls −1.3 lb
Jean-Baptiste et al,[54] 2007	Weekly group behavioral sessions, food replacement (by reimbursement)	18	16 wk	Intervention group −2.8 kg Controls +2.7 kg
Khazaal et al,[55] 2007	Weekly cognitive behavior therapy groups versus single nutrition education session	61	12 wk	Intervention group −2.9 kg Psychoeducation group −0.08 kg
Wu et al,[56] 2008	Lifestyle intervention (education, diet, exercise) versus usual care, versus metformin (Met) versus Met plus lifestyle	128	12 wk	Lifestyle group −1.4 kg Met group −3.2 kg Met + lifestyle group −4.7 kg Usual care group +3.1 kg

MEDICATION CHOICE TO REDUCE THE RISK OF DEVELOPING METABOLIC SYNDROME

Choice of antipsychotic medication may provide one of the rare opportunities for primary prevention in psychiatry. It is well established that the risk of weight gain and worsening of other metabolic parameters, such as dyslipidemia, varies between various antipsychotic agents.[63] For example, data from the registration trials show that the risk for clinically significant weight gain (using >7% gain more than baseline as the cutoff) was about 10 times greater when comparing olanzapine with placebo, although for drugs such as ziprasidone, aripiprazole, and paliperidone it was only about twice the risk of placebo. **Fig. 1** shows the proportions of subjects who gained 7% or more weight in short-term trials when randomized to antipsychotics or placebo. Thus, if the initial choice of antipsychotic is based on the associated risk of metabolic abnormalities, there is a compelling argument to be made for choosing a low-risk agent to start with. If the initial choice does not prove to be efficacious, the clinician can always switch to another agent after explaining the risk to the patient and obtaining their agreement to the choice. The results of the CATIE[28] and CTULASS[64] pragmatic clinical trials found that some of the older antipsychotics, such as perphenazine, were also associated with low risk of worsening metabolic indicators, such as weight and lipid levels. The older antipsychotics are generally thought to carry a greater risk of tardive dyskinesia compared with the newer agents, and this hazard needs to be discussed with the patient and caregivers if the prescriber is recommending one of the older agents. Ideally, decisions about choice of medication need to be made in collaboration with the patient who should be informed of the competing risks of the various choices so they can participate in the choice of medications in a well-informed manner.

Children and youth are particularly susceptible to weight gain when treated with antipsychotics.[63,65] For this reason, and because any metabolic abnormalities experienced at a young age are likely to have an adverse influence on risk for a long time, the choice of drug in children needs to be considered with even greater thought toward future consequences than in adults. The recently completed TEOSS study found that molindione, another older agent, had a more benign metabolic profile than olanzapine, but equivalent efficacy in youth with early onset schizophrenia.[66]

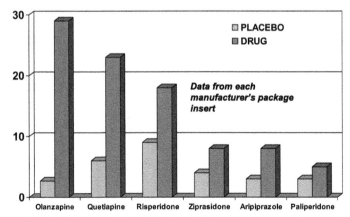

Fig. 1. Proportion of subjects gaining ≥7% of weight in short-term randomized clinical trials involving novel antipsychotics.

SWITCHING ANTIPSYCHOTIC MEDICATION

Patients who experience weight gain in the course of treatment present opportunities for secondary prevention of metabolic syndrome. Because there are well-established differences in the weight gain liability of the different antipsychotics, patients who gain weight on one of the agents known to be associated with a high risk of weight gain might be candidates for a switch to an agent with a lower risk. Several recent studies have indeed shown that a significant proportion of patients might show improvement in metabolic syndrome components after such a switch. Reductions in body weight and lipids occurred when patients were switched from olanzapine or risperidone to ziprasidone,[67] from olanzapine to aripiprazole,[68] or from aripiprazole to usual care (ie, olanzapine, quetiapine, risperidone).[69] Effect sizes of weight loss and metabolic improvements are in line with what can be expected from an adjunct pharmacological weight loss intervention.[67,68] Antipsychotic efficacy and side effect profile considerations need to be carefully balanced because the greater efficacy of some of the antipsychotics[28] are also associated with higher risk of metabolic side effects.[70] Clozapine presents a particularly difficult dilemma for patients and clinicians when other antipsychotics have not been efficacious, because it has consistently been shown to have both higher efficacy and higher risk of metabolic complications than other antipsychotics.[28,71] These decisions are best approached in collaboration with a well-informed patient and his/her caregivers.

INFLAMMATION IN METABOLIC SYNDROME

Because antipsychotic-induced weight gain in patients with schizophrenia may preferentially manifest as an increase in central body fat content rather than muscle mass or intercellular water,[72,73] this increased central adiposity renders patients with schizophrenia especially prone to metabolic adverse events.[74] This is because the accumulation of excess fat in central adipose tissue is often accompanied by a chronic subacute state of inflammation, shown by changes in both inflammatory cells and biochemical markers of inflammation.[75] These changes can be seen systematically in the tissues involved, in terms of increased circulating levels of inflammatory markers. In particular, increased levels of C-reactive protein (CRP), tumor necrosis factor-alpha (TNF-α), and interleukin-6 promote vascular endothelial damage through modulation of vascular nitric oxide and superoxide release, thus providing an important link between obesity and CVD[76,77]; they also mediate common denominators of cardiometabolic risk, including liver and muscle insulin resistance, lipid metabolism, and hypertension, thereby contributing to the increased prevalence of the metabolic syndrome in central obesity.[78] At the same time, the potentially protective adipokine, adiponectin, is reduced. All these changes have been implicated as cause of the metabolic risk factors.[16] It is possible that, in the future, indices of inflammation will be added to the criteria for metabolic syndrome.

METABOLIC MONITORING

As the prescribers of most psychotropic medications that may initiate or accelerate the development of metabolic syndrome, psychiatrists have been urged or, in some situations, mandated to monitor adverse metabolic changes their in patients. An influential recommendation appeared recently from a consensus panel convened by the American Psychiatric Association, the American Diabetes Association, the American Association of Clinical Endocrinologists, and North American Association for the Study of Obesity.[30] The recommendations of this consensus meeting are summarized in **Table 3**. Despite these recommendations, the rate of monitoring for various components of metabolic syndrome remains low in treatment settings. Some community settings, in which most individuals with serious mental illness receive treatment, do not have facilities for monitoring lipids and blood sugar.[79] The obvious solution is to increase the capabilities of the community treatment providers. However, this may not occur as rapidly as necessary, but some elements of metabolic monitoring can be implemented in most settings. Because weight gain and central adiposity are so closely correlated with changes in lipids and blood sugar, a minimum requirement could be weight and waist circumference monitoring in all settings. The authors also believe that blood pressure should be monitored at least once a year. Blood pressure can be measured by an automated device if a physician is not available, willing and/or skilled in taking blood pressure. Once adverse changes are detected using these simple clinical tools, affected patients could be referred to settings where blood work and interventions, if necessary, can be performed. Although these latter recommendations may fall short of the current official recommendations, the authors believe that, from a public health perspective, more individuals at risk may receive interventions if these measures were in place than is currently the case.

TREATMENT OF COMPONENTS OF THE METABOLIC SYNDROME

When metabolic syndrome is present, or when any one of the risk factors appears, treatment to reduce or normalize the level of the risk factor is the obvious medical response. Primary goals in the clinical management of individuals who have developed the metabolic syndrome are to reduce the risks for clinical atherosclerotic disease and diabetes. First-line therapy should be directed toward the major risk factors: LDL-C, hypertension, and diabetes. Prevention of type 2 diabetes mellitus is another important goal when it is not present in a person with the metabolic syndrome. The prime emphasis in management of the metabolic syndrome is to mitigate the modifiable, underlying risk factors (obesity, physical inactivity, and atherogenic diet) through lifestyle changes.[16]

Weight reduction has already been discussed; lifestyle changes aimed at weight reduction are the recommended initial approach to mild increases of metabolic syndrome components in all influential guidelines including the Adult Treatment Panel (ATP)-III recommendations, NHLBI,[16] and Canadian Cardiovascular Society.[29] Weight loss predictably lowers cholesterol, blood pressure, blood glucose, and insulin resistance.[16]

Treatment of Hyperglycemia and Type 2 Diabetes Mellitus

Recent efforts in the mental healthy population have centered around preventing the onset of type 2 diabetes mellitus, including preemptive lifestyle changes and early

Table 3
Consensus guidelines for monitoring patients on novel antipsychotics (ADA/APA)

	Baseline	4 Weeks	8 Weeks	12 Weeks	Every 3 Months	Yearly	5 Years
Personal/family history	x					x	
Weight (BMI)	x	x	x	X	x		
Waist circumference	x					x	
Blood pressure	x			x		x	
Fasting plasma glucose	x			x		x	
Fasting lipid profile	x			x			x

detection using Homoestatic Model Assessment (HOMA) of insulin resistance incorporating fasting glucose and insulin to detect increasing insulin resistance before hyperglycemia becomes manifest. However, such efforts highlight the complexity of discerning between diabetes prevention and early intervention.[80] Primary prevention may be difficult to achieve, especially if metabolically active antipsychotic medications are prescribed and secondary prevention becomes paramount. However, as with obesity, weight reduction, increased physical activity, or both will delay (or prevent) onset of type 2 diabetes. Several available studies on nonpsychiatric populations have demonstrated a reduction or delay in the development of type 2 diabetes, focusing on metformin, thiazolidinediones, and acarbose.[81–83] In addition, orlistat, acarbose, and lifestyle modification have been shown to reduce adverse cardiovascular outcomes but manifestation of type 2 diabetes.[80,84–86] Neither metformin nor thiazolidinediones are recommended solely for the prevention of diabetes because their cost-effectiveness and long-term safety have not been documented. For patients with established type 2 diabetes, a reduction in CVD risk from treatment of dyslipidemia and hypertension has been reported.[16]

Thiazolidinediones are peroxisome proliferator-activated receptor gamma (PPARγ) agonists that improve insulin sensitivity and stimulate adipogenesis. Thiazolidinediones for antipsychotic-induced hyperglycemia are under study.[87] Because of their action at the cellular level, mediated via an increase in PPAR gene expression, which, as a nuclear steroid hormone receptor, induces transcriptional upregulation of fatty acid transport proteins, they facilitate fatty acid entry into cells and the enzymes involved in the β-oxidation of fatty acids, potentially causing an increase in body fat. Hepatic dysfunction and cardiovascular risk are associated with this class of medications.[88] Cardiovascular benefits with glitazones are uncertain because of possible adverse cardiovascular events associated with these agents, and decisions to treat with these agents should be made on a case-by-case basis.

Metformin inhibits hepatic gluconeogenesis, reduces gastrointestinal glucose absorption, induces peripheral glucose uptake, and decreases the release of fatty acids via feedback regulation. Metformin has recently garnered some attention because a small trial showed that it attenuated olanzapine-induced weight gain and moderated insulin resistance. In this 12-week, double-blind, placebo-controlled trial, 128 newly treated Chinese patients with schizophrenia receiving antipsychotics were randomized to 4 arms after gaining more than 10% of preintervention body weight: placebo, metformin 750 mg daily, metformin 750 daily plus lifestyle changes, or lifestyle changes alone. The combination treatment of metformin and lifestyle changes showed the greatest benefit for weight loss, and, as expected, insulin sensitivity improved with metformin and lifestyle changes, and metformin alone.[62]

Adjunctive Therapy for Hyperlipidemia

Consistent with ATP-III and American Diabetes Association (ADA) guidelines, patients should have their cholesterol levels (total cholesterol, LDL-C, and HDL-C) and triglycerides measured on a regular basis. Established criteria allow for further stratification of CVD risk categories according to LDL and HDL levels. ATP-III recommends that atherogenic dyslipidemia can become a target for lipid-lowering therapy after the goal for LDL-C has been attained. That is, as long as LDL-C remains increased, it is the primary target of therapy, even in the metabolic syndrome, and other lipid risk factors are secondary.[16] If indicated, initial steps call for therapeutic lifestyle changes that include a low-fat and high-fiber diet, increased physical activity, and weight management. If unsuccessful, drug therapies including statins, bile acid sequestrants, niacin, and fibric acid may be initiated. Referral to a primary care or internal medicine physician is recommended.

Statins

Statins have proven efficacy for the prevention of CVD morbidity and mortality. Statins preferentially lower LDL-C and triglyceride levels, and have minor positive effects on HDL levels. The mode of action is interference with 3-hydroxy-3-methylglutaryl-con-zyme A reductase (HMG-COA), a key enzyme for cholesterol synthesis preferentially located in the liver. The net effect is lower cholesterol content in hepatocytes, and secondary stimulation of LDL receptor expression and increased LDL removal. Statins show benefits in managing the metabolic syndrome in several studies,[89] confirmed by a randomized controlled trial using rosuvastatin and atorvastatin.[90,91] In addition to their lipid-lowering potency, these outcomes suggest that statins improve other aspects of the metabolic syndrome than hyperlipidemia through modulation of inflammatory and thrombogenic responses.[92] Statins have a relatively benign safety profile. Myotoxicity, ranging from mild increase in creatine kinase levels to rhabdomyolysis, as well as hepatotoxicity can occur. The incidence of rhabdomyolysis is low, less than 0.1%. Most statins are metabolized by cytochrome P-450 isoenzymes and require close monitoring if administered with clozapine, olanzapine, and risperidone. Statins do differ in their absorption, plasma protein binding, excretion, solubility, and perhaps efficacy, and choice of medication should be made on an individual basis. Few trials have specifically assessed the safety of statins in schizophrenia.[89]

Treatment of High Blood Pressure

The goal for antihypertensive therapy without the presence of diabetes is a blood pressure less than 140/90 mm Hg, and in the presence of diabetes the goal is less than 130/80 mm Hg.[93] Lifestyle changes deserve increased emphasis in people with metabolic syndrome; the goal should be to reduce blood pressure as much as possible even in the absence of overt hypertension and to gain other metabolic benefits of lifestyle changes.[16] Effective lifestyle changes can include weight control, more physical activity, alcohol moderation, sodium reduction, and increased consumption of fresh fruits, vegetables, and low-fat dairy products.[93] Angiotensin-converting enzyme (ACE) inhibitors are first-line therapy for hypertension in the metabolic syndrome, especially when type 2 diabetes is present. Alternatives include angiotensin receptor blockers, which may lower the risk for diabetes,[94] and diuretics, or a combination thereof.

INTEGRATION OF PSYCHIATRIC AND NONPSYCHIATRIC MEDICAL CARE

Psychiatrists may accept the responsibility for monitoring the presence or appearance of hypertension, dyslipidemia, or insulin resistance, but, at the present time, they are not likely to undertake to treat these conditions, nor would this be the best care for the patient. The data available show that patients with severe mental illnesses typically receive lower quality primary medical care and have worse outcomes than those without mental illness,[95] that survival after a myocardial infarction was reduced by 35% if the individual had schizophrenia, and that these individuals were less likely to have received evidence-based interventions such as ACE inhibitors, aspirin, and reperfusion. In the CATIE trial, at baseline, 30% of those with diabetes, 62% of those with hypertension, and 88% of those with abnormal lipids, were not receiving treatment for these abnormalities. A Canadian study of rehospitalization after a cardiac event found that those with schizophrenia were significantly more likely than those with no mental illness to be rehospitalized (adjusted hazard ratio 1.43, 95%

confidence interval [CI] 1.22–1.69) for a cardiac event in the following 4 years.[96] These differences in outcome for heart disease treatment suggest that there are problems with access or delivery of care to people with severe mental illnesses, and that it is likely that this difference in the quality of care contributes to worse nonpsychiatric medical outcomes.

It has been proposed that a system that integrates the practitioners of both psychiatric and nonpsychiatric care might result in improved health outcomes for the seriously mentally ill. Druss and colleagues[95] randomized patients to either an integrated clinic in which both primary care and psychiatry were colocated, or to usual care in which there was no direct integration of psychiatric and nonpsychiatric medical services. They were able to show that there were improvements in ease of access to primary medical and preventative services. A recent study[97] tested the benefits of a medical case management model, using nurse case managers, in a randomized, controlled clinical trial. At the end of a year, the intervention group were found to have received significantly more recommended preventive services compared with the controls (58.7% vs 21.8%); have received more "evidence-based services for cardiometabolic conditions" (34.9% vs 27.7%); were more likely to have a primary care provider (71.2% vs 51.9%). A subset of subjects had sufficient data to calculate the Framingham Cardiovascular Risk Index and, in this subset, those in case management had significantly lower risk (6.9) than the controls (9.8). Kilbourne and colleagues[98] studied a self-management program for patients with bipolar disorder in a randomized, controlled clinical trial of persons recruited from a Veterans Administration hospital. The psychoeducational program (BCM) addressed symptom management and behavior change related to both mood disorder and risk factors for cardiovascular disease. They found that the controls showed worsening of both the mental and physical components of the SF-12, whereas those randomized to BCM showed some improvement in both components. These studies demonstrate the tantalizing possibility that the mortality gap between people with serious mental illness and the rest of the population might be narrowed or even eliminated by a variety of measures focusing on their nonpsychiatric health issues and integrating them into the overall treatment approach. It is disappointing that there has not been more funding to systematically study these approaches. To determine whether there is an effect on actual CVD outcomes will also require funding of long-term studies, because such outcomes take years to develop. Persons with serious mental illness have also been systematically excluded from large trials involving prevention of CVD and diabetes, thus data on the efficacy of those interventions on the risk in these highly vulnerable individuals are not available.

SUMMARY

The metabolic syndrome is highly prevalent in schizophrenia and other serious mental illnesses, and represents a constellation of risk factors for cardiovascular disease and type 2 diabetes mellitus. Genetic factors, treatment with antipsychotic medication, socioeconomic status, and lifestyle likely interact to account for the high risk of metabolic syndrome, diabetes, heart disease, and premature mortality in people with serious mental illness. Although some newer medications do seem to be more metabolically benign than their predecessors, others, like clozapine, have no substitute. Within a preventative framework, minimizing risk by choosing a low-risk medication if possible and regular monitoring of risk factors should allow for intervention before comorbidities become manifest. If any components of metabolic syndrome appear, lifestyle management to reduce weight and increase physical activity and fitness is the initial intervention recommended. These interventions should be available in the usual settings of care for persons with serious mental illness. If not sufficient, antipsychotic medication can be changed if this is clinically indicated and agreed to by the patient. If the prior measures fail to reduce the risk factors for diabetes and heart disease, specific pharmacological interventions must be considered in collaboration with a primary care practitioner. Given the high risk of developing diabetes and cardiovascular disease in persons with serious mental illness, psychiatrists who treat these individuals need to ensure they are familiar with these risks, monitor metabolic parameters in their patients, and educate their patients (and caregivers) about the risks and how to prevent them. Mental health treatment facilities, including community mental health centers, need to offer their patients/clients access to evidence-based lifestyle interventions and to adequate primary care. The National Institutes of Health and other national agencies responsible for studying innovations in health care need to ensure that persons with serious mental illness are included in trials of interventions aimed at heart disease and diabetes, and also fund interventions specifically for the mentally ill. Our collective failure to follow these recommendations will probably mean no reduction in the 20- to 25-year mortality gap between people with serious mental illness and the rest of the population, in the near future.

REFERENCES

1. Kraepelin E, Barclay RM, Robertson GM. Dementia praecox and paraphrenia. Edinburgh (UK): E. & S. Livingstone; 1919.
2. Colton CW, Manderscheid RW. Congruencies in increased mortality rates, years of potential life lost, and causes of death among public mental health clients in eight states. Prev Chronic Dis 2006;3(2):A42.
3. Hennekens CH, Hennekens AR, Hollar D, et al. Schizophrenia and increased risks of cardiovascular disease. Am Heart J 2005;150(6):1115–21.
4. Tsuang MT, Woolson RF, Fleming JA. Premature deaths in schizophrenia and affective disorders. An analysis of survival curves and variables affecting the shortened survival. Arch Gen Psychiatry 1980;37(9):979–83.
5. Mortensen PB, Juel K. Mortality and causes of death in first admitted schizophrenic patients. Br J Psychiatry 1993;163:183–9.
6. Felker B, Yazel JJ, Short D. Mortality and medical comorbidity among psychiatric patients: a review. Psychiatr Serv 1996;47(12):1356–63.
7. Brown S. Excess mortality of schizophrenia. A meta-analysis. Br J Psychiatry 1997;171:502–8.
8. Osby U, Correia N, Brandt L, et al. Mortality and causes of death in schizophrenia in Stockholm county, Sweden. Schizophr Res 2000;45(1–2):21–8.
9. Osby U, Brandt L, Correia N, et al. Excess mortality in bipolar and unipolar disorder in Sweden. Arch Gen Psychiatry 2001;58(9):844–50.
10. Laursen TM, Munk-Olsen T, Nordentoft M, et al. Increased mortality among patients admitted with major psychiatric disorders: a register-based study comparing mortality in unipolar depressive disorder, bipolar affective disorder, schizoaffective disorder, and schizophrenia. J Clin Psychiatry 2007;68(6):899–907.
11. McEvoy JP, Meyer JM, Goff DC, et al. Prevalence of the metabolic syndrome in patients with schizophrenia: baseline results from the Clinical Antipsychotic Trials of Intervention Effectiveness (CATIE) schizophrenia trial and comparison with national estimates from NHANES III. Schizophr Res 2005;80(1):19–32.

12. Meyer J, Loh C, Leckband SG, et al. Prevalence of the metabolic syndrome in veterans with schizophrenia. J Psychiatr Pract 2006;12(1):5–10.
13. Ford ES, Giles WH, Dietz WH. Prevalence of the metabolic syndrome among US adults: findings from the third National Health and Nutrition Examination Survey. JAMA 2002;287(3):356–9.
14. Fagiolini A, Frank E, Scott JA, et al. Metabolic syndrome in bipolar disorder: findings from the Bipolar Disorder Center for Pennsylvanians. Bipolar Disord 2005; 7(5):424–30.
15. Taylor V, Macdonald K, McKinnon MC, et al. Increased rates of obesity in first-presentation adults with mood disorders over the course of four-year follow-up. J Affect Disord 2008;109(1–2):127–31.
16. Grundy SM, Cleeman JI, Daniels SR, et al. Diagnosis and management of the metabolic syndrome: an American Heart Association/National Heart, Lung, and Blood Institute Scientific Statement. Circulation 2005;112(17):2735–52.
17. Gami AS, Witt BJ, Howard DE, et al. Metabolic syndrome and risk of incident cardiovascular events and death: a systematic review and meta-analysis of longitudinal studies. J Am Coll Cardiol 2007;49(4):403–14.
18. Galassi A, Reynolds K, He J. Metabolic syndrome and risk of cardiovascular disease: a meta-analysis. Am J Med 2006;119(10):812–9.
19. Meigs JB, Wilson PW, Fox CS, et al. Body mass index, metabolic syndrome, and risk of type 2 diabetes or cardiovascular disease. J Clin Endocrinol Metab 2006; 91(8):2906–12.
20. Kahn JG, Kronick R, Kreger M, et al. The cost of health insurance administration in California: estimates for insurers, physicians, and hospitals. Health Aff (Millwood) 2005;24(6):1629–39.
21. Lawrence D, Mitrou F, Zubrick SR. Smoking and mental illness: results from population surveys in Australia and the United States. BMC Public Health 2009;9:285.
22. Gregg EW, Cheng YJ, Cadwell BL, et al. Secular trends in cardiovascular disease risk factors according to body mass index in US adults. JAMA 2005;293(15): 1868–74.
23. Pi-Sunyer FX. The medical risks of obesity. Postgrad Med 2009;121(6):21–33.
24. Hubert HB, Feinleib M, McNamara PM, et al. Obesity as an independent risk factor for cardiovascular disease: a 26-year follow-up of participants in the Framingham Heart Study. Circulation 1983;67(5):968–77.
25. Manson JE, Colditz GA, Stampfer MJ, et al. A prospective study of obesity and risk of coronary heart disease in women. N Engl J Med 1990;322(13):882–9.
26. Allison DB, Mentore JL, Heo M, et al. Antipsychotic-induced weight gain: a comprehensive research synthesis [see comment]. Am J Psychiatry 1999; 156(11):1686–96.
27. Dickerson FB, Brown CH, Daumit GL, et al. Health status of individuals with serious mental illness. Schizophr Bull 2006;32(3):584–9.
28. Lieberman JA, Stroup TS, McEvoy JP, et al. Effectiveness of antipsychotic drugs in patients with chronic schizophrenia [see comment]. N Engl J Med 2005; 353(12):1209–23.
29. Genest J, McPherson R, Frohlich J, et al. 2009 Canadian Cardiovascular Society/ Canadian guidelines for the diagnosis and treatment of dyslipidemia and prevention of cardiovascular disease in the adult - 2009 recommendations. Can J Cardiol 2009;25(10):567–79.
30. American Diabetes Association, American Psychiatric Association, American Association of Clinical Endocrinologists, et al. Consensus development

conference on antipsychotic drugs and obesity and diabetes [see comment]. J Clin Psychiatry 2004;65(2):267–72.

31. Diabetes Prevention Program Research Group. The Diabetes Prevention Program (DPP): description of lifestyle intervention. Diabetes Care 2002; 25(12):2165–71.

32. Tuomilehto J, Lindstrom J, Eriksson JG, et al. Prevention of type 2 diabetes mellitus by changes in lifestyle among subjects with impaired glucose tolerance [see comment]. N Engl J Med 2001;344(18):1343–50.

33. Redmon JB, Bertoni AG, Connelly S, et al. Effect of the look AHEAD study intervention on medication use and related cost to treat cardiovascular disease risk factors in individuals with type 2 diabetes. Diabetes Care 2010;33(6):1153–8.

34. Klein S, Burke LE, Bray GA, et al. Clinical implications of obesity with specific focus on cardiovascular disease: a statement for professionals from the American Heart Association Council on Nutrition, Physical Activity, and Metabolism: endorsed by the American College of Cardiology Foundation. Circulation 2004; 110(18):2952–67.

35. Despres JP. Is visceral obesity the cause of the metabolic syndrome? Ann Med 2006;38(1):52–63.

36. You T, Nicklas BJ. Chronic inflammation: role of adipose tissue and modulation by weight loss. Curr Diabetes Rev 2006;2(1):29–37.

37. Goldstein DJ. Beneficial health effects of modest weight loss. Int J Obes Relat Metab Disord 1992;16(6):397–415.

38. Pasanisi F, Contaldo F, de Simone G, et al. Benefits of sustained moderate weight loss in obesity. Nutr Metab Cardiovasc Dis 2001;11(6):401–6.

39. Lee M, Aronne LJ. Weight management for type 2 diabetes mellitus: global cardiovascular risk reduction. Am J Cardiol 2007;99(4A):68B–79B.

40. Kelley DE, Wing R, Buonocore C, et al. Relative effects of calorie restriction and weight loss in noninsulin-dependent diabetes mellitus. J Clin Endocrinol Metab 1993;77(5):1287–93.

41. Wing RR, Koeske R, Epstein LH, et al. Long-term effects of modest weight loss in type II diabetic patients. Arch Intern Med 1987;147:1749–53.

42. Dattilo AM, Kris-Etherton PM. Effects of weight reduction on blood lipids and lipoproteins: a meta-analysis. Am J Clin Nutr 1992;56(2):320–8.

43. Eckel RH, Yost TJ. HDL subfractions and adipose tissue metabolism in the reduced-obese state. Am J Physiol 1989;256(6 Pt 1):E740–6.

44. Wadden TA, Anderson DA, Foster GD. Two-year changes in lipids and lipoproteins associated with the maintenance of a 5% to 10% reduction in initial weight: some findings and some questions. Obes Res 1999;7(2):170–8.

45. Rossner S, Bjorvell H. Early and late effects of weight loss on lipoprotein metabolism in severe obesity. Atherosclerosis 1987;64(2–3):125–30.

46. The Trials of Hypertension Prevention Collaborative Research Group. Effects of weight loss and sodium reduction intervention on blood pressure and hypertension incidence in overweight people with high-normal blood pressure. The Trials of Hypertension Prevention, Phase II. Arch Intern Med 1997;157:657–67.

47. Ganguli R, Cohn T, Faulkner G. Behavioural treatments for weight management in schizophrenia. In: Meyer J, Nasrallah H, eds. Medical illness and schizophrenia. Arlington (VA): American Psychiatric Publishing, Inc; 2009. p. 203–20.

48. Harmatz MG, Lapuc P. Behavior modification of overeating in a psychiatric population. J Consult Clin Psychol 1968;32(5):583–7.

49. Rotatori AF, Fox R, Wicks A. Weight loss with psychiatric residents in a behavioral self control program. Psychol Rep 1980;46(2):483–6.

50. Littrell KH, Hilligoss NM, Kirshner CD, et al. The effects of an educational intervention on antipsychotic-induced weight gain. J Nurs Scholarsh 2003;35(3):237–41.
51. Evans S, Newton R, Higgins S. Nutritional intervention to prevent weight gain in patients commenced on olanzapine: a randomized controlled trial. Aust N Z J Psychiatry 2005;39(6):479–86.
52. Brar JS, Ganguli R, Pandina G, et al. Effects of behavioral therapy on weight loss in overweight and obese patients with schizophrenia or schizoaffective disorder [see comment]. J Clin Psychiatry 2005;66(2):205–12.
53. Weber M, Wyne K. A cognitive/behavioral group intervention for weight loss in patients treated with atypical antipsychotics. Schizophr Res 2006;83(1):95–101.
54. Jean-Baptiste M, Tek C, Liskov E, et al. A pilot study of a weight management program with food provision in schizophrenia. Schizophr Res 2007;96(1–3): 198–205.
55. Khazaal Y, Fresard E, Rabia S, et al. Cognitive behavioural therapy for weight gain associated with antipsychotic drugs. Schizophr Res 2007;91(1–3):169–77.
56. Wu JC, Gillin JC, Buchsbaum MS, et al. Effect of sleep deprivation on brain metabolism of depressed patients. Am J Psychiatry 1992;149(4):538–43.
57. Cavazzoni P, Tanaka Y, Roychowdhury SM, et al. Nizatidine for prevention of weight gain with olanzapine: a double-blind placebo-controlled trial. Eur Neuropsychopharmacol 2003;13(2):81–5.
58. Poyurovsky M, Tal V, Maayan R, et al. The effect of famotidine addition on olanzapine-induced weight gain in first-episode schizophrenia patients: a double-blind placebo-controlled pilot study. Eur Neuropsychopharmacol 2004;14(4):332–6.
59. Baptista T, Hernandez L, Prieto LA, et al. Metformin in obesity associated with antipsychotic drug administration: a pilot study. J Clin Psychiatry 2001;62(8): 653–5.
60. Morrison JA, Cottingham EM, Barton BA. Metformin for weight loss in pediatric patients taking psychotropic drugs. Am J Psychiatry 2002;159(4):655–7.
61. Baptista T, Martinez J, Lacruz A, et al. Metformin for prevention of weight gain and insulin resistance with olanzapine: a double-blind placebo-controlled trial. Can J Psychiatry 2006;51(3):192–6.
62. Wu RR, Zhao JP, Jin H, et al. Lifestyle intervention and metformin for treatment of antipsychotic-induced weight gain: a randomized controlled trial. JAMA 2008; 299(2):185–93.
63. Newcomer JW. Second-generation (atypical) antipsychotics and metabolic effects: a comprehensive literature review. CNS Drugs 2005;19(Suppl 1):1–93.
64. Jones PB, Barnes TR, Davies L, et al. Randomized controlled trial of the effect on Quality of Life of second- vs first-generation antipsychotic drugs in schizophrenia: Cost Utility of the Latest Antipsychotic Drugs in Schizophrenia Study (CUtLASS 1). Arch Gen Psychiatry 2006;63(10):1079–87.
65. Correll CU, Manu P, Olshanskiy V, et al. Cardiometabolic risk of second-generation antipsychotic medications during first-time use in children and adolescents. JAMA 2009;302(16):1765–73.
66. Sikich L, Frazier JA, McClellan J, et al. Double-blind comparison of first- and second-generation antipsychotics in early-onset schizophrenia and schizo-affective disorder: findings from the treatment of early-onset schizophrenia spectrum disorders (TEOSS) study. Am J Psychiatry 2008;165(11):1420–31.
67. Weiden PJ, Newcomer JW, Loebel AD, et al. Long-term changes in weight and plasma lipids during maintenance treatment with ziprasidone. Neuropsychopharmacology 2008;33(5):985–94.

68. Newcomer JW, Campos JA, Marcus RN, et al. A multicenter, randomized, double-blind study of the effects of aripiprazole in overweight subjects with schizophrenia or schizoaffective disorder switched from olanzapine. J Clin Psychiatry 2008;69(7):1046–56.
69. Kolotkin RL, Corey-Lisle PK, Crosby RD, et al. Changes in weight and weight-related quality of life in a multicentre, randomized trial of aripiprazole versus standard of care. Eur Psychiatry 2008;23(8):561–6.
70. Fenton WS, Chavez MR. Medication-induced weight gain and dyslipidemia in patients with schizophrenia. Am J Psychiatry 2006;163(10):1697–704 [quiz: 1858–9].
71. Fontaine KR, Heo M, Harrigan EP, et al. Estimating the consequences of anti-psychotic induced weight gain on health and mortality rate. Psychiatry Res 2001;101(3):277–88.
72. Zhang ZJ, Yao ZJ, Liu W, et al. Effects of antipsychotics on fat deposition and changes in leptin and insulin levels. Magnetic resonance imaging study of previously untreated people with schizophrenia. Br J Psychiatry 2004;184:58–62.
73. Graham KA, Perkins DO, Edwards LJ, et al. Effect of olanzapine on body composition and energy expenditure in adults with first-episode psychosis [see comment]. Am J Psychiatry 2005;162(1):118–23.
74. Newcomer JW. Medical risk in patients with bipolar disorder and schizophrenia. J Clin Psychiatry 2006;67(Suppl 9):25–30 [discussion: 36–42].
75. Shoelson SE, Herrero L, Naaz A. Obesity, inflammation, and insulin resistance. Gastroenterology 2007;132(6):2169–80.
76. Eckel RH, Grundy SM, Zimmet PZ. The metabolic syndrome. Lancet 2005; 365(9468):1415–28.
77. Dervaux N, Wubuli M, Megnien JL, et al. Comparative associations of adiposity measures with cardiometabolic risk burden in asymptomatic subjects. Atherosclerosis 2008;201(2):413–7.
78. Fox CS, Massaro JM, Hoffmann U, et al. Abdominal visceral and subcutaneous adipose tissue compartments: association with metabolic risk factors in the Framingham Heart Study. Circulation 2007;116(1):39–48.
79. Druss BG, Marcus SC, Campbell J, et al. Medical services for clients in community mental health centers: results from a national survey. Psychiatr Serv 2008;59(8):917–20.
80. Southwood RL. Have clinical studies demonstrated diabetes prevention or delay of diabetes through early treatment? Am J Ther 2010;17(2):201–9.
81. Buchanan TA, Xiang AH, Peters RK, et al. Preservation of pancreatic beta-cell function and prevention of type 2 diabetes by pharmacological treatment of insulin resistance in high-risk Hispanic women. Diabetes 2002;51(9): 2796–803.
82. Azen SP, Peters RK, Berkowitz K, et al. TRIPOD (TRoglitazone In the Prevention Of Diabetes): a randomized, placebo-controlled trial of troglitazone in women with prior gestational diabetes mellitus. Control Clin Trials 1998;19(2):217–31.
83. Gerstein HC, Yusuf S, Bosch J, et al. Effect of rosiglitazone on the frequency of diabetes in patients with impaired glucose tolerance or impaired fasting glucose: a randomised controlled trial. Lancet 2006;368(9541):1096–105.
84. Chiasson JL, Josse RG, Gomis R, et al. Acarbose for prevention of type 2 diabetes mellitus: the STOP-NIDDM randomised trial. Lancet 2002;359(9323): 2072–7.
85. Torgerson DJ, Hauptman J, Boldrin MN, et al. Xenixal in the prevention of diabetes in obese subjects (XENDOS) study. Diabetes Care 2004;27:155–61.

86. Ratner R, Goldberg R, Haffner S, et al. Impact of intensive lifestyle and metformin therapy on cardiovascular disease risk factors in the diabetes prevention program. Diabetes Care 2005;28(4):888–94.
87. Baptista T, Rangel N, El Fakih Y, et al. Rosiglitazone in the assistance of metabolic control during olanzapine administration in schizophrenia: a pilot double-blind, placebo-controlled, 12-week trial. Pharmacopsychiatry 2009;42(1):14–9.
88. Nissen SE, Wolski K. Effect of rosiglitazone on the risk of myocardial infarction and death from cardiovascular causes. N Engl J Med 2007;356(24):2457–71.
89. Hanssens L, De Hert M, Kalnicka D, et al. Pharmacological treatment of severe dyslipidaemia in patients with schizophrenia. Int Clin Psychopharmacol 2007; 22(1):43–9.
90. Schuster H, Fox JC. Investigating cardiovascular risk reduction–the Rosuvastatin GALAXY Programme. Expert Opin Pharmacother 2004;5(5):1187–200.
91. Stalenhoef AF, Ballantyne CM, Sarti C, et al. A comparative study with rosuvastatin in subjects with metabolic syndrome: results of the COMETS study. Eur Heart J 2005;26(24):2664–72.
92. Vaughan CJ, Gotto AM Jr. Update on statins: 2003. Circulation 2004;110(7): 886–92.
93. Chobanian AV, Bakris GL, Black HR, et al. The Seventh Report of the Joint National Committee on Prevention, Detection, Evaluation, and Treatment of High Blood Pressure: the JNC 7 report. JAMA 2003;289(19):2560–72.
94. Scheen AJ. Prevention of type 2 diabetes mellitus through inhibition of the Renin-Angiotensin system. Drugs 2004;64(22):2537–65.
95. Druss BG, Rohrbaugh RM, Levinson CM, et al. Integrated medical care for patients with serious psychiatric illness: a randomized trial [see comment]. Arch Gen Psychiatry 2001;58(9):861–8.
96. Callahan RC, Boire MD, Lazo RG, et al. Schizophrenia and incidence of cardiovascular morbidity: a population-based longitudinal study in Ontario, Canada. Schizophr Res 2009;115:325–32.
97. Druss BG, von Esenwein SA, Compton MT, et al. A randomized trial of medical care management for community mental health settings: the Primary Care Access, Referral, and Evaluation (PCARE) study. Am J Psychiatry 2010;167(2): 151–9.
98. Kilbourne AM, Post EP, Nossek A, et al. Improving medical and psychiatric outcomes among individuals with bipolar disorder: a randomized controlled trial. Psychiatr Serv 2008;59(7):760–8.

Prevention of Dementia

Rodolfo Savica, MD, MSc[a],*, Ronald C. Petersen, PhD, MD[b]

KEYWORDS

- Dementia • Alzheimer disease • Mild cognitive impairment
- Risk factors

Dementia is a neurological condition that results in decline in multiple cognitive domains and is accompanied by a functional impairment. Individuals eventually lose their independence and will be unable to perform typical activities of daily living. Dementia is generally characterized by a decline in memory and at least one other cognitive function, and these difficulties are of sufficient magnitude to compromise daily function. Dementia is often the umbrella term under which there are several subcategories. Alzheimer disease (AD) is the most common form of dementia in aging and is a degenerative disorder.[1,2] The pathological hallmarks of AD include the deposition of amyloid in the brain producing amyloid plaques and the extracellular amyloid plaques in accompaniment with the intracellular misprocessed tau protein producing neurofibrillary tangles.[3,4]

AD was first described in 1906 by Alois Alzheimer. His index case was a 51-year-old woman with memory loss, behavioral difficulties, and language problems. She ultimately progressed to death and her autopsy revealed what are now called the beta-amyloid plaques and neurofibrillary tangles.

At present, AD can only be characterized definitively at the time of autopsy. However, a great deal of research is being conducted to define biomarkers characteristic of the underlying pathological process that can be identified in life.[3,5,6] It is not uncommon, especially in late life, to have the changes of AD accompanied by other neuropathologies such as concomitant Lewy bodies and vascular disease.[3] Currently, the neuropathological changes seen at the time of autopsy need to be accompanied by the clinical progression producing a dementia.[7–9] In the future, the clinical spectrum leading to the dementia of AD and the pathological spectrum may be separated to allow a more complete characterization of each continuum.

This work was supported by grants from the National Institute on Aging; P50-AG016754, U01 AG006786, and the Robert H. and Clarice Smith and Abigail Van Buren Alzheimer's Disease Research Program.

[a] Department of Neurology, Mayo Clinic, Gonda 8 South, 200 First Street SW, Rochester, MN 55905, USA

[b] Department of Neurology, Mayo Clinic Study of Aging, Mayo Alzheimer's Disease Research Center, Mayo Clinic, Rochester, MN 55905, USA

* Corresponding author.
E-mail address: savica.rodolfo@mayo.edu

Psychiatr Clin N Am 34 (2011) 127–145
doi:10.1016/j.psc.2010.11.006
0193-953X/11/$ – see front matter © 2011 Published by Elsevier Inc.

Currently, the cognitive decline associated with AD likely has a prodromal phase whereby individuals are affected by the underlying neuropathologic process, but the clinical manifestation does not reach the threshold for dementia. The construct of mild cognitive impairment (MCI) has come to represent this symptomatic predementia stage of the Alzheimer process.[10–14] MCI typically represents memory impairment beyond what one would expect for age, yet other cognitive processes and daily functions are relatively well preserved. There has been an increase in literature accumulating on MCI over the last decade. This research will likely influence future direction of the characterization of AD.

Vascular cognitive impairment also represents a continuum from mild impairment through the fully developed dementia phase of vascular disease.[15–18] The prevalence of pure vascular disease producing dementia is relatively low, but the combination of vascular disease and neuropathological entities is quite common. The cognitive profile of vascular cognitive impairment can be quite variable, depending upon the specific location of the ischemic lesions. In general, there is more executive dysfunction from frontal lobe involvement of vascular disease, and gait disorder and urinary incontinence occur earlier in the dementing process than they do in AD.[17,19]

Dementia associated with Lewy bodies is also becoming increasingly well recognized. Individuals with this type of dementing disorder have features of parkinsonism, dream-enactment behavior, daytime hallucinations, fluctuating cognition and behavior, and may have a somewhat different cognitive profile than AD.[20–22] Typically, in the early features of dementia with Lewy bodies, an individual may exhibit diminished speed of cognitive processing and visuospatial deficits early in the course. The extrapyramidal features are somewhat similar to parkinsonism and a tremor is less common.[22–24] The combination of Lewy bodies and Alzheimer changes is quite common, and the overlap of the two diseases is well recognized.[20–22]

Parkinson's disease in its advanced stages may be accompanied by cognitive and memory problems and, in many respects, share much of the neuropathologic features of dementia with Lewy bodies. The distinction between Parkinson's disease, dementia, and dementia with Lewy bodies tends to revolve around the timing of the onset of the motor and cognitive symptoms. If these clinical features manifest themselves within approximately 12 months in duration, the picture is more likely associated with dementia with Lewy bodies. In Parkinson's disease dementia, the dementia occurs years after the onset of the parkinsonian motor features.[25]

Frontotemporal lobar dementia (FTLD) is a degenerative disorder primarily involving the frontal and temporal lobes.[19,26–28] These individuals present with early behavioral changes such as inappropriate behavior, apathy, or hyperactive behavioral disorders constituting the behavioral variant of FTLD.[29] There are also language presentations of FTLD that present with primary progressive aphasia.[30,31] This is a neurodegenerative disorder often with abnormalities in the tau protein.[27]

The combination of these disorders is common in aging and presents a significant problem for aging societies around the world. At present, there is a great deal of research going forward trying to understand the underlying nature of these disorders with the intention of developing disease modifying treatments. Many pharmacologic approaches are being entertained, as well as the assessment of lifestyle factors. This article addresses this literature.

PREVALENCE OF DEMENTIA OR AD

The prevalence of a dementia refers to the number of events, in this instance dementia, in a given population at a designated point in time. The incidence of the disease is defined as the number of new cases of a given disease during a defined period of time in a specified population.[32] The incidence of dementia has been reported to be 34.2 per 100,000 person-years for all dementias and 5 to 8 per 1000 person-years for AD.[33–37] These data would imply that there are 10 to 15 new cases of dementia for every 1000 persons in the population during 1 year and more than half of these cases are due to AD. In the United States, 14% of all people age 71 years and older have some form of dementia. The Alzheimer's Association estimates that there are 5.3 million Americans who currently have AD.[1,38,39] Approximately 10% to 13% of individuals over age 65 have AD and age is the most prominent risk factor for AD, such that, by the time people reach their mid 80s, they have a one in three chance of having AD. The risk of AD doubles every 5 years after 65 years of age. In general, many studies indicate that there are more women than men with AD, largely due to the greater longevity for women. When age adjustments are used, there does not appear to be a significant age effect with regard to the trends in AD over the past several decades.[2,37,40,41] The Framingham study has calculated lifetime risks of AD in the general population. The risk of having AD was higher for women then men (about 17% vs 9%, respectively) and increased with age.[2] The projection for the number of cases of dementia and AD in the coming years is staggering and speaks to the importance of continued research with the development of therapeutic interventions. The worldwide prevalence of AD in 2010 was estimated to be 35.6 million and will likely increase to more than 65 million by the year 2030.[42]

Prevention

Prevention can be considered as all actions that are performed to eradicate, eliminate, or minimize the impact of an event. In medical science, this event is usually a disease or disability. When none of the approaches to prevention are effective, a secondary goal of delaying or reducing the frequency of the disease or reducing disability can be entertained. Typically, prevention in medical science can be defined as levels of prevention: primary, secondary, and tertiary.[32,43]

Primary prevention refers to the efforts in public health to prevent the disease before symptom onset. True prevention would mean that the disease would never manifest itself later in life. In many respects, prevention may not be a realistic outcome but can serve as a goal with intermediate targets being delay of onset or slowing of progression.[44] In neurodegenerative diseases, these actions would be performed to prevent the symptomatic phase and reduce the risk of disease. Medications and lifestyle factors are currently being investigated to determine their effectiveness at preventing disease onset.

Secondary prevention refers to the reduction or cessation of symptom progression once the symptoms have appeared. Again, the goal is to reduce the disability of the disease once the disease process has begun. In degenerative dementias, the secondary prevention stage might apply to the phase of MCI since, at this point, symptoms are present but are not sufficiently severe to constitute dementia. Therefore, treatment trials aimed at subjects with MCI could be considered secondary prevention studies.

Tertiary prevention refers to a treatment designed to halt the progression of the disease once it has been established. The goal, again, is to reduce the disability and improve the long-term prognosis for individuals with the manifest disease. Currently, although tertiary prevention would maintain in an individual with a neurodegenerative disease in an impaired state, it is still worth pursuing.

Implicit in the discussion of, in particular, primary and secondary prevention is the concept of biomarkers. That is, since the disease process has not manifested itself clinically, such as in primary prevention, the clinical signals are absent. As such, the field needs to develop biomarkers as surrogates of the underlying disease process to allow the impact of the prevention.[45,46] Clearly, reducing the likelihood that a person would progress to the symptomatic stage such as that seen in secondary and tertiary prevention studies would be a laudable goal, but biomarkers would be quite useful in characterizing the effects on the underlying disease process. When dealing with an underlying continuum of clinical progression and pathologic processes, these distinctions among primary, secondary, and tertiary prevention are somewhat arbitrary.

This approach to prevention has been questioned in previous years. Geoffrey Rose[47] supports the theory that current prevention is reductionistic and that a more efficacious strategy would be to act on the early causes of the disease in an entire population, appreciating the so-called "prevention paradox."[43] The paradox is present when the measure that produces a benefit to a subset of the population offers little benefit to the overall population. For example, reducing cigarette smoking will likely improve the quality of life of some individuals but have no effect on others. Yet, the elimination of cigarette smoking is an example of prevention.

A challenge in the field of neurodegenerative diseases concerns the timing of the putative prevention strategy. That is, when potentially effective therapies are initiated too late in the underlying disease process, even in the asymptomatic stage, the true impact of prevention may not be appreciated. However, if one were to initiate therapies earlier in life, the overall effect of the prevention might be more appropriately realized. This is a theoretical dilemma since many studies that involve pure prevention would need to be initiated early in the lives of individuals, and the studies would need to continue for many years. As such, many investigators are choosing to address the disease in the secondary prevention stage (eg, MCI) in an effort to exert some type of a disease-modifying effect on the underlying pathology.

This can be applied to the degenerative process of Parkinson's disease. Currently, it is believed that Parkinson's disease begins 20 to 30 years before the motor manifestations are apparent and spreads gradually.[48,49] Tremor, bradykinesia, and rigidity are the hallmarks of Parkinson's disease, but they may not become manifest until many years after the degenerative process was initiated.[48,50] At times, there are subtle symptoms such as constipation,[51,52] anosmia,[53] anxiety,[54,55] autonomic dysfunction, or sleep disturbances[56] that may appear decades before the classic motor symptoms; but they are likely indices of the onset of the degenerative process. Therefore, in this case, primary preventions start very early in life rather than close to the time of symptom onset.

One can imagine a similar problem in dementing disorders where true primary prevention would need to be initiated very early in life. Most investigators believe that the neuropathological process that characterizes AD begins years, if not decades, before clinical symptoms appear. This may also be true for MCI insofar as the MCI stage is accompanied by significant pathology when it is described.[57] Once again, this speaks for the utility of biomarkers as assessing early stages of the disease process.

In summary, although true prevention is an ideal goal, intermediary targets such as delaying the onset and slowing the progression of the degenerative process might be more reasonable. As such, numerous studies have been performed and others are planned aimed at altering the trajectory of the clinical symptoms that constitute the onset of the disorder. A postponement in the onset of the clinical symptoms would have a significant impact on individuals and families, as well as the health care in society. Similarly, reducing the rate of progression of the disease, even though the symptoms are present, will have a significant impact on improving the quality of life of the individuals and their families, and will reduce the costs to health care systems.

Therefore, numerous strategies are being investigated with the goal of altering the trajectory of the clinical course and the underlying pathology.

PHARMACOLOGICAL APPROACHES
Acetylcholinesterase Inhibitors

There is a reduction in the cholinergic system in the brains of patients with AD.[58] Acetylcholinesterase is the enzyme that breaks down acetylcholine and the inhibition of this enzyme can help increase cholinergic activity. There are currently three drugs that are cholinesterase inhibitors that have been approved for the treatment of AD: donepezil, rivastigmine, and galantamine. In general, these three compounds have similar efficacy and are approved for either mild-to-moderate AD or the entire AD spectrum. The drugs have a modest effect at improving symptoms in the disease but can be useful in individual patients. The compounds have similar side effect profiles, largely increasing gastrointestinal system motility, but generally are well tolerated. However, none of these drugs delays the ultimate underlying progression of the AD process.[59] When these drugs were used in secondary prevention studies, particularly in MCI, none of them was demonstrated to reduce the rate at which individuals progressed to the dementia stage of AD.[59–63] One study involving donepezil and high-dose vitamin E demonstrated that donepezil was shown to reduce the risk of progressing from MCI to AD for 12 months in all subjects and up to 24 months in subjects who were apolipoprotein E4 carriers.[63] However, over the 36-month duration of the study, none of the interventions was documented to be effective.

N-methyl-ᴅ-aspartate Antagonists

The N-methyl-ᴅ-aspartate (NMDA) antagonists have been studied in AD and have been approved for the treatment of moderate to severe AD.[64,65] Memantine is the only approved drug at this time in the United States and it acts on the glutamate receptors. If NMDA receptors are upregulated, the release of glutamate leads to neuronal toxicity and neuronal damage. NMDA receptors are thought to play a role in the pathologic cascade of AD. NMDA antagonists may act as neuroprotectors, preventing this cascade.[65] There have not been any trials that have demonstrated that memantine is effective at reducing the risk of developing either MCI or AD.[66] Some studies have shown that the combination of memantine with an acetylcholinesterase inhibitor may improve functional abilities.[67] Nevertheless, the combination has not been shown to have a disease modifying effect on the underlying pathologic process.

All four of these drugs have been approved for symptomatic treatment of the dementia phase of AD, but none has been demonstrated to alter the disease process itself. Therefore, although somewhat useful in treating individuals with AD, these compounds do not appear to have any effect on prevention of the symptomatic phase of AD.[59]

Vitamins

Numerous studies have been conducted concerning the possible protective role of vitamins in treating or preventing dementia.[68] Many vitamins are considered to be antioxidant agents that may prevent or reduce the oxidative stress that has been described as part of the neuronal degeneration.[69,70] The biochemical cascade that starts in the brain during AD leads to the increase of oxygen-free radicals and reactive oxygen species (ROS).[71] Several different components of the neurodegenerative cascade may contribute to generating ROS. Furthermore, the tissue injury itself can produce these compounds.[72–74] To retard this mechanism, the use of antioxidants was a reasonable strategy to treat AD and cognitive decline.[71] Various vitamins, including B-12, folate,[75–79] B-6, B-3,[78] vitamin E, and others, have been extensively investigated. However, the studies do not show consistent results in the reduction of AD or cognitive decline. Most studies have used the fully developed dementia of AD and followed the cohort for variable periods of time to see if there was a reduced risk of progression in AD. The measurement of the vitamins was performed either directly by pill counts or by blood sample tests or, occasionally, inferred from responses to food questionnaires.

Some preliminary evidence indicated that low folate levels may be associated with an increased risk of AD.[75,79] One study reported a possible reduced risk of AD in a population that used the high intake of folate[73]; however, these results were not confirmed in another study.[76] There is a good deal of methodological variability in these studies and, consequently, the relation between B-12 and AD was uncertain. A higher intake of Niacin (B-3) was suggested to reduce the risk of AD in one study; however, these findings have not been replicated subsequently.[78] Other studies have suggested the possible reduction in the risk of AD or cognitive decline with the use of vitamin C, vitamin E, or the combination.[70,73,80–84] However, once again, there have not been consistent results from these. As mentioned above, in one study comparing donepezil and vitamin E in the MCI stage of the disease process, no benefit of vitamin E was determined to slow the rate of progression from MCI to AD.[63] However, another study by the same group did show that vitamin E might be effective at slowing the rate of progression in the fully developed dementia phase of AD[85]; these findings were also recently confirmed by other investigators.[86] There has been some discrepancy between studies that have used supplemental vitamin E and vitamin E in dietary intake, indicating that the latter may be preferable.

Therefore, although experimental and laboratory models suggest that the oxidative cascade may play a role in AD, the currently clinical trials do not provide strong support for the role of vitamins in reducing the risk of dementia or its prodromal phases. Again, the time of intervention may be critical in that, perhaps, the reduction of ROS at an earlier point in life may be beneficial rather than waiting until symptoms appear.

PHYSICAL ACTIVITY

Physical activity has been associated with a reduced risk of developing cognitive disorders and mental diseases (ANN of General Psychiatry).[87] Several observational studies have reported that people who are physically active were at lower risk of developing cognitive impairment or AD later in life.[88–94] Abbott and colleagues[88] observed that men who walk for at least two miles per day were less likely to develop dementia over a 6-year period. These findings were confirmed in the Nurses' Health Study that showed that increased physical activity was associated with higher cognitive scores.[95] Subsequent prospective studies have supported the role of physical activity in protecting against AD and cognitive decline.[88,89,92,93,96–100] Most of these studies use physical exercise in self-reported questionnaires of frequency of these activities, such as swimming, hiking, and running. There was a reduction of risk of AD in those subjects who exercised regularly as opposed to those people who did not exercise on a routine bases.[89] Moreover, these investigators reported that the protective effect was increased as the number of activities increased; that is, the risk was lower when four activities were performed as opposed to fewer. In addition, the protective effect of physical exercise in dementia or cognitive decline was also present when exercise was limited to later in life.

There have also been a number of clinical trials involving physical exercise. In the Fitness for Aging Brain Study, individuals older than 50 years of age were randomly allocated to 24 weeks of physical exercise or to an educational program.[101] The subjects in the exercise group had better cognitive scores compared with the subjects in the educational program over the 18 months of followup.[101] The mechanism by which physical activity may improve cognition in older subjects is unknown,[87] but a study involving transgenic mice indicated that exercise may increase the metabolism of the amyloid beta protein and actually reduce its deposition in animals predisposed to Alzheimer's-like lesions in the Brain.[102] It is possible that physical activity increases synaptogenesis, plasticity, and neural response to stress through the induction of endorphins, brain derived growth factor, insulin-like growth factors, and vascular endothelial growth factor.[103–106] Another proposed mechanism includes the possible stimulation of angiogenesis and brain perfusion.[107] Colcombe and colleagues[108,109] demonstrated that, in humans, physical exercise increases blood perfusion of brain regions that modulate attention.

There is a prominent body of research demonstrating possible positive effect of exercise in aging. One of the major aims of physical exercise is to decrease morbidity and mortality and increase the quality of life in individuals. Spirduso and Cronin[110] reviewed the literature on this topic and demonstrated that physical activity is consistently associated with a better quality of life. Higher physical activity increased independence and improved activities of daily living.

An impressive study on the role of physical activity and cognitive function in older adults has recently been reported from Australia.[101] This study was a randomized control trial of 24-week physical activity intervention conducted on individuals who reported memory problems but did not meet criteria for dementia. This was a double-blinded study and participants were randomly assigned to an education or usual care group for a 24-week home-based program of physical activity. An intent-to-treat analysis reveals that the intervention group improved over the usual care group on a typical scale used in AD clinical trials: the Alzheimer's Disease Assessment Scale-Cognitive subscale. At 18 months, the participants in the intervention group improved on the scale to a greater extent than those in the usual care group. This study demonstrated that, in subjects with a subjective memory impairment, a 6-month program of physical activity provided modest improvement in cognition over 18 months.

The National Institute on Aging encourages the use of exercise to prevent diseases, to maximize independence, and improve mobility while reducing depression. The National Institute on Aging suggests exercise programs such as 30 minutes of endurance activity, strength exercises, exercise to improve balance, and stretching exercises. They encouraged participation in these activities on a regular basis to promote quality of life.[111]

INTELLECTUAL ACTIVITIES

Several recent studies have suggested that there is a positive association between intellectual activity and reduction of the risk for cognitive decline or AD.[91,92,112–118] The Seattle Longitudinal Study explored a possible link between higher intellectual activities in AD.[119,120] The Seattle Longitudinal Study included over 5000 subjects in 1956 and followed them for more than 4 decades. The study found that higher levels of intellectual activities and an intellectually stimulating environment may reduce the risk of cognitive decline later in life, and suggested that reducing mental activities might be a risk factor for subsequent cognitive decline. In addition, several studies have documented the role of higher education in reducing a risk for cognitive decline in AD and numerous observational studies have supported this contention.[33,115–118,121–126]

A systematic review of the literature indicated that several quality studies associated education and risk for AD.[127] These investigators concluded that a lower level of education increases the risk of having AD by approximately 30%.[127] In addition, some studies explored the possible role of higher education in subjects who were carriers of the apolipoprotein E4 allele, but these studies have often showed inconsistent results.[128–130] Higher education may be a protective factor but may also be related to higher socioeconomic status and perhaps a healthier lifestyle, so the association may not be straightforward.

There is also the construct of cognitive reserve, indicating that individuals with higher education may be able to compensate for a considerable neuropathological burden and may be able to postpone the diagnosis for a greater period of time.[131,132] However, when these individuals eventually reach the stage of dementia, their cognitive decline may be more precipitous.[132] A recent neuropathological study suggested that the education does provide an element of reserve such that the clinical expression of cognitive impairment was delayed.[133] Therefore, education or cognitively stimulating activities may be somewhat protective against cognitive decline and dementia later in life.[133]

COGNITIVE TRAINING

Mental exercise and training have been described as a possible strategy to increased so-called "brain reserve" later in life.[134] Several clinical trials have been performed to assess the role of cognitive training in delaying or even preventing subsequent cognitive decline.[135–140] The Advanced Cognitive Training for Independent and Vital Elderly (ACTIVE) study has been influential in defining the role of cognitive training. This trial investigated the effect of 10 weekly sessions of cognitive exercises on 2,832 elderly individuals using four tasks: memory, reasoning, processing, and wait-and-see controls. After 5 years of follow up, this study demonstrated that specific mental activities can produce benefits not only on cognitive performance but also on instrumental activities of daily living.[136,137,141] The reasoning task was reasonably protective against decline in instrumental activities of daily living.

Moreover, some studies have assessed the complex relationship between cognitive training and quality of life and depression. One study showed that cognitive training was more helpful at maintaining mood rather than enhancing cognitive abilities.[142] Apparently, the Study of Mental Activity and Regular Training for the Prevention of Cognitive Decline in at Risk Individuals: The SMART trial demonstrated that progressively increasing the level of training over time was more efficacious at delaying cognitive decline than using a fixed and standardized training regimen.[143]

The biological mechanism underlying the effect of cognitive training is unknown. However, some experimental evidence indicates that in animals there is actually an increase in brain volume after prolonged mental activity.[144] In humans, there is some evidence that mental activities related to a decrease in atrophy of the hippocampal formations and indicates a complex time-dependent change in cortical function as revealed by functional MRI.[145,146] Some animal models have indicated that cognitive training may be associated with a reduction in amyloid pathology, which could imply a disease modifying effect of these activities.[102,147] In humans, it has also been described that mental activity may reduce the establishment of alternative compensatory pathways in spite of a certain burden of pathology.[148]

MEDITERRANEAN DIET

The Mediterranean Diet involves certain nutritional and behavioral recommendations that have been inspired by the food and lifestyle of the coastal regions of the Mediterranean areas (southern Italy, Crete, and Greece) in the 1960s. In addition to regular physical activity, the diet consists of fresh fruit, plant foods, olive oil, dairy products, fish, and poultry with limited amounts of eggs and red meat. A moderate amount of wine is also included in this diet.

Some cohort studies have examined the association between the Mediterranean Diet and cognitive decline of AD.[149-152] The exposure to the diet was assessed with self-recorded food questionnaires and one study reported that a higher adherence to the Mediterranean Diet was associated with a lower risk of progression from cognitively normal to MCI.[149] The other study showed that subjects exposed to the Mediterranean Diet had better scores on the Mini-Mental State Examination and less decline on a memory test.[151] The mechanisms of risk reduction are thought to be related to role of antioxidants present in this diet and its potential relationship at reducing reactive oxygen species.

SOCIAL NETWORKS

Social engagement can be defined as the participation in social activities and maintenance of social connections. Martial status, loneliness, participation in social and political events in the community, and contact with family and friends have been used by several studies to measure and quantify the degree of social engagement and its association with AD or cognitive decline. A number of cohort studies in the United States and Europe have explored social engagement as a possible risk for the future development of AD.[90,153-161] Through observing populations for several years and following them longitudinally, these studies indicated that self-reported questionnaires tended to imply that social activities may be protective against developing a cognitive decline. In particular, being single and not cohabiting with partner in life has been associated with an increased risk of AD; however, these findings could not be applied to individuals who were divorced or widowed. The latter result, however, was not confirmed in a study that showed that being widowed in mid-life or later life was associated with a higher risk of AD as compared with people who were cohabitating either in mid-life or later life.[156] Moreover, the degree of loneliness, decreased social networking, and activities seem to be associated with a higher risk.[162]

Some caution is warranted to interpret these findings because a reduction in social engagement can be an early sign of AD rather than a risk factor. Patients with early AD may have reduced social activity because they are less functional and are tending to withdraw. Although evidence is not definitive with respect to social activity, there seems to be a reasonable degree of support for maintaining social networks. Consequently, this recommendation is often provided by health care workers as a means of maintaining a high quality of life.

META-ANALYSIS

The Agency for Healthcare Research and Quality (AHRQ) prepared a systematic review of the available literature and a meta-analysis to better understand the current evidence on cognitive decline and AD.[162] The investigators prepared a list of inclusion criteria excluding small-to-moderate observational studies and randomized control trials and studies with less than 1 year of observation. A challenging problem in this type of study pertains to the lack of homogeneity across the studies in defining AD or cognitive decline; there was not a consistent diagnostic definition provided in many of these studies.

In the analysis, 25 systematic reviews and 250 primary research studies were included. Most factors did not show a significant and consistent association with a reduction in the risk of AD or cognitive decline. Alternatively, physical activities and cognitive engagements seem to be factors that were more consistently associated with a reduction in AD and cognitive decline, although a strict length with causality was not found. The reduction of the risk was small to moderate in AD and small in cognitive decline. Although there was some evidence for a reduction in late-life cognitive loss, there appeared to be insufficient evidence to draw definite conclusions. However, it must be realized that some of the issues addressed in this type of analysis may not be amenable to randomized control trials, and consequently, the available data were based on relatively short-term observational studies. As such, this type of analysis may not be entirely appropriate for these topics. The investigators concluded that further research needs to be done to better understand factors associated with a risk of AD and cognitive decline and suggested that a more homogeneous definition of the diagnostic entities would be helpful.

COMMENTS ON META-ANALYSES

A meta-analysis is a "quantitative approach for systematically assessing the previous research to arrive at conclusions about the body of research."[163] In other words, this is a research technique that tries to combine different studies on the same topic to provide a quantitative result that might address the questions under study. The unit of a meta-analysis is not the population of subjects but rather individuals. An important step in initiating a meta-analysis is to perform an extremely thorough review of the current literature on the selected topic to find all of the relevant papers. Moreover, it is necessary to clearly state the inclusion criteria to define studies that would be used for the analysis. It is difficult to interpret studies using different designs and combining studies that may have had different foci. For example, combining cohort studies and case control studies may lead to uninterpretable results. Meta-analyses are very helpful to provide a quick and easy interpretation for a large body of literature pertaining to clinical practice or for addressing certain scientific issues. However, there are limitations of meta-analyses. The variable quality of the different studies may severely impact the quantitative meta-analytical result. It is not always possible to have high quality studies across the field, yet often meta-analyses combine these various investigations as if they were done equally well. This may lead to results that are difficult to interpret. The ideal studies for meta-analyses are randomized clinical trials. These studies have defined onsets and ends, and the criteria for inclusion are clearly defined. However, observational studies are less precise by nature and, consequently, often do not meet the strict criteria that are observed in randomized clinical trials. Nevertheless, some of the issues that are very important to address can only be done adequately through observational studies. However, the techniques used in meta-analyses downgrade the quality of a study if it is purely observational.

Another concern with meta-analyses pertains to the sample sizes of the studies. Meta-analyses tend to place a great deal of weight on studies with large sample sizes. As discussed above, the quality of the study might not be in direct proportion to the size of the study. For example, a study with a large sample size but of marginal clinical assessment might be combined with a smaller study with a better clinical assessment and the larger study will carry more weight in the analysis in spite of the rather cursory clinical features. This can compromise the interpretation of the results. Finally, meta-analyses tend to be more effective when a specific question is being addressed rather than a more general scientific issue. As noted above, the randomized control trial addressing a particular question carries the greatest amount of weight in a meta-analysis, and studies that are addressing more diffuse issues are more difficult to conduct.

NATIONAL INSTITUTES OF HEALTH STATE-OF-THE-SCIENCE CONFERENCE

The National Institutes of Health recently organized a meeting to assess the available scientific evidence related to the prevention of AD and cognitive decline. In this meeting, there was an independent panel of health professionals and public representatives who evaluated the results of a systematic literature review and considered the presentations of investigators in the field of aging and dementia. The meeting focused on the identification of risk factors that may be associated with AD and cognitive decline, including the therapeutic effects of any medications that are available. The focus was to determine if there are any factors that may maintain or improve cognitive function over the lifespan and the relationship between those factors and AD in cognitive decline.[164]

Although the panel recognized the magnitude of the progress and knowledge over the past decades, they did not draw any firm conclusions about modifiable risk factors for AD or cognitive decline. Moreover, they indicated that there was inconsistent evidence regarding the diagnoses of AD, MCI, and cognitive decline and concluded that no pharmaceutical agents or dietary supplements were noted to be preventive. They suggested that additional randomized control trials should be performed in a representative population to identify factors that might delay the onset or slow the progression of cognitive decline or AD.

The feedback concerning the State-of-the-Science report was mixed. Critics felt that the panel failed to recognize the distinction between causal relationships and associations. There are numerous studies that indicate that there is an association between exercise and AD, for example, but since definitive clinical trials were unavailable to document this distinction, the panel rejected this information. On the one hand, certain factors may be associated with increasing a risk of getting AD but not definitely indicate that those factors cause the disorder. Nevertheless, the relationship between several of the factors involving exercise and intellectual activity were underestimated. All agreed that additional research needs to be conducted in this area.

SUMMARY

The importance of defining factors that may delay the onset, slow the progression, or even prevent AD and cognitive decline cannot be overestimated. With the aging of world populations, the burden of individuals with all degrees of cognitive impairment on societies will be enormous. A great deal of research has been conducted concerning these factors over the past decades. Although it is true that there are no definitive interventions that have been defined to prevent or slow the cognitive decline in aging, there are very strong trends in the literature. The available evidence suggests that physical activity, intellectual activity, and social engagement are the most helpful factors at reducing AD and cognitive decline and, at the same time, these factors may be helpful for enhancing quality of life. Clearly, further studies are needed to better understand the early pathological changes related to the symptoms of AD and cognitive decline, and these studies need to be conducted in a prospective fashion in representative populations. There is optimism in the field with respect to possible disease-modifying effects that can be achieved through a variety of nutritional, pharmacological, and lifestyle modifications.

REFERENCES

1. Hebert LE, Scherr PA, Bienias JL, et al. Alzheimer disease in the US population: prevalence estimates using the 2000 census. Arch Neurol 2003; 60(8):1119–22.
2. Bachman DL, Wolf PA, Linn RT, et al. Incidence of dementia and probable Alzheimer's disease in a general population: the Framingham study. Neurology 1993;43:515–9.

3. Duyckaerts C, Delatour B, Potier MC. Classification and basic pathology of Alzheimer disease. Acta Neuropathol 2009;118(1):5–36.

4. Bennett DA, Schneider JA, Wilson RS, et al. Neurofibrillary tangles mediate the association of amyloid load with clinical Alzheimer disease and level of cognitive function. Arch Neurol 2004;61(3):378–84.

5. Dickson DW, Davies P, Bevona C, et al. Hippocampal sclerosis: a common pathological feature of dementia in very old (>80 year of age) humans. Acta Neuropathol 1994;88:212–21.

6. Boeve BF, Braak H, Parisi JE, et al. Memory function and neurofibrillary degeneration in the medial temporal lobe. Neurology 1998;50(S4):A61.

7. McKhann G, Drachman D, Folstein M, et al. Clinical Diagnosis of Alzheimer's Disease: report of the NINCDS-ADRDA work group under the auspices of Department of Health and Human Services Task Force on Alzheimer's Disease. Neurology 1984;34:939–44.

8. World Health Organization. International statistical classification of diseases and related health problems. 10th edition. Geneva (Switzerland): World Health Organization; 1992. categories F00–99.

9. American Psychiatry Association. Diagnostic and statistical manual of mental disorders. Revised. 3rd edition. Washington, DC: American Psychiatric Association; 1987.

10. Petersen RC. Mild cognitive impairment: transition between aging and Alzheimer's disease. Neurologia 2000;15:93–101.

11. Bozoki A, Giordani B, Heidebrink JL, et al. Mild cognitive impairments predict dementia in nondemented elderly patients with memory loss. Arch Neurol 2001;58:411–6.

12. Petersen RC, Smith GE, Waring SC, et al. Mild cognitive impairment: clinical characterization and outcome. Arch Neurol 1999;56:303–8.

13. Petersen RC, Negash S. Mild cognitive impairment: an overview. CNS Spectr 2008;13(1):45–53.

14. Petersen R, Knopman D, Boeve B, et al. Mild cognitive impairment: ten years later. Arch Neurol 2009;66(22):1447–55.

15. Knopman DS, Parisi JE, Boeve BF, et al. Vascular dementia in a population-based autopsy study. Arch Neurol 2003;60:569–76.

16. del Ser T, Bermejo F, Protera A, et al. Vascular dementia. A clinicopathologic study. J Neurol Sci 1990;96:1–17.

17. Murray ME, Knopman DS, Dickson DW. Vascular dementia: clinical, neuroradiologic and neuropathologic aspects. Panminerva Med 2007;49(4):197–207.

18. Hachinski V, Iadecola C, Petersen RC, et al. National Institute of Neurological Disorders and Stroke-Canadian Stroke Network vascular cognitive impairment harmonization standards. Stroke 2006;37(9):2220–41.

19. Boeve BF. A review of the non-Alzheimer dementias. J Clin Psychiatry 2006; 67(12):1985–2001 [discussion: 1983–4].

20. Forstl H, Burns A, Luthert P, et al. The Lewy-body variant of Alzheimer's disease. Clinical and pathological findings. Br J Psychiatry 1993;162:385–92.

21. Hansen L, Salmon D, Galasko D, et al. The Lewy body variant of Alzheimer's disease: a clinical and pathologic entity. Neurology 1990;40:1–8.

22. Cercy SP, Bylsma FW. Lewy bodies and progressive dementia: a critical review and meta-analysis. J Int Neuropsychol Soc 1997;3(2):179–94.

23. Boeve BF, Silber MH, Ferman TJ, et al. REM sleep behavior disorder and degenerative dementia: an association likely reflecting Lewy body disease. Neurology 1998;51:363–70.

24. Boeve BF, Silber MH, Petersen RC, et al. REM sleep behavior disorder and degenerative dementia with or without Parkinsonism: a syndrome predictive of Lewy body disease? Neurology 1997;48(Suppl A):A358.
25. Boeve BF. Parkinson-related dementias. Neurol Clin 2007;25(3):761–81, vii.
26. Rosen HJ, Lengenfelder J, Miller B. Frontotemporal dementia. In: DeKosky ST, editor. Neurologic clinics. Philadelphia: WB Saunders; 2000. p. 979–92.
27. Grossman M. Frontotemporal dementia: a review. J Int Neuropsychol Soc 2002; 8:566–83.
28. Neary D, Snowden JS, Gustafson L, et al. Frontotemporal lobar degeneration: a consensus on clinical diagnostic criteria. Neurology 1998;51(6):1546–54.
29. Chow TW. Frontotemporal dementias: clinical features and management. Semin Clin Neuropsychiatry 2003;8:58–70.
30. Mesulam MM. Primary progressive aphasia: differentiation from Alzheimer's disease. Ann Neurol 1987;22:533–4.
31. Mesulam MM. Primary progressive aphasia—a language-based dementia. N Engl J Med 2003;349:1535–42.
32. Last JM. International epidemiological association. A dictionary of epidemiology. 4th edition. New York: Oxford University Press; 2001.
33. Di Carlo A, Baldereschi M, Amaducci L, et al. Incidence of dementia, Alzheimer's disease, and vascular dementia in Italy. The ILSA Study. J Am Geriatr Soc 2002;50(1):41–8.
34. Bermejo F, Morales JM. Dementia and door-to-door studies in Spain. J Neurol Neurosurg Psychiatry 1994;57(7):874.
35. Ruitenberg A, Ott A, van Swieten JC, et al. Incidence of dementia: does gender make a difference? Neurobiol Aging 2001;22(4):575–80.
36. Knopman DS, Petersen RC, Cha RH, et al. Incidence and causes of nondegenerative nonvascular dementia: a population-based study. Arch Neurol 2006; 63(2):218–21.
37. Rocca WA, Cha RH, Waring SC, et al. Incidence of dementia and Alzheimer's disease: a reanalysis of data from Rochester, Minnesota, 1975–1984. Am J Epidemiol 1998;148(1):51–62.
38. Plassman BL, Langa KM, Fisher GG, et al. Prevalence of dementia in the United States: the aging, demographics, and memory study. Neuroepidemiology 2007; 29(1–2):125–32.
39. Alzheimer's Association. 2009 Alzheimer's disease facts and figures. Alzheimers Dement 2009;5:234–70.
40. Fillenbaum GG, Heyman A, Huber MS, et al. The prevalence and 3-year incidence of dementia in older Black and White community residents. J Clin Epidemiol 1998;51(7):587–95.
41. Fitzpatrick A, Kuller LH, Ives DG, et al. Incidence and prevalence of dementia in the cardiovascular health study. J Am Geriatr Soc 2004;52:195–204.
42. Alzheimer's Disease International. World Alzheimer Report 2009. Available at: http://www.alz.co.uk/research/files/World%20Alzheimer%20Report.pdf. Accessed September 30, 2009.
43. Szklo M, Nieto FJ. Epidemiology: beyond the basics. 2nd edition. Sudbury (MA): Jones and Bartlett Publishers; 2007.
44. Sloane PD, Zimmerman S, Suchindran C, et al. The public health impact of Alzheimer's disease, 2000–2050: potential implication of treatment advances. Annu Rev Public Health 2002;23:213–31.
45. Shaw LM, Korecka M, Clark CM, et al. Biomarkers of neurodegeneration for diagnosis and monitoring therapeutics. Nat Rev Drug Discov 2007;6(4):295–303.

46. Shaw LM, Vanderstichele H, Knapik-Czajka M, et al. Cerebrospinal fluid biomarker signature in Alzheimer's disease neuroimaging initiative subjects. Ann Neurol 2009;65(4):403–13.

47. Rose G. The strategy of preventive medicine. New York: Oxford University Press; 1994.

48. Savica R, Rocca WA, Ahlskog JE. When does Parkinson disease start? Arch Neurol 2010;67(7):798–801.

49. Braak H, Ghebremedhin E, Rub U, et al. Stages in the development of Parkinson's disease-related pathology. Cell Tissue Res 2004;318(1):121–34.

50. Wolters EC, Francot C, Bergmans P, et al. Preclinical (premotor) Parkinson's disease. J Neurol 2000;247(Suppl 2):II103–9.

51. Savica R, Carlin JM, Grossardt BR, et al. Medical records documentation of constipation preceding Parkinson disease: a case-control study. Neurology 2009; 73(21):1752–8.

52. Abbott RD, Petrovitch H, White LR, et al. Frequency of bowel movements and the future risk of Parkinson's disease. Neurology 2001;57(3):456–62.

53. Ross GW, Petrovitch H, Abbott RD, et al. Association of olfactory dysfunction with risk for future Parkinson's disease. Ann Neurol 2008;63(2):167–73.

54. Shiba M, Bower JH, Maraganore DM, et al. Anxiety disorders and depressive disorders preceding Parkinson's disease: a case-control study. Mov Disord 2000;15(4):669–77.

55. Bower JH, Grossardt BR, Maraganore DM, et al. Anxious personality predicts an increased risk of Parkinson's disease. Mov Disord 2010;25(13):2105–13.

56. Claassen DO, Josephs KA, Ahlskog JE, et al. REM sleep behavior disorder preceding other aspects of synucleinopathies by up to half a century. Neurology 2010;75(6):494–9.

57. Petersen RC, Parisi JE, Dickson DW, et al. Neuropathology of amnestic mild cognitive impairment. Arch Neurol 2006;63:665–72.

58. Francis PT, Palmer AM, Snape M, et al. The cholinergic hypothesis of Alzheimer's disease: a review of progress. J Neurol Neurosurg Psychiatry 1999;66(2):137–47.

59. Hansen RA, Gartlehner G, Webb AP, et al. Efficacy and safety of donepezil, galantamine, and rivastigmine for the treatment of Alzheimer's disease: a systematic review and meta-analysis. Clin Interv Aging 2008;3(2):211–25.

60. Thal LJ, Ferris SH, Kirby L, et al. A randomized, double-blind, study of rofecoxib in patients with mild cognitive impairment. Neuropsychopharmacology 2005;30: 1204–15.

61. Winblad B, Gauthier S, Scinto L, et al. Safety and efficacy of galantamine in subjects with mild cognitive impairment. Neurology 2008;70(22):2024–35.

62. Feldman HH, Ferris S, Winblad B, et al. Effect of rivastigmine on delay to diagnosis of Alzheimer's disease from mild cognitive impairment: the InDDEx study. Lancet Neurol 2007;6(6):501–12.

63. Petersen RC, Thomas RG, Grundman M, et al. Vitamin E and donepezil for the treatment of mild cognitive impairment. N Engl J Med 2005;352(23): 2379–88.

64. Reisberg B, Doody R, Stoffler A, et al. Memantine in moderate-to-severe Alzheimer's disease. N Engl J Med 2003;348(14):1333–41.

65. McKeage K. Spotlight on memantine in moderate to severe Alzheimer's disease. Drugs Aging 2010;27(2):177–9.

66. McKeage K. Memantine: a review of its use in moderate to severe Alzheimer's disease. CNS Drugs 2009;23(10):881–97.

67. Tariot PN, Farlow MR, Grossberg GT, et al. Memantine treatment in patients with moderate to severe Alzheimer disease already receiving donepezil: a randomized controlled trial. JAMA 2004;291(3):317–24.
68. Balk E, Chung M, Raman G, et al. B vitamins and berries and age-related neurodegenerative disorders. Evid Rep Technol Assess (Full Rep) 2006;134:1–161.
69. Frei B. Reactive oxygen species and antioxidant vitamins: mechanisms of action. Am J Med 1994;97(3A):5S–13S [discussion: 22S–8S].
70. Morris MC, Evans DA, Bienias JL, et al. Dietary intake of antioxidant nutrients and the risk of incident Alzheimer disease in a biracial community study. JAMA 2002;287(24):3230–7.
71. Pratico D, Clark CM, Liun F, et al. Increase of brain oxidative stress in mild cognitive impairment: a possible predictor of Alzheimer disease. Arch Neurol 2002; 59:972–6.
72. McGeer PL, Rogers J. Anti-inflammatory agents as a therapeutic approach to Alzheimer's disease. Neurology 1992;42:447–9.
73. Luchsinger JA, Tang MX, Shea S, et al. Antioxidant vitamin intake and risk of Alzheimer disease. Arch Neurol 2003;60(2):203–8.
74. Gray SL, Anderson ML, Crane PK, et al. Antioxidant vitamin supplement use and risk of dementia or Alzheimer's disease in older adults. J Am Geriatr Soc 2008; 56(2):291–5.
75. Ravaglia G, Forti P, Maioli F, et al. Homocysteine and folate as risk factors for dementia and Alzheimer disease. Am J Clin Nutr 2005;82(3):636–43.
76. Morris MC, Evans DA, Schneider JA, et al. Dietary folate and vitamins B-12 and B-6 not associated with incident Alzheimer's disease. J Alzheimers Dis 2006; 9(4):435–43.
77. Luchsinger JA, Tang MX, Miller J, et al. Relation of higher folate intake to lower risk of Alzheimer disease in the elderly. Arch Neurol 2007;64(1):86–92.
78. Morris MC, Evans DA, Bienias JL, et al. Dietary niacin and the risk of incident Alzheimer's disease and of cognitive decline. J Neurol Neurosurg Psychiatry 2004;75(8):1093–9.
79. Wang HX, Wahlin A, Basun H, et al. Vitamin B(12) and folate in relation to the development of Alzheimer's disease. Neurology 2001;56(9):1188–94.
80. Fillenbaum GG, Kuchibhatla MN, Hanlon JT, et al. Dementia and Alzheimer's disease in community-dwelling elders taking vitamin C and/or vitamin E. Ann Pharmacother 2005;39(12):2009–14.
81. Laurin D, Masaki KH, Foley DJ, et al. Midlife dietary intake of antioxidants and risk of late-life incident dementia: the Honolulu-Asia Aging Study. Am J Epidemiol 2004;159(10):959–67.
82. Masaki KH, Losonczy KG, Izmirlian G, et al. Association of vitamin E and C supplement use with cognitive function and dementia in elderly men. Neurology 2000;54:1265–72.
83. Morris MC, Beckett LA, Scherr PA, et al. Vitamin E and vitamin C supplements use and risk of incident Alzheimer disease. Alzheimer Dis Assoc Disord 1998; 12:121–6.
84. Zandi PP, Anthony JC, Khachaturian AS, et al. Reduced risk of Alzheimer disease in users of antioxidant vitamin supplements. Arch Neurol 2004;61:82–8.
85. Sano M, Ernesto C, Thomas RG, et al. A controlled trial of selegiline, alpha-tocopherol, or both as treatment for Alzheimer's disease. The Alzheimer's Disease Cooperative Study. N Engl J Med 1997;336(17):1216–22.
86. Devore EE, Grodstein F, van Rooij FJ, et al. Dietary antioxidants and long-term risk of dementia. Arch Neurol 2010;67(7):819–25.

87. Lautenschlager NT, Almeida OP, Flicker L, et al. Can physical activity improve the mental health of older adults? Ann Gen Hosp Psychiatry 2004;3(1):12.
88. Abbott RD, White LR, Ross GW, et al. Walking and dementia in physically capable elderly men. JAMA 2004;292(12):1447–53.
89. Larson EB, Wang L, Bowen JD, et al. Exercise is associated with reduced risk for incident dementia among persons 65 years of age and older. Ann Intern Med 2006;144(2):73–81.
90. Yaffe K, Barnes D, Nevitt M, et al. A prospective study of physical activity and cognitive decline in elderly women: women who walk. Arch Intern Med 2001;161(14):1703–8.
91. Verghese J, LeValley A, Derby C, et al. Leisure activities and the risk of amnestic mild cognitive impairment in the elderly. Neurology 2006;66(6):821–7.
92. Verghese J, Lipton RB, Katz MJ, et al. Leisure activities and the risk of dementia in the elderly. N Engl J Med 2003;348(25):2508–16.
93. Lytle ME, Vander Bilt J, Pandav RS, et al. Exercise level and cognitive decline: the MoVIES project. Alzheimer Dis Assoc Disord 2004;18(2):57–64.
94. Schuit AJ, Feskens EJ, Launer LJ, et al. Physical activity and cognitive decline, the role of the apolipoprotein e4 allele. Med Sci Sports Exerc 2001;33(5):772–7.
95. Weuve J, Kang JH, Manson JE, et al. Physical activity, including walking, and cognitive function in older women. JAMA 2004;292(12):1454–61.
96. Laurin D, Verreault R, Lindsay J, et al. Physical activity and risk of cognitive impairment and dementia in elderly persons. Arch Neurol 2001;58(3):498–504.
97. Andel R, Crowe M, Pedersen NL, et al. Physical exercise at midlife and risk of dementia three decades later: a population-based study of Swedish twins. J Gerontol A Biol Sci Med Sci 2008;63(1):62–6.
98. Rovio S, Kareholt I, Helkala EL, et al. Leisure-time physical activity at midlife and the risk of dementia and Alzheimer's disease. Lancet Neurol 2005;4(11):705–11.
99. Rovio S, Kareholt I, Viitanen M, et al. Work-related physical activity and the risk of dementia and Alzheimer's disease. Int J Geriatr Psychiatry 2007;22(9):874–82.
100. Baker LD, Frank LL, Foster-Schubert K, et al. Effects of aerobic exercise on mild cognitive impairment: a controlled trial. Arch Neurol 2010;67(1):71–9.
101. Lautenschlager NT, Cox KL, Flicker L, et al. Effect of physical activity on cognitive function in older adults at risk for Alzheimer disease: a randomized trial. JAMA 2008;300(9):1027–37.
102. Costa DA, Cracchiolo JR, Bachstetter AD, et al. Enrichment improves cognition in AD mice by amyloid-related and unrelated mechanisms. Neurobiol Aging 2007;28(6):831–44.
103. Stranahan AM, Khalil D, Gould E. Social isolation delays the positive effects of running on adult neurogenesis. Nat Neurosci 2006;9(4):526–33.
104. Cotman CW, Berchtold NC. Exercise: a behavioral intervention to enhance brain health and plasticity. Trends Neurosci 2002;25(6):295–301.
105. Kronenberg G, Bick-Sander A, Bunk E, et al. Physical exercise prevents age-related decline in precursor cell activity in the mouse dentate gyrus. Neurobiol Aging 2006;27(10):1505–13.
106. Uda M, Ishido M, Kami K, et al. Effects of chronic treadmill running on neurogenesis in the dentate gyrus of the hippocampus of adult rat. Brain Res 2006;1104(1):64–72.
107. Swain RA, Harris AB, Wiener EC, et al. Prolonged exercise induces angiogenesis and increases cerebral blood volume in primary motor cortex of the rat. Neuroscience 2003;117(4):1037–46.

108. Colcombe SJ, Kramer AF, Erickson KI, et al. Cardiovascular fitness, cortical plasticity, and aging. Proc Natl Acad Sci U S A 2004;101(9):3316–21.
109. Colcombe SJ, Kramer AF, McAuley E, et al. Neurocognitive aging and cardiovascular fitness: recent findings and future directions. J Mol Neurosci 2004; 24(1):9–14.
110. Spirduso WW, Cronin DL. Exercise dose-response effects on quality of life and independent living in older adults. Med Sci Sports Exerc 2001;33(6 Suppl): S598–608 [discussion: S9–10].
111. Health NIo. National Institute of Health. 2010. Available at: http://nihseniorhealth. gov/exerciseforolderadults/toc.html. Accessed January 9, 2010.
112. Wilson RS, Bennett DA, Bienias JL, et al. Cognitive activity and incident AD in a population-based sample of older persons. Neurology 2002;59(12):1910–4.
113. Wilson RS, Bennett DA, Bienias JL, et al. Cognitive activity and cognitive decline in a biracial community population. Neurology 2003;61:812–6.
114. Wilson RS, Mendes de Leon CF, Barnes LL, et al. Participation in cognitively stimulating activities and risk of incident Alzheimer disease. JAMA 2002;287: 742–8.
115. Alvarado BE, Zunzunegui MV, Del Ser T, et al. Cognitive decline is related to education and occupation in a Spanish elderly cohort. Aging Clin Exp Res 2002;14(2):132–42.
116. Koster A, Penninx BW, Bosma H, et al. Socioeconomic differences in cognitive decline and the role of biomedical factors. Ann Epidemiol 2005;15(8):564–71.
117. Lee S, Buring JE, Cook NR, et al. The relation of education and income to cognitive function among professional women. Neuroepidemiology 2006;26(2): 93–101.
118. Lee S, Kawachi I, Berkman LF, et al. Education, other socioeconomic indicators, and cognitive function. Am J Epidemiol 2003;157(8):712–20.
119. Schaie KW. Intellectual development in adulthood: the Seattle Longitudinal Study. New York: Cambridge University Press; 1996.
120. Schaie KW. Developmental influences on adult intelligence: the Seattle Longitudinal Study. New York: Oxford University Press; 2005.
121. Yoshitake T, Kiyohara Y, Kato I, et al. Incidence and risk factors of vascular dementia and Alzheimer's disease in a defined elderly Japanese population: the Hisayama Study. Neurology 1995;45(6):1161–8.
122. Karp A, Kareholt I, Qiu C, et al. Relation of education and occupation-based socioeconomic status to incident Alzheimer's disease. Am J Epidemiol 2004; 159(2):175–83.
123. Letenneur L, Gilleron V, Commenges D, et al. Are sex and educational level independent predictors of dementia and Alzheimer's disease? Incidence data from the PAQUID project. J Neurol Neurosurg Psychiatry 1999;66(2): 177–83.
124. Stern Y, Gurland B, Tatemichi TK, et al. Influence of education and occupation on the incidence of Alzheimer's disease. JAMA 1994;271(13):1004–10.
125. Scarmeas N, Levy G, Tang MX, et al. Influence of leisure activity on the incidence of Alzheimer's disease. Neurology 2001;57(12):2236–42.
126. Kukull WA, Higdon R, Bowen JD, et al. Dementia and Alzheimer disease incidence: a prospective cohort study. Arch Neurol 2002;59(11):1737–46.
127. Caamano-Isorna F, Corral M, Montes-Martinez A, et al. Education and dementia: a meta-analytic study. Neuroepidemiology 2006;26(4):226–32.
128. Manly JJ, Schupf N, Tang MX, et al. Cognitive decline and literacy among ethnically diverse elders. J Geriatr Psychiatry Neurol 2005;18(4):213–7.

129. Wilson RS, Hebert LE, Scherr PA, et al. Educational attainment and cognitive decline in old age. Neurology 2009;72(5):460–5.
130. Karlamangla AS, Miller-Martinez D, Aneshensel CS, et al. Trajectories of cognitive function in late life in the United States: demographic and socioeconomic predictors. Am J Epidemiol 2009;170(3):331–42.
131. Stern Y, Alexander GE, Prohovnik I, et al. Relationship between lifetime occupation and parietal flow: implications for a reserve against Alzheimer's disease pathology. Neurology 1995;45(1):55–60.
132. Stern Y. What is cognitive reserve? Theory and research application of the reserve concept. J Int Neuropsychol Soc 2002;8:448–60.
133. Brayne C, Ince PG, Keage HA, et al. Education, the brain and dementia: neuroprotection or compensation? Brain 2010;133(Pt 8):2210–6.
134. Valenzuela MJ, Sachdev P. Brain reserve and dementia: a systematic review. Psychol Med 2006;36(4):441–54.
135. Valenzuela MJ, Sachdev P. Brain reserve and cognitive decline: a non-parametric systematic review. Psychol Med 2006;36(8):1065–73.
136. Ball K, Berch DB, Helmers KF, et al. Effects of cognitive training interventions with older adults: a randomized controlled trial. JAMA 2002;288(18):2271–81.
137. Jobe JB, Smith DM, Ball K, et al. ACTIVE: a cognitive intervention trial to promote independence in older adults. Control Clin Trials 2001;22(4):453–79.
138. Oswald WD, Rupprecht R, Gunzelmann T, et al. The SIMA-project: effects of 1 year cognitive and psychomotor training on cognitive abilities of the elderly. Behav Brain Res 1996;78(1):67–72.
139. Scogin F, Bienias JL. A three-year follow-up of older adult participants in a memory-skills training program. Psychol Aging 1988;3(4):334–7.
140. Neely AS, Backman L. Long-term maintenance of gains from memory training in older adults: two 3 1/2-year follow-up studies. J Gerontol 1993;48(5):P233–7.
141. Willis SL, Tennstedt SL, Marsiske M, et al. Long-term effects of cognitive training on everyday functional outcomes in older adults. JAMA 2006;296(23):2805–14.
142. Olazaran J, Muniz R, Reisberg B, et al. Benefits of cognitive-motor intervention in MCI and mild to moderate Alzheimer disease. Neurology 2004;63(12): 2348–53.
143. Valenzuela MJ. Brain reserve and the prevention of dementia. Curr Opin Psychiatry 2008;21(3):296–302.
144. Rosenzweig MR, Bennett EL. Effects of differential environments on brain weights and enzyme activities in gerbils, rats, and mice. Dev Psychobiol 1969;2(2):87–95.
145. May A, Hajak G, Ganssbauer S, et al. Structural brain alterations following 5 days of intervention: dynamic aspects of neuroplasticity. Cereb Cortex 2007;17(1): 205–10.
146. Westerberg H, Klingberg T. Changes in cortical activity after training of working memory—a single-subject analysis. Physiol Behav 2007;92(1–2):186–92.
147. Lazarov O, Robinson J, Tang YP, et al. Environmental enrichment reduces Abeta levels and amyloid deposition in transgenic mice. Cell 2005;120(5):701–13.
148. Valenzuela MJ, Breakspear M, Sachdev P. Complex mental activity and the aging brain: molecular, cellular and cortical network mechanisms. Brain Res Rev 2007;56(1):198–213.
149. Scarmeas N, Stern Y, Mayeux R, et al. Mediterranean diet and mild cognitive impairment. Arch Neurol 2009;66(2):216–25.
150. Scarmeas N, Stern Y, Tang MX, et al. Mediterranean diet and risk for Alzheimer's disease. Ann Neurol 2006;59(6):912–21.

151. Feart C, Samieri C, Rondeau V, et al. Adherence to a Mediterranean diet, cognitive decline, and risk of dementia. JAMA 2009;302(6):638–48.
152. Scarmeas N, Luchsinger JA, Schupf N, et al. Physical activity, diet, and risk of Alzheimer disease. JAMA 2009;302(6):627–37.
153. Helmer C, Damon D, Letenneur L, et al. Marital status and risk of Alzheimer's disease: a French population-based cohort study. Neurology 1999;53(9):1953–8.
154. Wilson RS, Krueger KR, Arnold SE, et al. Loneliness and risk of Alzheimer disease. Arch Gen Psychiatry 2007;64(2):234–40.
155. Fratiglioni L, Wang HX, Ericsson K, et al. Influence of social network on occurrence of dementia: a community-based longitudinal study. Lancet 2000; 355(9212):1315–9.
156. Hakansson K, Rovio S, Helkala EL, et al. Association between mid-life marital status and cognitive function in later life: population based cohort study. BMJ 2009;339:b2462.
157. Saczynski JS, Pfeifer LA, Masaki K, et al. The effect of social engagement on incident dementia: the Honolulu-Asia Aging Study. Am J Epidemiol 2006; 163(5):433–40.
158. Barnes LL, Mendes de Leon CF, Wilson RS, et al. Social resources and cognitive decline in a population of older African Americans and whites. Neurology 2004; 63(12):2322–6.
159. Holtzman RE, Rebok GW, Saczynski JS, et al. Social network characteristics and cognition in middle-aged and older adults. J Gerontol B Psychol Sci Soc Sci 2004;59(6):P278–84.
160. Green AF, Rebok G, Lyketsos CG. Influence of social network characteristics on cognition and functional status with aging. Int J Geriatr Psychiatry 2008;23(9): 972–8.
161. Seeman TE, Lusignolo TM, Albert M, et al. Social relationships, social support, and patterns of cognitive aging in healthy, high-functioning older adults: MacArthur studies of successful aging. Health Psychol 2001;20(4):243–55.
162. Williams JW, Plassman BL, Burke J, et al. Preventing Alzheimer's Disease and Cognitive Decline. Evidence Report/Technology Assessment No 193 (Prepared by the Duke Evidence-based Practice Center under Contract No HHSA 290-2007-10066-I)AHRQ Publication No 10-E005. Rockville (MD): Agency for Healthcare Research and Quality; 2010. p. 193.
163. Petitti DB. Meta analysis, decision analysis, and cost-effectiveness analysis: methods for quantitave syntesis in medicine. 2nd edition. New York: Oxford University Press; 2000.
164. State NIoH. National Institutes of Health State of the Science Conference statement: preventing Alzheimer's Disease and Cognitive Decline. Bethesda (MD), April 26–28, 2010.

Genomics for Disease Treatment and Prevention

Cinnamon S. Bloss, PhD[a], Dilip V. Jeste, MD[b],
Nicholas J. Schork, PhD[c],*

KEYWORDS

- Genomics • Genetic testing • Genetic risk assessment
- Public health genomics • Pharmacogenomics

The last decade has brought with it enormous advances in genetics and genomics. In parallel, there has been a growing sense that genomic technologies and discoveries will, sooner rather than later, revolutionize the practice of medicine and bring about a paradigm shift in the way we think of health care, including mental health care, for the individual. Specifically, it has been anticipated that these advances will eventually lead to a new model of health care centered on disease prevention and reinforced by disease treatments that are tailored to the individual. This vision of health care is in stark contrast to our current model, which is largely geared toward acute crisis intervention once disease is present and often progressed to the point of being irreversible. These facts raise several important questions. For example, where do things stand in terms of our ability to harness the fruits of genetic and genomic discovery for disease treatment and prevention? In terms of the science, what are the current research priorities? Furthermore, although few would, in theory, oppose the adoption of an improved health care system based on personalized medicine, are there social, economic, and policy barriers to moving forward on this front, in particular regarding adoption of policies centered on disease prevention?

This work was supported, in part, by the Stein Institute for Research on Aging, the Scripps Genomic Medicine Division of Scripps Health, the Scripps Translational Science Institute Clinical and Translational Science Award [grant number U54 RR0252204-01], and the UCSD Translational Science Institute Clinical and Translational Science Award [grant number 1UL1RR031980-01].

[a] The Scripps Translational Science Institute, 3344 North Torrey Pines Court, Suite 300, La Jolla, CA 92037, USA

[b] Department of Psychiatry and Neurosciences, Sam and Rose Stein Institute for Research on Aging, University of California, San Diego, 9500 Gilman Drive #0664, San Diego, CA 92093, USA

[c] Department of Molecular and Experimental Medicine, The Scripps Research Institute and the Scripps Translational Science Institute, 3344 North Torrey Pines Court, Suite 300, La Jolla, CA 92037, USA

* Corresponding author. The Scripps Research Institute, 3344 North Torrey Pines Court, Suite 300, La Jolla, CA 92037.

E-mail address: nschork@scripps.edu

Psychiatr Clin N Am 34 (2011) 147–166
doi:10.1016/j.psc.2010.11.005
0193-953X/11/$ – see front matter © 2011 Elsevier Inc. All rights reserved.

In brief, genomic medicine is the use of information from the genome to guide clinical decision making. Personalized medicine is a broader concept that refers to a model of health care emphasizing the use of each individual's unique clinical, genetic, genomic, and environmental information for disease prevention and treatment.[1] The state of science and technology is such that we can now examine and measure an individual's entire genome. Hence, individualized risk predictions and treatment decisions based on genomic information are theoretically possible, and in some instances, actually taking place. Personalized medicine draws on genomic medicine to leverage our knowledge of genetics and genomics for preventive health care, as well as administration of personalized, targeted therapies for individuals with existing conditions.

This article begins by providing a brief history of genetics followed by a review of heritability estimates for major chronic diseases as a way of highlighting the putative importance of genetics for disease treatment and prevention. It then provides a brief primer on genetics, genomics, and genome-wide association studies (GWAS), followed by an assessment of the extent to which advances in genetics and genomics are currently being applied clinically, both broadly and specifically in the context of mental health care. The authors attempt to pinpoint where (sometimes sizable) gaps in the science exist that ultimately preclude additional clinical applications. Next, priority research areas are proposed that ultimately will be of critical importance to fully harnessing genetics and genomics for disease treatment and prevention. Finally, the authors review the current social, economic, and public policy environments, which in some cases do not seem to be conducive to the adoption of genomic and personalized medicine, and suggest possible areas in which changes may be encouraged.

A BRIEF HISTORY OF GENETICS AND GENOMICS

It is important to be aware that genetics and genomics are complementary but different disciplines. Whereas genetics is the study of inheritance, or the way traits are passed down from one generation to another, genomics refers to the study of all the genes and gene products in an individual, as well as how those genes interact with one another and the environment.[2] In 1866, Gregor Mendel published his theories of inheritance based on hybridization experiments in garden peas. Although largely ignored until the early 1900s, his work is considered to form the basic theory of modern genetics. Mendel discovered that when he crossed a white flower and a purple flower plant, rather than being a mix of the two, the offspring were purple flowered. From several successive crosses, he developed the ideas of dominant and recessive inheritance in which dominant factors (purple flowered) will hide recessive factors (white flowered). Later, in the early 1900s, Sir Archibald Garrod described several human diseases that he termed "inborn errors of metabolism" (eg, albinism), which showed a similar pattern of inheritance to that of the white color in Mendel's hybridization experiments and thus suggested a genetic basis for these diseases.[3] Garrod described the nature of autosomal recessive inheritance (where two copies of an abnormal genetic variant or "allele" are needed to express the disease) with respect to these conditions, and using Mendelian principles illustrated that two parents heterozygous for the disease allele (ie, who carry only one copy) have a 1-in-4 chance of producing a child having both disease alleles and, hence, the unwanted disorder.

In 1909 Wilhelm Johannsen coined the term "gene," and in 1915 Thomas Morgan Hunt showed that genes, which exist on chromosomes, are the basic units of inheritance.[4] Over the next several years, many additional examples of diseases inherited in an autosomal recessive manner were discovered, including phenylketon-uria and cystic fibrosis. Autosomal dominant diseases (where only one copy of an abnormal allele is needed to express the disease) were also described, including Huntington's disease and Marfan's syndrome. X-linked recessive and X-linked domi-nant traits (see Glossary of Terms Appendix) were also discovered and described. Of importance is that disorders following these patterns of inheritance, termed "Mendelian disorders," have been among the easiest to analyze and the best under-stood. These disorders and modes of inheritance arguably have also led to a common fatalistic view among lay people that genes are deterministic and that if one inherits a disease allele, one will inherit an unwanted disorder. This view stands in opposition to more recent notions of the "susceptibility allele," based in large part on findings from the field of genomics, specifically GWAS, in which inheritance of a specific genetic variant does not guarantee the emergence of a disease, but merely confers some envi-ronmentally and/or other genetic factor mediated probability of developing a disease.[5]

In 1920 Hans Winkler coined the term "genome" to refer to all the genes in an organism by combining the words gene and chromosome.[6] Building on evidence that DNA, or deoxyribonucleic acid, was the primary component of chromosomes and genes, in 1953 James Watson and Francis Crick, with the help of Rosalind Franklin, discovered the double-helix structure of DNA, and in 1966 Marshall Niren-berg was credited with "cracking the genetic code" and describing how it operates to make proteins.[7] From these important discoveries, several downstream events occurred that began to reflect progression from the study of inheritance to the study of how genomic profiles could be used in medicine and in other arenas. For instance, in 1978 the biotechnology company Genentech, Inc. genetically engineered bacteria to produce human insulin (the first drug made through the use of recombinant DNA technology) for the treatment of diabetes,[8] and in 1983 scientists identified the gene responsible for Huntington's disease, which led to the first genetic test for a disease. In 1984, Sir Alec John Jeffreys developed DNA profiling or "fingerprinting" to be used in paternity testing and forensics, and in 1986 Richard Buckland was the first person acquitted of a crime based on DNA evidence. In 1989 Stephen Fodor, who later cofounded the gene chip company Affymetrix, developed the first DNA "microarray" and scanner, which would eventually lead to a method for testing hundreds of thou-sands of genetic variants simultaneously and thus foreshadowing the upcoming era of GWAS.[9]

More recently, two major research initiatives have led to the present-day "post-genomics" era: the Human Genome Project and the International HapMap Project. The goal of the Human Genome Project was to draft a reference human genome delin-eating the sequence of chemical base pairs that make up DNA, as well as to determine the location of the roughly 25,000 genes thought to populate the human genome. In 2000 a draft sequence was released[10,11] and in 2003 the final version was published. Related to this, the goal of the International HapMap Project[12,13] was to create a genome-wide database cataloging patterns of common human sequence variation within and across both individuals and populations. Of note, an explicit aim of the Hap-Map was to facilitate identification of commonly occurring, complex (ie, non-Mende-lian) disease-causing genetic variants based on the "common disease, common variant" hypothesis,[14] a hypothesis that incidentally has been called into question for explaining the genetic contributions to mental illness.[15] This hypothesis suggests that genetic influences on complex diseases are attributable to common allelic vari-ants present in more than 5% of the population. These variants represent "risk factors" or "susceptibility variants" for disease, as opposed to the more deterministic variants governed by Mendel's principles. Taken together with technological developments enabling cost-effective applications of DNA microarrays capable of measuring hundreds of thousands of genetic variants at once, these two initiatives led to the first[16] of many GWAS to be published. Although GWAS have some weaknesses, to be discussed in later sections of this article, it is this research paradigm (now together with whole-genome sequencing) that has generally been thought of as laying the groundwork for the era of genomic and personalized medicine.

HERITABILITY OF MAJOR CHRONIC DISEASES

It is important to make explicit the reasons for considering genetics and genomics to have substantial utility for disease treatment and prevention, especially given the obvious role of environmental (including behavioral) factors in the etiology of many conditions (eg, the role of smoking in the development of lung cancer), including neuropsychiatric disorders. Essentially, from family, twin, and adoption studies, researchers have been able to estimate the proportion of variance due to genetics (ie, "heritability") and the proportion of variance due to environment for a range of chronic diseases and other phenotypes. A heritability estimate of 1.0 indicates that all of the variation in a trait can be accounted for by genetics, and a heritability estimate of 0 indicates that all of the variation in a trait can be accounted for by nongenetic factors (eg, environment). **Table 1** gives heritability estimates for chronic disorders of aging, aging phenotypes, and major neuropsychiatric disorders. These estimates range from 0.25 for human longevity[17,18] to 0.85 for bipolar disorder,[19,20] indicating a strong genetic component with respect to many chronic diseases and phenotypes relevant for human health, including mental health. Ultimately, the large extent to which human disease can be attributable to genetic factors underscores the importance of genetics and genomics research and its impact on health care.[21]

GENETICS, GENOMICS, AND GWAS PRIMER

There are many study designs that have been successfully applied to genetic analyses. Here, however, the authors provide a primer that is primarily focused on GWAS, given that it is this paradigm that has recently provided a means of assessing

Table 1
Heritability estimates for chronic disorders of aging, aging phenotypes, and neuropsychiatric disorders

Disorder/Phenotype	Heritability Estimate	References
Obesity	0.77	84,85
Coronary heart disease	0.57	86
Type II diabetes	0.64	87
Colorectal cancer	0.35	88
Prostate cancer	0.42	88
Breast cancer	0.27	88
Alzheimer disease	0.74	89
Longevity	0.25	17,18
Schizophrenia	0.81	90
Bipolar disorder	0.85	19,20
Unipolar depression	0.37	91,92
Anxiety disorders	0.32	93,94

the entire genome to identify specific genetic differences among human beings that contribute to variation in disease susceptibility.

The human genome sequence comprises roughly 3 billion nucleotide bases (6 billion if one considers its diploid nature). Although more than 99% of that sequence does not differ from person to person, it is the differences in sequence that are of interest because it is these differences that, along with environmental/behavioral differences, contribute to phenotypic divergence. Variation in the DNA sequence can take different forms. By far the most common form of variation is characterized by sites in the sequence where individuals differ by a single base. These differences are known as single nucleotide polymorphisms or SNPs, and they occur, on average, at about 1 site per 300 bases.[22] More than 10 million SNPs are thought to be present in the human genome. SNPs are also relatively common such that, by definition, the minor allele of any given SNP is present in at least 5% of individuals. GWAS have traditionally focused on using high-throughput genotyping to assess SNP variation across the genome to identify sites where frequency differences exist between individuals with and without disease (or with and without a certain phenotype). One can imagine that genotyping 10 million sites in the genome could potentially be very expensive and time consuming. The genome, however, exhibits a structural property known as linkage disequilibrium, whereby large sections of DNA sequence within a given chromosome are highly correlated. This structural property allows a shortcut that makes GWAS cost-effective and feasible, in that representative SNPs (ie, "tag" SNPs) from each section of a correlated sequence can be genotyped and then used to infer genotypes at other unmeasured bases within the same section of sequence. These sections of correlated sequence are known as haplotypes. This method of genotyping tag SNPs across known haplotypes means that GWAS studies are possible with genotyping of only 500,000 to 1 million SNPs. Indeed, using this method, over the past 5 years or so more than 400 GWAS have been published identifying more than 150 risk variants for more than 60 common diseases and traits.[23]

Missing Heritability

GWAS have been a powerful tool for conducting unbiased scans of the genome to identify SNPs implicated in common, complex diseases, and represent an important advance compared with candidate gene studies. There is a wide gap, however, between the proportion of variance in disease susceptibility explained by the results of GWAS (usually between 1% and 10%) and the proportion of variance in disease susceptibility thought to be caused by genetics based on heritability estimates (see **Table 1**),[24,25] which can be as high as 50% or more. Furthermore, this is particularly true for neuropsychiatric disorders where GWAS have been less successful relative to studies of other common chronic aging-related diseases.[26] Many reasons for this missing heritability have been proposed, including the need for much larger sample sizes to detect additional SNPs of smaller effect that are yet to be found. In addition, rare variation (<1% frequency) and structural variation (eg, copy number variants, insertions, deletions, inversions, and translocations), forms of variation that are not well captured with most genotyping chips currently in use, likely account for some fraction of the unexplained genetic variability. Finally, low power to detect gene-gene interactions, inadequate examination of gene-environment interactions, phenotypic heterogeneity or imprecise phenotypic definition, and epigenomic alterations such as imprinting or parent-of-origin effects have also all been proposed as explanations for missing heritability.[25] Some of these explanations (eg, phenotypic heterogeneity) may be particularly relevant for explaining missing heritability in neuropsychiatric disorders. Furthermore, as mentioned previously, with regard to mental illness in particular, the "common disease, common variant" hypothesis has been called into question, and it has been proposed that an alternative evolution-informed framework, characterized by the importance of gene-environment interactions and rare variants, is more tenable for these types of disorders.[15] To some extent, it is this issue of unexplained genetic variance that has hindered the use of genomic information from GWAS for the development of clinically useful predictive tests for common, complex (non-Mendelian) diseases. In turn, this has limited the development of more targeted prevention strategies. The authors propose that one priority research area for leveraging genomics for disease prediction and prevention should be development of new strategies for finding and investigating the remaining heritability, especially in the area of neuropsychiatric diseases.

Sequencing and Other Research Strategies

DNA sequencing, which involves measuring each nucleotide base as opposed to just SNP variation and tag SNPs, is one approach for finding missing heritability that has wide support in the genetics community. This approach has the enormous benefit of providing information about all the different forms of common, as well as rare, genetic variation within the genome, including SNPs, copy number variations, insertion/deletions, inversions, and unique de novo single base mutations. Furthermore, although sequencing is currently limited to candidate genes, it is rapidly becoming more refined and cost-effective, such that whole-genome sequencing will likely become more widely available and feasible in the near future. In the aging and neuropsychiatric literature, there is little precedent for sequencing on a large scale; however, one recent example of this approach is a study by Halaschek-Wiener and colleagues[27] in which they sequenced 24 candidate aging genes in healthy adults aged 85 years or older. Of note, 41% of the genetic variants they identified were not previously recorded in existing genetic reference databases. This finding suggests that previous genetic strategies such as GWAS and candidate gene studies are likely unable to detect much of the genetic variation that underlies complex diseases and phenotypes, and that DNA sequencing will be critical in this regard. Several studies using this approach for studying neuropsychiatric diseases are also ongoing, including studies in schizophrenia, bipolar disorder, and anorexia nervosa.[28] In addition to sequencing, meta- and combined data set analysis (ie, "mega-analysis") of comparable, and in many cases publically available data,[29,30] can be leveraged to increase sample sizes and power to detect variants of smaller effect. Also, future GWAS can be improved by including more precisely measured phenotypes rather than the common "case-control" design, as well as measures of environmental exposures. Gene-gene interactions can also be investigated via a priori hypothesis testing. Finally, family data can be leveraged to better elucidate gene-environment interactions as well as parent-of-origin effects. The authors propose that accounting for the missing heritability in common chronic diseases, including neuropsychiatric diseases, will be an important hurdle to overcome in the use of genomics for making reliable and valid individual disease risk predictions and designing complementary targeted disease prevention strategies.

APPLICATIONS OF GENETICS AND GENOMICS IN DISEASE PREVENTION AND TREATMENT

This section discusses some of the major areas in which genetics and genomics are poised to make (and in some cases already have made) strong impacts on the practice of medicine.

Pharmacogenomics and Treatment Response

Pharmacogenomics is the study of genetic variation that is associated with the variable responses of individuals to any given drug treatment,[1] including individual differences in drug efficacy and susceptibility to adverse effects. This area of genomics provides possibly the best and clearest example of how genomics can be used to bring about more targeted and individualized treatments and actually influence clinical care. This area has already made a number of significant impacts in this regard. Specifically, over the past several years many associations between genetic variants and drug response have been discovered, including, for example, the now well-known association between CYP2C9 and VKORC1 gene variants and warfarin.[31]

Warfarin is one of the most commonly used anticoagulant medications, prescribed worldwide to prevent stroke and venous thromboembolism.[32] Unfortunately, however, dosing of warfarin is highly complex due to many factors that affect its metabolism, including clinical (drug-drug interactions, dietary interactions, age, and body surface area) and genetic factors, in particular variants in the genes CYP2C9 and VKORC1.[33,34] In fact, it is estimated that consideration of combined genotypes across variants in these genes, together with factors such as age and body size, account for 35% to 60% of the variability in warfarin dosing requirements. Evidence for the importance of these variants in influencing warfarin metabolism led the US Food and Drug Administration (FDA) to update the labeling of warfarin in 2007 to include a statement acknowledging the importance and potential of genotyping during the early phase of dosing.[35] This particular update, however, did not dictate how physicians should change the dosage based on genotype. Based on additional research since then, the FDA again updated its warfarin labeling in 2010 to include specific ranges of initial doses assigned to each genotype representing the expected steady-state maintenance doses.

To the extent that pharmacogenomic research efforts and resulting label updates by the FDA lead to improved drug safety and efficacy, this represents a real step forward in the use of genomics for disease treatment (and prevention of adverse effects) and for ushering in a new era of personalized medicine. Other examples of pharmacogenomic associations and FDA label updates are included in **Table 2**.[35] In brief, azathioprine and 6-mercaptopurine (6-MP) are immunosuppressants used to treat some cancers, as well as autoimmune diseases such as rheumatoid arthritis and Crohn's disease. Genetic testing for variants in the TPMT gene have been found to be associated with adverse side effects, including severe myelotoxicity, and the 6-MP label was the first label to be updated in the last decade based on pharmacogenomic information. A similar association was found between irinotecan, an anticancer chemotherapy drug, and variations in the gene UGT1A1. This label update was the first to recommend a specific dosing reduction based on pharmacogenomics because of an increased risk of neutropenia in patients with certain genotypes. In terms of mental health and applications to neurological disorders, carbamazepine, an anticonvulsant and mood stabilizer used in the treatment of epilepsy, bipolar disorder, trigeminal neuralgia, and other neuropsychiatric disorders, has shown an association with variants in HLA-B*1502. Specifically, genotyping of variants in HLA-B*1502 can identify individuals at risk for Stevens-Johnson syndrome and toxic epidermal necrolysis, 2 forms of rare but potentially fatal skin diseases.[36] Similarly, associations between abacavir and variants in HLA-B*5701 have also been shown to predict adverse drug effects. Finally, another notable pharmacogenomic association is that between genetic variants in CYP2C19 and metabolism of clopidogrel, which is used in at-risk patients to prevent strokes and heart attacks. In 2010, the label of clopidogrel was

Table 2
Select pharmacogenomic medication label updates by the Food and Drug Administration in the past 10 years

Genetic Variant	Medication	Rationale for Testing and Label Update
TPMT	Azathioprine/ 6-mercaptopurine	Can identify individuals at increased risk for severe, life-threatening myelotoxicity
UGT1A1	Irinotecan	Can identify individuals at increased risk of neutropenia
CYP2C9 & VKORC1	Warfarin	Can more precisely identify appropriate initial doses for individuals to avoid well-known risks of minor and major bleeding
HLA-B*1502	Carbamazepine	Can identify individuals at increased risk for potentially life-threatening dermatological side effects
HLA-B*5701	Abacavir	Can identify individuals with increased risk of hypersensitivity reaction
CYP2C19	Clopidogrel	Can identify individuals who are less responsive and may not receive full protection from heart attacks, stroke, and cardiovascular death

Data from Lesko LJ, Zineh I. DNA, drugs and chariots: on a decade of pharmacogenomics at the US FDA. Pharmacogenomics 2010;11(4):507–12; and Table of valid genomic biomarkers in the context of approved drug labels. 2010. Available at: http://www.fda.gov/Drugs/ScienceResearch/ResearchAreas/Pharmacogenetics/ucm083378.htm. Accessed July 20, 2010.

updated with a warning that patients carrying variants associated with poor metabolism of the drug may be less responsive to the medication and thus fail to receive full protection from heart attacks, stroke, and cardiovascular death.[37]

While pharmacogenomic research and findings have led the FDA to take major steps forward in translating genomic findings into better, individualized disease treatments, there is still much work to be done. For example, with respect to pharmacogenomics in psychiatry, limited evidence from twin and family studies suggests that response to antipsychotic and antidepressant medications are heritable traits. Specifically, studies on single pairs of monozygotic twins observed similar response to treatment with antipsychotics[38] and similar levels of drug-induced weight gain,[39] and studies on siblings and first-degree relatives observed similarities in treatment-induced tardive dyskinesia and response to antidepressants.[40,41] Furthermore, genetic variants in the HLA complex have been associated with risk of drug-induced agranulocytosis, which led a biotechnology company to develop and offer a genetic test for the determination of high (1.5%) or low (0.5%) risk in conjunction with prescription of clozapine.[42] This test, however, has not been widely adopted by physicians,[43] and the FDA has not updated labels of major antidepressants or antipsychotics, in part because of difficulties replicating findings in this area and a lack of large-scale controlled studies. Another issue that may inhibit translation of pharmacogenomic findings into the clinic is a lack of adequate training of community physicians in pharmacogenomics. Furthermore, the clinical availability of genetic testing for pharmacogenomic variants is still limited in many areas, and there remain important questions with respect to insurance reimbursement and who will pay for testing.

Although not a pharmacogenomic association per se, another genetic association that may have implications for the treatment of unipolar depression is the well-studied gene-environment interaction between the promoter region of the serotonin transporter gene (5-HTTLPR) and stressful life events. In a large cohort, childhood abuse and stressful life events were associated with a high risk of becoming depressed in individuals with the short allele of the 5-HTTLPR, but had little effect on the development of depression among long-allele homozygotes.[44] Further work stemming from this initial report suggests that the finding has more general implications in that this variant is likely not directly associated with depression, but that the 5-HTTLPR, together with polymorphisms in other genes such as BDNF and CRHR1,[45] are more broadly associated with personal dispositions that are more or less sensitive to environmental surroundings. In terms of treatment for depression, psychological therapy and antidepressant medications have, on average, comparable efficacy in unselected groups of patients diagnosed with depression. Of importance, however, the potential gene-environment interaction involving 5-HTTLPR suggests that individuals who are more sensitive to environmental stimuli may respond better to psychological treatments than to antidepressant medication.[45,46] Although this particular gene-environment interaction has been called into question in recent years,[47] these findings illustrate the potential importance of further study of gene-environment interactions in other contexts, as well as the potential implications of such findings for disease treatment and prevention in psychiatry. Another issue particularly relevant for mental health conditions such as depression is that of placebo effects and the cyclical nature of the conditions themselves, which both have implications for drug and pharmacogenomic discovery in this particular disease area.

Predictive and Disease Susceptibility Testing

The clinical validity and utility of predictive testing for disease based on genetic information currently varies dramatically, depending on the mode of inheritance of the disease, what is known about the specific genetic variants implicated, and protective variants that may be important, as well as the degree of redundancy of genetic information with other traditional risk factors that are routinely, easily, and more inexpensively assessed clinically (eg, family history of disease). For instance, work that has uncovered the genetic variations involved in diseases that are inherited according to simple Mendelian principles has led to the development and availability of predictive genetic tests that have nearly 100% accuracy. Thus, a decade after the Huntington's disease gene was mapped to chromosome 4, the pathogenic mutation was localized and identified as a CAG-repeat expansion[48] for which testing is now available to offspring of individuals with the disease. This predictive test has high reliability, validity, and clinical utility given the mode of inheritance of the disease and the fact that the causal mutation is known and can be measured. Furthermore, test results indicating the presence of the CAG-repeat provide information that is not redundant with standard clinical risk factors such as family history (ie, one can have a family history and still not inherit Huntington's disease), and therefore has high clinical and personal utility.

Similarly, genetic linkage studies in families with hereditary breast, ovarian, and colon cancers have identified several important high-penetrance genetic variants, which are now currently being used for screening, disease risk counseling, and preventive treatment programs for breast cancer.[49] For example, although breast cancer is a complex disease (ie, non-Mendelian), the high-penetrance susceptibility genetic variations identified, specifically variations in the BRCA1 and BRCA2 genes, confer a 50% to 80% chance of developing breast cancer by age 70 years.[50] Thus, a positive test result in this case provides critical additional information (beyond clinical risk factors) with respect to degree of disease risk. Furthermore, based on genetic test results, changes in surveillance practices (eg, frequency of mammography) or even decisions as to whether to undergo prophylactic surgery to decrease risk are often recommended[51] by health care providers.

By contrast, susceptibility testing in the case of common, complex diseases for which no high-penetrance risk variants have been identified is highly controversial (though currently performed in some contexts). As alluded to previously, it is likely that most complex diseases are caused by multiple environmental factors and multiple low-penetrance common genetic factors, possibly together with rare variations that are yet to be identified. This etiology is illustrated by the fact that most of the risk variants underlying complex diseases that have been identified through GWAS thus far have been characterized by effect sizes that are small, with odds ratios typically between 1.1 and 1.5. In addition, for most diseases, the variants identified explain little of the total genetic variance known from heritability estimates (see **Table 1**). Nevertheless, work in this area continues to determine the feasibility of combining information from many small-effect risk variants to develop more complex algorithms that can accurately predict an individual's genetic risk for common, complex diseases,[52] including risk for neuropsychiatric disease.[53] Early studies suggest, however, that while the use of combined genotypes of small-effect variants identified to date is informative, this approach does not necessarily confer improved risk predictions when compared with traditional clinical risk factors alone,[54] as there is often much redundancy. Thus, this hinders, to some extent, broader-scale preventive efforts based on susceptibility testing for complex diseases using genomic information derived from GWAS.

Susceptibility testing using genomic information may also benefit from utilization of protective genetic variants; however, research to discover such variants is incomplete. For example, although much work is ongoing to identify variants associated with healthy aging, findings are controversial[55] and, to the authors' knowledge, broadly applicable algorithms to predict longevity that take into account the frequency of the phenotype have not been constructed. In addition, identification of genetic variants associated with protective traits such as optimism and resilience[56] may serve to further clarify risk predictions, particularly for neuropsychiatric disorders; however, to date there has been a lack of needed studies in this area.

Personal/Consumer Genomics

Although highly controversial,[57] leveraging recent findings from GWAS together with high-throughput SNP genotyping technology, several companies[58–61] now offer commercially available tests that aim to calculate an individual's genetic risk for between 20 and 40 common, complex diseases using genome-wide genotyping. The purchase of these tests is ultimately initiated by consumers without the obligatory involvement of a health care provider.[62] Costs currently range from $100 to more than $2000 per individual, depending on the specific test and the company from which the test is purchased. Neurological/neuropsychiatric disorders that are represented across testing panels for the major personal genetic testing companies include Alzheimer's disease, multiple sclerosis, and amyotrophic lateral sclerosis.

This type of testing is hotly debated for the aforementioned reasons as well as the small effect sizes of SNP variants identified from GWAS, and the fact that these variants explain only a small fraction of the total genetic variance and only confer small increases in disease risk. Even so, personal genetic testing proponents argue that providing this type of information directly to consumers can empower them to take control of their health by improving their compliance with health screening practices and by making more healthful lifestyle choices (ie, make efforts to modify their disease risk). On the other hand, critics are concerned that there is a lack of research on how best to present this type of risk information to individual consumers to ensure adequate understanding of the results,[63] as well as on how individual consumers are likely to respond to their results. Researchers focusing on the ethical, legal, and social implications of such testing have noted that it is an open question as to whether this type of susceptibility testing would lead consumers to (a) make positive health behavior changes in response to their results; (b) adopt more fatalistic attitudes and/or experience high levels of anxiety in response to estimates of high risk; or perhaps worse yet, (c) be falsely reassured by inaccurate or incomplete estimates of low risk. This possibility becomes particularly problematic in light of recent evidence calling into question the consistency and accuracy of the risk estimates provided.[64,65] In fairness to genetic studies, however, it is important to emphasize that all clinical testing and health care guidance from physicians and other health care providers (eg, routine blood chemistries) suffer from some degree of variability and inconsistency. Studies are ongoing, including the authors' Scripps Genomic Health Initiative, to shed light on some of these issues, in particular the behavioral and psychological response to testing[66] and genomic risk disclosure.

Diagnosis, Prognosis, and Monitoring

In addition to DNA sequence-based testing, which is stable and does not change over the course of a person's lifetime, genomic biomarkers such as whole-genome gene expression are now starting to be used in diagnosis, prognosis, and monitoring of disease. Such transcriptomic, proteomic, and/or metabolomic profiles, combined with other testing and clinical factors, may provide assistance in diagnosing individuals at the earliest possible subclinical stages of disease when preventive strategies can be employed and treatments are more effective, or after a diagnosis has been made but differentiation of disease subtype is needed to guide intervention and drug treatment plans. The use of such markers for diagnosis and subtype differentiation in neuropsychiatric disorders may be particularly useful given the difficulties often encountered in differential diagnosis.

There are some instances in which genomic biomarkers are currently being used in clinical care. For instance, whole-genome gene expression data are now being used routinely to identify subtypes of cancer, including new subclasses of tumors within acute myeloid leukemia,[67] as well as distinguishing between Burkitt lymphoma and diffuse B-cell lymphoma.[68] Moreover, in the clinical management of cancer, genomic signatures are even moving beyond classification and diagnosis and are further being used to predict prognosis and response to therapy. For example, gene expression signatures have been used to develop profiles that can predict prognosis in early-stage non-small-cell lung cancer,[69] as well as predict sensitivity and response to individual chemotherapeutic drugs, which can help with monitoring and guide the use of these drugs alone and in combination with existing therapies.[70,71] Additional work with respect to disease monitoring has involved the use of gene expression in peripheral blood mononuclear cells for predicting graft rejection in the area of solid organ transplantation.[72]

In many ways, cancer provides an ideal opportunity for the use of biomarkers such as those obtained from whole-genome gene expression data, because the disease lesion usually resides in an accessible tissue (ie, the tumor) that can be biopsied and measured directly. In general, affected tissues in neuropsychiatric and other diseases that affect mental health (eg, the brain) are less accessible and more difficult to measure in living patients, making the development of preventive and treatment opportunities based on such biomarkers difficult. The general strategy regarding the development of biomarkers for neuropsychiatric disorders is to measure gene expression or other markers in surrogate tissues, such as blood or cerebrospinal fluid. For example, artificial neural networks analysis of blood gene expression patterns was recently used to classify 52 antipsychotics-free schizophrenia patients and 49 controls with almost 88% accuracy,[73] suggesting that blood-based gene expression may have utility as a diagnostic tool for schizophrenia. In addition, similar studies have been performed in Parkinson's disease,[74] Huntington's disease,[75] and Alzheimer's disease[76]; however, to the authors' knowledge none of these expression profiles are currently being used clinically. Recently, telomeres, which are DNA sequences at the ends of chromosomes that are thought to protect chromosomes from damage, have also been studied within the context of disorders of aging, and to some extent in neuropsychiatric disease. For instance, leukocyte telomere length has been associated with many diseases and phenotypes, including risk of Alzheimer's disease, cognitive aging, cardiovascular disease, and poststroke mortality.[77]

SOCIAL, ECONOMIC, AND POLICY ISSUES FOR GENOMIC MEDICINE

As described thus far, there are significant scientific challenges that still need to be overcome for the vision of genomic and personalized medicine to become a reality, and this is true to an even greater degree for the area of mental health. In addition, however, it is important to consider other issues outside of genomic science that may be involved, such as social, economic, and policy issues.

Pharmaceutical, Biotechnology, and Insurance Companies

Early in the drug development process, pharmaceutical and biotechnology companies often use genomic and other biomarkers to aid in research and development; however, it is only in some cases that they develop these markers as commercially available companion diagnostics that can be used to identify a patient's likelihood of responding to a drug or experiencing an adverse event. Although there are several reasons for this and the process of drug development is complex, one primary reason is that there is often considerable risk in the development of such personalized medicine tests for a given drug because these tests can serve to divide the treatable patient population into subsegments, which can then decrease market share[78] and potential profits. Some research has suggested that companies are most likely to include companion diagnostics for "later-to-market" drugs that enter into crowded markets. For instance, if two drugs are already on the market and are relatively undifferentiated, the third drug on the market is likely to capture a relatively small market share. A companion diagnostic for the third drug, however, that identifies a segment of the patient population that will respond particularly well or experience fewer adverse events, could generate higher pricing and thus added value.[79]

Similarly, although it has been widely predicted that personalized medicine will dramatically reduce health care costs, insurance companies have been reluctant to provide reimbursements for "personalized medicine tests." Several reasons have been put forth for this reluctance,[78] including an inability to easily identify tests that truly reduce costs. In brief, per patient savings (ie, the difference between the cost of treating the disease and the cost of the treatment intervention indicated by the test), as well as the likelihood that a test suggests an intervention for any particular patient, are two primary factors that determine a test's cost-effectiveness. Tests that help to avoid the use of expensive therapies, minimize costly adverse events, or delay expensive procedures can be cost-effective; however, tests that only save a small amount per patient or that have a low probability of identifying patients requiring an intervention (eg, testing all-comers for a rare disease) are not cost-effective. In addition, adoption is further complicated by the high customer turnover experienced by many insurance companies in the United States, which is particularly salient in terms of reimbursement for prophylactic tests and preventive interventions. Specifically, this high turnover makes it less economical for companies to reimburse for tests and interventions that minimize the likelihood of conditions that will occur much later in life (ie, when customers may have switched their coverage to another company). Other concerns that have been expressed by payers include difficulties in enforcing standard protocols to ensure that physicians follow through with appropriate patient care based on test results, and potential misuse of test information (particularly in the early stages of development) in ways that could harm patients.[78] Further, companies are affected by the fact that agencies like the FDA often struggle with what constitutes evidence that a drug should really only be given to a certain group of individuals. For instance, are restricted trials required or is retrospective data sufficient?

There are clearly some instances in which there are incentives for both pharmaceutical/biotechnology and insurance companies to invest in personalized medicine; however, it is also apparent that there are several situations in which it is currently economically disadvantageous for them to do so. It is an open question as to whether these relevant "stakeholders" will be willing to work together and with regulatory bodies to reshape incentive structures.

Physicians and Legislation

Potential issues have also been raised regarding provider (eg, physician) incentives/disincentives for adopting personalized medicine. In particular, there are concerns raised by the fact that the current, procedure-based reimbursement system confers economic rewards to providers based on performing increasing numbers of procedures. As such, providers may be more likely to adopt personalized medicine tests that increase the number of procedures performed after testing (eg, they may be more likely to adopt genetic susceptibility testing for colon cancer if it might lead to more frequent colonoscopies for a given patient).[78] Tests that ultimately decrease the likelihood of future procedures (or are neutral), however, may be less likely to be adopted. Another potential issue concerning physicians is reflected by recent findings that only 1 in 10 physicians felt he or she had the necessary training and knowledge in genomics[80] to provide adequate care in this area to their patients. Thus, lack of appropriate training and education in genomics may be a significant hindrance to adoption of personalized medicine tests as well, although it is encouraging that there are some recent initiatives to bring about changes in this area.[81]

In terms of legislative initiatives, there is evidence that personalized medicine is a priority health care issue for the United States (**Table 3**). For instance, recent enactment of the Genetic Information Non-Discrimination Act (GINA) to ensure genetic privacy, the Health and Human Services Personalized Health Care Initiative to support research addressing individual aspects of disease prevention, and the Genomics and Personalized Medicine Act introduced in Congress, all suggest the support of many policy makers for personalized medicine.[1] In addition, it is notable that the Ethical, Legal, and Social Issues branch of the Human Genome Project[82] was initiated specifically to deal with outcomes and "fall-out" from this large-scale initiative. There are few other areas of science where similar programs have been initiated for such reasons. However, more work is needed, especially to the extent that government-sponsored

Table 3
Legislative acts and initiatives supporting genomic medicine

Legislative Acts/Initiatives	Description	References
Genetic Information Non-Discrimination Act	Protects against discrimination based on genetic information regarding health insurance and employment	95
Health and Human Services Personalized Health Care Initiative	Provides federal leadership supporting research addressing individual aspects of disease and disease prevention. Goal is to shape preventive and diagnostic care to match each person's unique genetic characteristics	96
Genomics and Personalized Medicine Act	A bill to improve access to and appropriate use of valid, reliable, and accurate molecular genetic tests by all populations	97
Ethical, Legal, and Social Issues (ELSI) Research in Genomics	The US Department of Energy and the National Institutes of Health devote 3%–5% of their annual Human Genome Program budgets toward studying the ELSI surrounding availability of genetic information. This represents the world's largest bioethics program	82

Data from Ginsburg GS, Willard HF. Genomic and personalized medicine: foundations and applications. Transl Res 2009;154(6):277–87.

initiatives can encourage other relevant stakeholders (eg, insurance companies) to work together to update existing policies.

Public Health Genomics

While the pace of genetic and genomic technology has been rapid, many have noted that the complementary work in behavioral and public health arenas needed to translate findings into clinical applications for disease treatment and prevention has lagged far behind.[83] One obvious reason for this is that there is much disagreement about whether genomic discovery is at a point where translation into clinical applications is appropriate (eg, the controversial "personal genetic testing" described previously). To begin to address this gap, in 2008 the National Human Genome Research Institute (NHGRI) convened a 2-day workshop that brought together a group of 50 scientists representing a broad range of disciplines including public health, communication, behavioral and social sciences, genetics, epidemiology, medicine, and public policy. When asked to recommend forward-looking priorities for translational research, the group identified three priority research areas: (1) improving the public's "genetic literacy" to enhance consumer skills; (2) gauging whether genomic information improves risk communication and adoption of healthier behaviors more than current approaches and public health interventions; and (3) exploring whether genomic discovery in concert with emerging technologies can elucidate new behavioral intervention targets.[83] It is anticipated that these themes may help inform development of funding priorities, and this effort on the part of the NHGRI underscores the attention being given to and importance being placed on development of behavioral and public health efforts needed for translation of genomic discoveries.

SUMMARY AND FUTURE DIRECTIONS

In summary, this article has reviewed the status of genomic scientific discovery, current applications of genomics for disease treatment and prevention, and relevant social, economic, and policy issues in genomics. Through this, an attempt has been made to highlight exciting areas where genetic and genomic discoveries are already being used in the clinic to improve health care, including mental health care (eg, pharmacogenomics). However, the authors have tried to pinpoint where sizable gaps in the science exist that ultimately preclude additional clinical applications (eg, lack of validity and utility of susceptibility testing for common, complex disease based on information derived from GWAS) and to suggest priority areas for further research (eg, DNA sequencing in neuropsychiatric disease, public health genomics). Also noted is the important role of nonscientific issues (eg, insurance reimbursement policies, level of physician education in the area of genomics) that will no doubt play a pivotal role in the speed with which genetics and genomics are, and continue to be, harnessed to bring about personalized medicine. In short, while the pace of genetic and genomic science, technology, and discovery has been rapid, more work is needed to fully realize the potential for impacting disease treatment and prevention generally, and mental health specifically.

APPENDIX: GLOSSARY OF TERMS

Allele – an alternative form of a genetic variant

Autosomal dominant – a pattern of inheritance in which an affected individual has one copy of an abnormal allele and one normal allele on a pair of nonsex chromosomes

Autosomal recessive – a pattern of inheritance in which an affected individual has 2 copies of an abnormal allele on a pair of nonsex chromosomes

Biomarker – a substance used as an indicator of a biological state (eg, DNA sequence, gene expression)

Copy number variant (CNV) – a DNA sequence of hundreds to thousands of base pairs that is present a variable number of times across individuals

Complex disorder – disorder with a genetic component, but without a clear-cut pattern of inheritance

DNA sequencing – refers to sequencing methods for measuring and determining the order of all the nucleotide bases in a molecule of DNA

Epigenomics – an emerging area of genomics that involves the study of changes in the regulation of gene activity and expression that are not dependent on gene sequence

Genomic medicine – the use of information from the genome to guide clinical decision making

Haplotype – a region of the genome on a given chromosome containing strongly correlated SNPs

Heritability – the proportion of phenotypic variation in a population that is attributable to genetic variation among individuals

Human Genome Project – a 13-year effort coordinated by the US Department of Energy and the National Institutes of Health to identify all the approximately 20,000 to 25,000 genes in human DNA, determine the sequences of the 3 billion chemical base pairs that make up human DNA, store this information in databases, improve tools for data analysis, transfer related technologies to the private sector, and address the ethical, legal, and social issues that may arise from the project

International HapMap Project – a multi-country effort to identify and catalog genetic similarities and differences in human beings across individuals and populations, and to identify chromosomal regions where genetic variants are shared

Linkage disequilibrium – the nonrandom association of alleles at 2 or more sites on the same chromosome

Mendelian disorder – disorder caused by a single gene defect, which tends to occur in either dominant or recessive inheritance patterns

Personal/consumer genomics – controversial genetic testing services in which Internet-based companies provide, for a fee, information on an individual's genomic makeup and risk for 20 to 40 common, complex diseases with varying levels of detail and interpretation

Personalized medicine – a broad concept that refers to a model of health care emphasizing the use of each individual's unique clinical, genetic, genomic, and environmental information for disease prevention and treatment

Pharmacogenomics – the branch of pharmacology and genomics that deals with the influence of genetic variation on drug response in patients by correlating DNA sequence variants or other biomarkers with a drug's efficacy or toxicity

Public health genomics – the branch of genomics that studies and promotes the integration of genomics into public health research, policy, and practice to prevent disease and improve the health of all people

Single nucleotide polymorphism (SNP) – a site within the genome that differs by a single nucleotide base across different individuals

X-linked dominant – a pattern of inheritance by which a dominant allele is carried on the X chromosome

X-linked recessive – a pattern of inheritance in which an allele on the X chromosome causes the phenotype to be expressed (1) in males and (2) in females who are homozygous for the allele

REFERENCES

1. Ginsburg GS, Willard HF. Genomic and personalized medicine: foundations and applications. Transl Res 2009;154(6):277–87.
2. Genomics frequently asked questions. 2008. Available at: http://www.ct.gov/dph/cwp/view.asp?a=3134&every=387810. Accessed July 18, 2010.
3. Nebert DW, Zhang G, Vesell ES. From human genetics and genomics to pharmacogenetics and pharmacogenomics: past lessons, future directions. Drug Metab Rev 2008;40(2):187–224.
4. Colby B. Outsmart your genes: online companion to the book and guide to predictive medicine. 2010. Available at: http://www.outsmartyourgenes.com/history.html. Accessed July 18, 2010.
5. Lander ES, Schork NJ. Genetic dissection of complex traits. Science 1994; 265(5181):2037–48.
6. Lederberg J, McCray AT. Ome sweet 'omics—a genealogical treasury of words. The Scientist 2001;15(7).
7. Leder P. Retrospective. Marshall Warren Nirenberg (1927–2010). Science 2010; 327(5968):972.
8. First successful laboratory production of human insulin announced. San Francisco (CA): Genentech, Inc; 1978.

9. Lander ES, Weinberg RA. Genomics: journey to the center of biology. Science 2000;287(5459):1777–82.

10. Venter JC, Adams MD, Myers EW, et al. The sequence of the human genome. Science 2001;291(5507):1304–51.

11. Lander ES, Linton LM, Birren B, et al. Initial sequencing and analysis of the human genome. Nature 2001;409(6822):860–921.

12. International HapMap Consortium. The International HapMap Project. Nature 2003;426(6968):789–96.

13. International HapMap Consortium. A haplotype map of the human genome. Nature 2005;437(7063):1299–320.

14. Collins FS, Guyer MS, Charkravarti A. Variations on a theme: cataloging human DNA sequence variation. Science 1997;278(5343):1580–1.

15. Uher R. The role of genetic variation in the causation of mental illness: an evolution-informed framework. Mol Psychiatry 2009;14(12):1072–82.

16. Klein RJ, Zeiss C, Chew EY, et al. Complement factor H polymorphism in age-related macular degeneration. Science 2005;308(5720):385–9.

17. Cournil A, Kirkwood TB. If you would live long, choose your parents well. Trends Genet 2001;17(5):233–5.

18. Gudmundsson H, Gudbjartsson DF, Frigge M, et al. Inheritance of human longevity in Iceland. Eur J Hum Genet 2000;8(10):743–9.

19. McGuffin P, Rijsdijk F, Andrew M, et al. The heritability of bipolar affective disorder and the genetic relationship to unipolar depression. Arch Gen Psychiatry 2003; 60(5):497–502.

20. Kieseppa T, Partonen T, Haukka J, et al. High concordance of bipolar I disorder in a nationwide sample of twins. Am J Psychiatry 2004;161(10):1814–21.

21. Feldman MW, Lewontin RC. The heritability hang-up. Science 1975;190(4220): 1163–8.

22. Manolio TA, Brooks LD, Collins FS. A HapMap harvest of insights into the genetics of common disease. J Clin Invest 2008;118(5):1590–605.

23. Manolio TA, Collins FS. The HapMap and genome-wide association studies in diagnosis and therapy. Annu Rev Med 2009;60:443–56.

24. Vineis P, Pearce N. Missing heritability in genome-wide association study research. Nat Rev Genet 2010;11(8):589.

25. Manolio TA, Collins FS, Cox NJ, et al. Finding the missing heritability of complex diseases. Nature 2009;461(7265):747–53.

26. Bloss CS, Schiabor KM, Schork NJ. Human behavioral informatics in genetic studies of neuropsychiatric disease: multivariate profile-based analysis. Brain Res Bull 2010;83(3–4):177–88.

27. Halaschek-Wiener J, Amirabbasi-Beik M, Monfared N, et al. Genetic variation in healthy oldest-old. PLoS One 2009;4(8):e6641.

28. Scott AA, Bloss CS, Murray SS, et al. Large scale candidate gene resequencing in anorexia nervosa. San Diego (CA): World Congress of Psychiatric Genetics; 2009.

29. Park JH, Wacholder S, Gail MH, et al. Estimation of effect size distribution from genome-wide association studies and implications for future discoveries. Nat Genet 2010;42(7):570–5.

30. dbGaP: genotypes and phenotypes. Available at: http://www.ncbi.nlm.nih.gov/gap. Accessed August 20, 2010.

31. PharmGKB: pharmacogenomics knowledge base. Available at: http://www.pharmgkb.org/. Accessed August 20, 2010.

32. Elias DJ, Topol EJ. Warfarin pharmacogenomics: a big step forward for individualized medicine: enlightened dosing of warfarin. Eur J Hum Genet 2008;16(5):532–4.

33. Carlquist JF, Horne BD, Muhlestein JB, et al. Genotypes of the cytochrome p450 isoform, CYP2C9, and the vitamin K epoxide reductase complex subunit 1 conjointly determine stable warfarin dose: a prospective study. J Thromb Thrombolysis 2006;22(3):191–7.
34. Rieder MJ, Reiner AP, Gage BF, et al. Effect of VKORC1 haplotypes on transcriptional regulation and warfarin dose. N Engl J Med 2005;352(22):2285–93.
35. Lesko LJ, Zineh I. DNA, drugs and chariots: on a decade of pharmacogenomics at the US FDA. Pharmacogenomics 2010;11(4):507–12.
36. Ferrell PB Jr, McLeod HL. Carbamazepine, HLA-B*1502 and risk of Stevens-Johnson syndrome and toxic epidermal necrolysis: US FDA recommendations. Pharmacogenomics 2008;9(10):1543–6.
37. Table of valid genomic biomarkers in the context of approved drug labels. 2010. Available at: http://www.fda.gov/Drugs/ScienceResearch/ResearchAreas/Pharmacogenetics/ucm083378.htm. Accessed July 20, 2010.
38. Vojvoda D, Grimmell K, Sernyak M, et al. Monozygotic twins concordant for response to clozapine. Lancet 1996;347(8993):61.
39. Wehmeier PM, Gebhardt S, Schmidtke J, et al. Clozapine: weight gain in a pair of monozygotic twins concordant for schizophrenia and mild mental retardation. Psychiatry Res 2005;133(2–3):273–6.
40. Muller DJ, Schulze TG, Knapp M, et al. Familial occurrence of tardive dyskinesia. Acta Psychiatr Scand 2001;104(5):375–9.
41. Franchini L, Serretti A, Gasperini M, et al. Familial concordance of fluvoxamine response as a tool for differentiating mood disorder pedigrees. J Psychiatr Res 1998;32(5):255–9.
42. Clinical data achieves validation of genetic biomarker for determining risk of clozapine induced agranulocytosis. 2006. Available at: http://www.clda.com/uploads/Clozapine-April19-FINAL.pdf. Accessed July 18, 2010.
43. Arranz MJ, Kapur S. Pharmacogenetics in psychiatry: are we ready for widespread clinical use? Schizophr Bull 2008;34(6):1130–44.
44. Caspi A, Sugden K, Moffitt TE, et al. Influence of life stress on depression: moderation by a polymorphism in the 5-HTT gene. Science 2003;301(5631):386–9.
45. Uher R. The implications of gene-environment interactions in depression: will cause inform cure? Mol Psychiatry 2008;13(12):1070–8.
46. Nemeroff CB, Heim CM, Thase ME, et al. Differential responses to psychotherapy versus pharmacotherapy in patients with chronic forms of major depression and childhood trauma. Proc Natl Acad Sci U S A 2003;100(24):14293–6.
47. Risch N, Herrell R, Lehner T, et al. Interaction between the serotonin transporter gene (5-HTTLPR), stressful life events, and risk of depression: a meta-analysis. JAMA 2009;301(23):2462–71.
48. Bates GP. History of genetic disease: the molecular genetics of Huntington disease—a history. Nat Rev Genet 2005;6(10):766–73.
49. Huang E, Huang A. Breast cancer and genomic medicine. In: Willard H, Ginsburg GS, editors. Genomic and personalized medicine. Durham (NC): Elsevier; 2009. p. 869–78.
50. Memorial Sloan-Kettering Cancer Center: breast/ovarian cancer: BRCA1 & BRCA2. 2010. Available at: http://www.mskcc.org/mskcc/html/8623.cfm#45826. Accessed July 22, 2010.
51. Schwartz GF, Hughes KS, Lynch HT, et al. Proceedings of the international consensus conference on breast cancer risk, genetics, risk management, April, 2007. Cancer 2008;113(10):2627–37.

52. Wray NR, Goddard ME, Visscher PM. Prediction of individual genetic risk of complex disease. Curr Opin Genet Dev 2008;18(3):257–63.
53. Purcell SM, Wray NR, Stone JL, et al. Common polygenic variation contributes to risk of schizophrenia and bipolar disorder. Nature 2009;460(7256):748–52.
54. Meigs JB, Shrader P, Sullivan LM, et al. Genotype score in addition to common risk factors for prediction of type 2 diabetes. N Engl J Med 2008;359(21): 2208–19.
55. Sebastiani P, Solovieff N, Puca A, et al. Genetic signatures of exceptional longevity in humans. Science 2010. DOI:10.1126/science.1190532.
56. Lamond AJ, Depp CA, Allison M, et al. Measurement and predictors of resilience among community-dwelling older women. J Psychiatr Res 2008;43(2):148–54.
57. Pollack A. F.D.A. Faults companies on unapproved genetic tests. New York: The New York Times; 2010.
58. Available at: http://www.navigenics.com/. Accessed June 4, 2009.
59. Available at: http://www.decodeme.com/. Accessed June 4, 2009.
60. Available at: https://www.23andme.com/. Accessed June 4, 2009.
61. Available at: http://www.pathway.com/. Accessed January 13, 2010.
62. Gurwitz D, Bregman-Eschet Y. Personal genomics services: whose genomes? Eur J Hum Genet 2009;17(7):883–9.
63. McBride CM, Alford SH, Reid RJ, et al. Putting science over supposition in the arena of personalized genomics. Nat Genet 2008;40(8):939–42.
64. Ng PC, Murray SS, Levy S, et al. An agenda for personalized medicine. Nature 2009;461(7265):724–6.
65. Direct-to-consumer genetic TESTS: misleading test results are further complicated by deceptive marketing and other questionable practices. 2010. Available at: http://www.gao.gov/new.items/d10847t.pdf. Accessed July 23, 2010.
66. Bloss CS, Ornowski L, Silver E, et al. Consumer perceptions of direct-to-consumer personalized genomic risk assessments. Genet Med 2010;12(9): 556–66.
67. Bullinger L, Valk PJ. Gene expression profiling in acute myeloid leukemia. J Clin Oncol 2005;23(26):6296–305.
68. Dave SS, Fu K, Wright GW, et al. Molecular diagnosis of Burkitt's lymphoma. N Engl J Med 2006;354(23):2431–42.
69. Potti A, Mukherjee S, Petersen R, et al. A genomic strategy to refine prognosis in early-stage non-small-cell lung cancer. N Engl J Med 2006;355(6):570–80.
70. Potti A, Dressman HK, Bild A, et al. Genomic signatures to guide the use of chemotherapeutics. Nat Med 2006;12(11):1294–300.
71. Andersen JN, Sathyanarayanan S, Di Bacco A, et al. Pathway-based identification of biomarkers for targeted therapeutics: personalized oncology with PI3K pathway inhibitors. Sci Transl Med 2010;2(43):43ra55.
72. Starling RC, Pham M, Valantine H, et al. Molecular testing in the management of cardiac transplant recipients: initial clinical experience. J Heart Lung Transplant 2006;25(12):1389–95.
73. Takahashi M, Hayashi H, Watanabe Y, et al. Diagnostic classification of schizophrenia by neural network analysis of blood-based gene expression signatures. Schizophr Res 2010;119(1–3):210–8.
74. Scherzer CR, Eklund AC, Morse LJ, et al. Molecular markers of early Parkinson's disease based on gene expression in blood. Proc Natl Acad Sci U S A 2007; 104(3):955–60.
75. Lovrecic L, Kastrin A, Kobal J, et al. Gene expression changes in blood as a putative biomarker for Huntington's disease. Mov Disord 2009;24(15):2277–81.

76. Fehlbaum-Beurdeley P, Jarrige-Le Prado AC, Pallares D, et al. Toward an Alzheimer's disease diagnosis via high-resolution blood gene expression. Alzheimers Dement 2010;6(1):25–38.

77. Oeseburg H, de Boer RA, van Gilst WH, et al. Telomere biology in healthy aging and disease. Pflugers Arch 2010;459(2):259–68.

78. Davis JC, Furstenthal L, Desai AA, et al. The microeconomics of personalized medicine: today's challenge and tomorrow's promise. Nat Rev Drug Discov 2009;8(4):279–86.

79. Papadopoulos N, Kinzler KW, Vogelstein B. The role of companion diagnostics in the development and use of mutation-targeted cancer therapies. Nat Biotechnol 2006;24(8):985–95.

80. Healy M. As genetic testing races ahead, doctors are left behind. Los Angeles (CA): Los Angeles Times; 2009.

81. Toner B. Scripps spearheads new association to create online 'genomic medicine university' to educate physicians. La Jolla (CA): Pharmacogenomics Reporter; 2010.

82. Ethical, legal, and social issues research. Available at: http://www.ornl.gov/sci/techresources/Human_Genome/research/elsi.shtml. Accessed August 20, 2010.

83. McBride CM, Bowen D, Brody LC, et al. Future health applications of genomics: priorities for communication, behavioral, and social sciences research. Am J Prev Med 2010;38(5):556–65.

84. Stunkard AJ, Foch TT, Hrubec Z. A twin study of human obesity. JAMA 1986; 256(1):51–4.

85. Stunkard AJ, Sorensen TI, Hanis C, et al. An adoption study of human obesity. N Engl J Med 1986;314(4):193–8.

86. Zdravkovic S, Wienke A, Pedersen NL, et al. Heritability of death from coronary heart disease: a 36-year follow-up of 20 966 Swedish twins. J Intern Med 2002; 252(3):247–54.

87. King R, Rotter J, Motulsky A, editors. The genetic basis of common diseases. New York: Oxford University Press; 2002. p. 457–80.

88. Lichtenstein P, Holm NV, Verkasalo PK, et al. Environmental and heritable factors in the causation of cancer—analyses of cohorts of twins from Sweden, Denmark, and Finland. N Engl J Med 2000;343(2):78–85.

89. Gatz M, Pedersen NL, Berg S, et al. Heritability for Alzheimer's disease: the study of dementia in Swedish twins. J Gerontol A Biol Sci Med Sci 1997;52(2):M117–25.

90. Sullivan PF, Kendler KS, Neale MC. Schizophrenia as a complex trait: evidence from a meta-analysis of twin studies. Arch Gen Psychiatry 2003;60(12):1187–92.

91. Sullivan PF, Neale MC, Kendler KS. Genetic epidemiology of major depression: review and meta-analysis. Am J Psychiatry 2000;157(10):1552–62.

92. McGuffin P, Katz R, Watkins S, et al. A hospital-based twin register of the heritability of DSM-IV unipolar depression. Arch Gen Psychiatry 1996;53(2):129–36.

93. Hettema JM, Prescott CA, Kendler KS. A population-based twin study of generalized anxiety disorder in men and women. J Nerv Ment Dis 2001;189(7):413–20.

94. Hettema JM, Neale MC, Kendler KS. A review and meta-analysis of the genetic epidemiology of anxiety disorders. Am J Psychiatry 2001;158(10):1568–78.

95. Genetic Information Nondiscrimination Act (GINA) of 2008. 2010. Available at: http://www.genome.gov/24519851. Accessed July 20, 2010.

96. Personalized health care. 2008. Available at: http://www.hhs.gov/myhealthcare/. Accessed July 20, 2010.

97. S. 3822: Genomics and Personalized Medicine Act 2006. Available at: http://www.govtrack.us/congress/bill.xpd?bill=s109-3822. Accessed July 18, 2010.

Internet-Based Depression Prevention over the Life Course: A Call for Behavioral Vaccines

Benjamin W. Van Voorhees, MD, MPH[a,b,c,*], Nicholas Mahoney[d],
Rina Mazo[d], Alinne Z. Barrera, PhD[e], Christopher P. Siemer, BS[d],
Tracy R.G. Gladstone, PhD[f,g,h], Ricardo F. Muñoz, PhD[i]

KEYWORDS

- Mental disorders • Prevention and control • Internet
- Intervention studies • Child

Funding: Supported by a career development award from the National Institutes of Mental Health (NIMH K-08 MH 072918-01A2).
Disclosures: Benjamin W. Van Voorhees has served as a consultant to Prevail Health Solutions, Inc, Mevident Inc, San Francisco and Social Kinetics, Palo Alto, CA, and the Hong Kong University to develop Internet-based interventions. To facilitate dissemination, the University of Chicago recently agreed to grant a no-cost license to Mevident Incorporated (3/5/2010) to develop a school-based version. Neither Dr Van Voorhees nor the university will receive any royalties or equity. Dr Van Voorhees has agreed to assist the company in adapting the intervention at the rate of $1000/day for 5.5 days. The CATCH-IT Internet site and all materials remain open for public use and is made freely available to health care providers at http://catchit-public.bsd.uchicago.edu/.

[a] Section of General Internal Medicine, Department of Medicine, The University of Chicago, 5841 South Maryland Boulevard, Chicago, IL 60637, USA
[b] Section of Child and Adolescent Psychiatry, Department of Psychiatry, The University of Chicago, 5841 South Maryland Avenue, MC 2007, Chicago, IL 60637, USA
[c] Section of Developmental and Behavioral Pediatrics, Department of Pediatrics, The University of Chicago, 5841 South Maryland Avenue, MC 2007, Chicago, IL 60637, USA
[d] Section of General Internal Medicine, Department of Medicine, The University of Chicago, 5841 South Maryland Avenue, MC 2007, Chicago, IL 60637, USA
[e] Pacific Graduate School of Psychology, Palo Alto University, 1791 Arastradero Road, Palo Alto, CA 94304-1337, USA
[f] Wellesley Centers for Women, Wellesley College, 106 Central Street, Wellesley, MA 02481, USA
[g] Department of Psychiatry, Children's Hospital, 300 Longwood Avenue, Boston, MA 02115, USA
[h] Judge Baker Children's Center, 53 Parker Hill Avenue, Boston, MA 02120, USA
[i] Department of Psychiatry, San Francisco General Hospital, University of California, 1001 Potrero Avenue, San Francisco, CA, USA
* Corresponding author. Section of General Internal Medicine, Department of Medicine, The University of Chicago, 5841 South Maryland Boulevard, Chicago, IL 60637.
E-mail address: bvanvoor@medicine.bsd.uchicago.edu

Psychiatr Clin N Am 34 (2011) 167–183
doi:10.1016/j.psc.2010.11.002
0193-953X/11/$ – see front matter © 2011 Elsevier Inc. All rights reserved.

SIGNIFICANCE

Major depression is the number one cause of disability worldwide.[1] The lifetime prevalence of major depression in the United States is 16.6%, but is as high as 19.8% for those in more recent birth cohorts.[2] Depression, known as a "life-course" disorder, usually has its first onset in mid-adolescence, and recurs every 5 to 7 years in 80% of individuals.[3] Most people with major depression do not obtain treatment[4]; of those who do obtain evidence-based treatment, approximately one-third do not improve.[5,6] Depression is associated with substantial impairment both during and after the episode. Many who suffer from depression face difficulties in various areas, including school, interpersonal relationships, occupational adjustment, and behavior (eg, substance abuse, suicide attempts). Depression affects both the individual and the nation, with a loss of $77.4 billion dollars per year attributed to depression in the United States alone.[7–9]

NEED FOR PREVENTIVE INTERVENTIONS

There are 121 million people with depression worldwide, yet fewer than 25% of them have access to effective treatments, and many of those in the developed world who do have access do not seek treatment.[10] For example, even in study settings such as Youth Partners in Care (YPIC) where youth received a comprehensive primary care intervention to facilitate treatment, less than one-third of depressed adolescents in primary care attended counseling referrals to mental health specialists.[11] Even within structured study settings, most individuals do not make full functional recoveries, warranting the use of both effective treatment and prevention strategies.[10,12] Prevention-focused efforts have the potential to make a major impact on global public health, particularly if they are highly scalable and easily disseminated.[10] Two recent meta-analyses indicate that clinical episodes of depression can be prevented, with a demonstrated mean incidence rate ratio of 0.78 (22% risk reduction) for all interventions.[13,14]

VALUE OF TECHNOLOGY-BASED APPROACHES IN PREVENTING DEPRESSION

The Institute of Medicine (IOM) has published 2 major reports on the prevention of mental, emotional, and behavioral disorders,[16,17] and has called for the development and rigorous evaluation of new technology based on new prevention strategies. Technology-based delivery offers considerable benefits including easy access (time and space), patient autonomy, and "nonconsumable" services that are autonomous from traditional (face-to-face) interventions.[10,17] In the IOM model (**Fig. 1**), interventions are deployed to prevent the onset of illness in individuals who do not already meet diagnostic criteria for these disorders. Such interventions can be universal (applied to the entire population), selected (applied to those with a risk factor for disorder), and indicated (applied to those with early symptoms of disorder). Ritterband and others have summarized key components for Internet interventions, such as the importance of the motivation of participants, participant use of interventions, Web site design, and support for participation.[18–20] However, technology-based interventions have important limitations, such as the difficulty motivating participants to completion, stigma, and limited availability of Internet access in economically distressed settings.[21,22]

"BEHAVIORAL VACCINE" MODEL

Effective vaccine strategies include several key components that relate closely to Internet-based prevention (**Fig. 2**). These elements include: (1) a schedule of vaccines

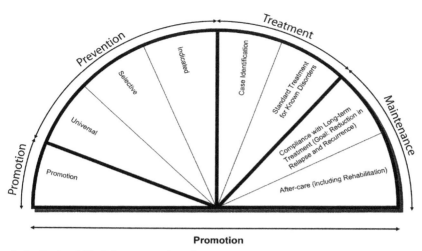

Fig. 1. Institute of Medicine prevention diagram.

across the life span to address specific threats; (2) an active ingredient (eg, an antigen or live attenuated organism) that is intended to protect against the disease; (3) an adjuvant to boost the immune system's natural response to active components; and (4) a structured implementation and delivery schedule that optimizes immunity The authors have previously worked to develop Internet interventions based on the frameworks proposed by Nation and colleagues[23] and Wandersman[24] for conventional, face-to-face effective community-based interventions,[25,26] and propose to integrate these models into a "behavioral vaccine model," which the authors believe is aptly applicable to technology-based delivery. Like vaccines, behavioral vaccines require 4 key components: (1) a life-course schedule that is theory-driven and includes booster doses; (2) information and training (active components) to encode responses

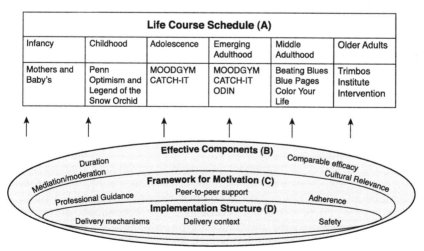

Fig. 2. Biological and behavioral vaccines across the life course with some examples of interventions.

to future threats that is theoretically and empirically grounded; (3) a motivational framework to boost response to behavior prescription ("motivation," "positive relationships," and "dose"); and (4) a structured implementation strategy, as one must intervene before the onset of disorder ("Web site design," "varied teaching methods," "effective training," "practitioner control").[20,23,24]

In this article the authors review the literature on Internet-based depression prevention programs using this behavioral vaccine development model, reviewing literature relevant to each component of the model in turn. Specifically, literature on effective components of Internet-based depression prevention programs across the life-course is examined, followed by a review of frameworks for motivation. Finally, the literature pertaining to implementation strategies associated with these Internet-based prevention programs is discussed. Cohen's D effect sizes (based on self-report symptoms) and number needed to treat (based on clinical assessments) were calculated for each age group.

The studies reviewed here were identified through a systematic search of Medline and PsycInfo databases for unique Internet depression intervention papers that met the authors' inclusion criteria. The great majority of articles identified did not meet the IOM criteria for a prevention study. Most of the studies were best characterized as "early intervention," encompassing mixed populations of those just below (indicated prevention) and above (case identification treatment) diagnostic threshold. Because only a limited number of true "prevention" studies are available for review, to provide a broad overview of this field this article includes early-intervention studies that reported at least 6 months of follow-up.

LIFE-COURSE SCHEDULE

The first component of an effective vaccine is a life-course schedule that is theory driven. This section reviews interventions in light of timing, life-course stage, and theoretical grounding of the intervention components (eg, problem-solving therapy vs cognitive behavioral psychotherapy).

Interventions Involving Mothers, Infants, and Children

While not identifying a published intervention, the authors are aware of several unpublished projects that suggest the prospect of progress in this life-course period, including Mothers and Babies, Legend of the Snow Orchid, and the Pennsylvania Optimism Study, for which some limited information is available.

The Mothers and Babies Internet Project (HealthyPregnancy.ucsf.edu and EmbarazoSaludable.ucsf.edu) is an unpublished pilot randomized controlled trial (RCT) examining an intervention intended to prevent postpartum depression in an international sample of pregnant women. The program uses an automated, self-help, web-adapted, cognitive behavioral therapy (CBT)-based intervention,[27] and recruited participants online using sponsored links over a 6-month period (January to July 2009). Participants were subsequently stratified based on depression status as baseline ("prevention" or "treatment"—depending on whether they are above or below the diagnostic threshold) and randomized to either the Mothers and Babies or information condition. Using automated email messages, depression status was assessed monthly up to 6 months postpartum, with subsequent deployment of a CBT-based intervention components focusing on reducing risk of depression during the peripartum transition. The sample, currently N>1000, consisted of primarily Latino women (81%) from 45 countries in their late twenties (mean = 27.6 years, standard deviation [SD] = 5.6). Half of the participants were married (50%), the majority were educated (83% completed college degrees or above), most were employed (60%), and many had no history of major depressive episodes (69%). Another novel project is the Legend of the Snow Orchid Internet site (https://www.roc-n-ash.com/imheportal/welcome/) developed by Daniel Fung for the Department of Mental Health, Singapore. The site uses a fantasy-based game to reduce anxiety and depressed mood.[28] The Pennsylvania Optimism Study program has been developed and deployed in multiple settings. The program focuses on creating a more favorable attributional style, and plans are under way to develop an Internet application.[29]

Adolescent and Emerging Adulthood Studies

Six Internet-based studies were identified that focused on the prevention of depression in adolescents and/or emerging adults. Combined, these sites observed a mean effect size of 0.32 between randomization groups, and a pre-/post-effect size of 0.65 at the latest follow-up.[30–35]

In a study of a problem-solving therapy (PST), which currently has no available data, approximately 210 participants between the ages of 12 and 18 years with mild to moderate depressive symptoms will be randomized into an active group and a control group.[31] This PST intervention uses a step-by-step approach to first triage problems based on their importance, and then to generate, implement, and evaluate trial solutions. The control group will receive no treatment except a link to a Web site with general information about depression and anxiety. The active group will undergo a PST Internet intervention for a total of 5 weeks, and follow-up assessments will occur at 3 weeks, 5 weeks, 4 months, and 8 months.

The program MoodGYM (http://www.moodgym.anu.edu.au) consists of 5 modules, ranging between 30 and 45 minutes each that focus on prevention, education, and treatment using CBT. An observational study of 2909 registrants (mean age = 35.5 years, SD = 13) and 71 university students demonstrated that the participants who completed more modules exhibited the best results, suggesting that more time on the site yields better outcomes. Its effectiveness in preventing depression was demonstrated through 3 randomized clinical trials that compared MoodGYM to the participation in a health class, using a universal prevention model. Initial early-intervention studies were completed in 2 single-gender schools (baseline depressed: male = 19.5%; female = 25%). In the single-gender study, males showed a lower likelihood of becoming depressed, and in the female-only study, those in the intervention group were less depressed than those in the control group at 20 weeks (moderate effect size).[32,33] In the larger RCT (N = 1477, mean age = 14.34; SD = 0.75; baseline depressed = 10.1%), the effectiveness of MoodGYM was compared with that of a wait-list control group who received a typical school curriculum health class. Only male participants showed a reduction in risk of depression (36.9% intervention, 48.5% control).[30]

The Web site Project CATCH-IT (http://catchit-public.bsd.uchicago.edu) provides an alternative source of depression intervention for youth. Project CATCH-IT is a primary care–based Web site that focuses on the prevention of depression in adolescents through the integration of CBT, interpersonal psychotherapy (IPT), and behavioral activation (BA). The Web site interacts with its users through homework assignments and short narratives. A pilot study of Project CATCH-IT with participants who were emerging adults (age range = 18–24 years) demonstrated moderate effect sizes (group effect = 0.81) for the site post intervention. In a preventative RCT study of Project CATCH-IT, 84 participants were recruited via screening in the primary care setting (subthreshold depressed mood to enter the study, indicated prevention model) and randomized into either a motivational interview group (MI group) or a brief advice group as preparation for the Internet component. Those included had a mean age of 17.39 years (SD = 2.04) and were from mostly moderate- to high-income families. The MI group visited the study Web site more often and had significantly fewer depressive episodes at the 3-month follow-up.[34,35]

Clarke and colleagues[36] conducted an early-intervention (includes those above and below diagnostic threshold) RCT of 160 participants (80% female, mean age = 22.5 [SD = 2.5], 44.9% depressed at baseline) in 2009. The unguided program consisted of 4 main sections with interactive exercises and a CBT tutorial based on the Coping with Depression Course. Internet intervention participants were recruited from a common Health Maintenance Organization (HMO), and demonstrated moderate reductions in depressed mood compared with treatment as usual at 32 weeks after enrollment.

Middle Adult

Nine Internet-based studies were identified that focused on middle-aged adults (mean age = 41.8 years), with a mean between-group effect size of 0.30.[37–46] BluePages (http://bluepages.anu.edu/au) is a depression literacy Web site that was designed to provide evidence-based information and treatment to a youth population. An early-intervention study (individuals above and below diagnostic threshold) was conducted to compare the results of using BluePages or MoodGYM. The study consisted of 525 participants (71% female) with a mean age of 36.43 years (SD = 9.40). The participants were randomized into 3 groups: MoodGYM, BluePages, and an attention placebo consisting of a weekly interview to discuss lifestyle factors. Both sites were effective in reducing symptoms of depression, showing similar results, but those with baseline Center for Epidemiological Studies Depression Scales (CES-D) scores above 16 evidenced significantly higher effect sizes.[39,43]

In a separate study, 299 adults (mean age = 43.3 years), 74.6% depressed at baseline, were used to measure the effectiveness of an Internet CBT program, ODIN (includes both focus on pleasurable activities and changing pessimistic cognitions), compared with a control group that received access to the Kaiser Permanente Online home page that provided noninteractive information about health concerns. The computer-generated invitation model included a mixed depressed/nondepressed sample (separate samples generated by query of health records), which could be described as early intervention. Of these participants (73% female), 74.6% were depressed at baseline. The 6-month follow-up provided a moderate pre-/post-effect size, but demonstrated a small between-group effect size compared with the control group.[41] (However, many individuals in both groups were under active treatment.)

Color Your Life (CYL) is a multimedia, interactive computer program for depression that was intended to intervene to reduce depressed mood in a heterogeneous population (some above and below diagnostic thresholds, early intervention). The program models an existing Coping with Depression course by Lewinsohn and colleagues,[47] which includes CBT-based lessons and incorporates a homework assignment following each of the 9 30-minute lessons. Originally CYL was designed for a targeted age group of those older than 50, but it was later adapted to suit a more expansive adult population (18–65 years). To test the program, 303 participants between 18 and 65 years (mean = 44, SD = 11.6) were divided into CYL, treatment as usual (TAU), or CYL+TAU. In this early-intervention study (mean baseline Beck Depression Index score = 27.8), 21% of the population had no previous major depressive episodes. The results showed medium to large improvement effect sizes in all 3 groups at the 6-month follow-up.[42]

Cavanagh and Geisler[48] studied the effectiveness of a self-help online CBT program called Beating the Blues, which consisted of an introductory video and 9 50-minute treatment sessions with corresponding homework assignments (computer-based approach in clinic at that time). In an observational study, 219 participants (mean age = 43 years, 60% female), 32% exhibiting depression symptoms, tested the site and showed significant improvements that were sustained after 6 months.[38] A separate study was conducted on Beating the Blues using a sample size of 310 participants (mean age = 44.7 years) with an average of 1.9 episodes of depression pretreatment. The researchers compared the effectiveness of this program with a TAU control group comprising patients who saw general practitioners for anxiety and/or depression (above and below diagnostic thresholds) recruited from 7 general practices in London and Southeast England. The results showed a significant decrease in scores for depression and anxiety among those assigned to the Beating the Blues condition, and the average of both depression and anxiety scores fell to the near-normal range.[46]

In a larger early-intervention study by Andersson and colleagues,[37] 117 adults (74% female) with a mean age of 36.1 years (SD = 10.57) and a baseline Beck Depression Inventory (BDI) score of 21.0 were randomized into either a CBT intervention or control group. The active group was directed through email to undergo an Internet self-help CBT program consisting of 5 modules with a total of 89 pages of text and a quiz following each module. Both groups exhibited a reduction in depression symptoms, but the active group showed greater improvements in their mood.[37]

In a prevention RCT (263 participants, age 18 years and older), CBT and PST programs were compared alongside a wait-list control group who received no treatment until 3 months after the intervention was completed. Both treatments differed in length (CBT = 8 weeks, PST = 5 weeks), but had similar design formats; only the CBT site offered video and audio options for its users. Both programs rendered moderate to high effect sizes immediately after intervention, which increased at the 12-month follow-up.[49]

Older Adult

Only one Internet-based depression prevention study targeting older adults was identified. In an early-intervention study conducted by Spek and colleagues[50,51] in 2007, 301 participants (63.5% female) (mean BDI baseline score = 18.4) with a mean age of 55 years (SD = 4.6) were randomly assigned to 1 of 3 groups: an Internet-based CBT intervention created at the Trimbos Institute in the Netherlands, a face-to-face CBT group, and a wait-list control. The CBT site consisted of 8 weekly modules comprising text, exercises, videos, and figures. The intervention produced moderate between-group effect sizes both at postintervention and after the 12-month follow-up.

EFFECTIVE COMPONENTS

To gauge the effectiveness of Internet-based behavioral vaccines, the active components of these prevention programs are reviewed by comparing results to similar, more traditional, face-to-face interventions. More specifically, the duration of benefits, the role of various components, mediating and moderating responses, and the ability of included interventions to demonstrate "socio-cultural relevance" are examined.

Comparable Effectiveness

Where data were available, the Internet interventions reviewed demonstrated similar effect sizes to face-to-face interventions using comparable curriculums. The youth Internet intervention studies yielded a mean between-group effect size of

0.25,[30,32–34,36] with the Van Voorhees study exhibiting a number needed to treat (NNT) value of 5.26.[34] Among face-to-face interventions for adolescents and emerging adults, Clarke and colleagues[52] and Garber and colleagues[53] both showed an overall mean effect size of 0.16, and NNTs of 5.13 and 8.85, respectively.[52,53] For adult Internet intervention studies, the mean between-group effect sizes at the last follow-up evaluation was 0.28[37–39,41–43,46,51] with the NNT values in 2 of the studies calculated to be 30.3 for Patten[45] and 4.26 for Meyer and colleagues.[44] Two adult face-to-face studies, focused on postpartum depression, produced a mean between-group effect size of 0.60 and had an NNT of 5.0 for Elliott and colleagues,[54] 6.25 for Zlotnick and colleagues,[55] and 6.66 for Lara and colleagues.[56]

Duration of Benefits

Most of the studies continued with a follow-up visit ranging from 2 months to a year later, with enduring reductions in depressed mood. When interpreting the effectiveness of Internet interventions, the positive outcomes seen directly after treatment should also be observed at the subsequent follow-up visits. In a study of older adults, the pre-/post-effect size of the Internet intervention was calculated to be 1.00 immediately post intervention.[50,51] Fifty-seven percent of the Internet CBT group completed the 1-year follow-up and the pre-/post-effect size increased to 1.20, providing evidence of long-term effectiveness.[51] In adult studies of CYL, MoodGYM, and CATCH-IT, depression scores continued to decline at each long-term follow-up.[32–34,42] These results are consistent with findings by Clarke and colleagues[52,57] of sustained reduction in depressed mood for up to 1 year of follow-up, but whether mood rebounds after 1 year cannot be known.

Moderators and Mediators

Moderators and mediators of effect have rarely been identified in the studies of focus. Higher levels of depressed mood and a greater number of prior episodes may predict poorer outcomes at follow-up, but this has not been consistently found.[34,41,46] In MoodGYM, those who completed a greater number of modules demonstrated larger changes in depressed mood than those who did not, but the relationship between adherence and outcome has been less clear in other studies.[41,58,59] Combining Internet-based approaches with other interventions may potentially enhance efficacy. For example, the combination of a motivational interview with an Internet site demonstrated an advantage in preventing depressive episodes.[35] Similarly, Andersson and colleagues[37,60] reported that CBT combined with a discussion group demonstrated a greater effect size than CBT alone. In a meta-analysis, guided interventions, CBT-based interventions, and experiencing major or clinical depression were associated with greater effectiveness.[59]

Sociocultural Relevance

In all but one mixed-gender experiment, a majority of the participants were females. Of the articles that listed gender as part of their demographics, 7 contained ratios of females over 60% of the study population.[33,37,39,41,45,50,51,60] One possible reason for this is that women, in general, account for a majority of the population suffering from depression, so recruitment appears to show a bias toward women. Three studies that provided ethnicity indicated that overall, approximately 61% of the participants were Caucasian and 25% African American.[34,35,61] Also, 7 adult studies indicated mostly mid to high levels of education,[37,39,41,42,45,50,51,60] and most of the youth population was recruited from moderate- to high-income families.[30,32–35,61] The studies spanned over many regions and to an extent reflected national cultures in Canada,[45] the United States,[34,35,41,61] Australia,[30,32,33,39] and Europe[31,37,42,49–51,60] (mainly the Netherlands[31,37,42,50,51,60] and one in Sweden[49]). However, the degree to which each intervention was tailored to meet the needs of ethnic minorities or cultural differences within each country was not clearly specified. CATCH-IT included stories intended to reflect the experiences of adolescents in varying social and cultural frameworks.[34,35]

Tailoring of interventions to personal profiles (ethnicity, form of motivation, attitudes) is supported both by theory and substantial empirical evidence. From the perspective of cognitive psychology, attention is increased with material relevant to either a "current concern" or if presented by a person with a similar life situation.[12,62] Several studies have compared tailored and standard depression and CBT-based interventions in ethnic minority populations.[12] Matching of intervention to motivational style, or providing external motivation (eg, incentives) for those who prefer external motivations and internal motivations (eg, linking behaviors to personal goals) for those who prefer internal motivations, may enhance adherence to health and diet recommendations in public health messages.[63] The PEN-3 (Persons, Environment, and Neighborhood) Model of Health Behaviors has been used to successfully adapt behavior-change interventions to meet the needs of diverse populations.[64] A rule-based or even an artificial intelligence model could be developed to facilitate tailoring.[65]

FRAMEWORK FOR MOTIVATION

Like vaccines that are "adjuvant" in enhancing immune response, behavior-change interventions often have a *motivational framework* to boost response to behavior prescription ("motivation," "positive relationships" [professional guidance and peer to peer], and an appropriate "dose" [eg, adherence]).

Degree of Professional Guidance

In most trials, support was provided to the users throughout the online interventions, but the methods varied considerably. Additional support serves several different purposes: (1) it monitors user progress on the site; (2) it provides weekly lessons; and (3) it determines if the users' emotional safety is maintained.[34] Support can be provided through email,[31,37,49] or by phone,[34,35,39,61] or no support can be given.[41,42,50,51] In 3 MoodGYM studies, support was given in the school environment by a supervising professional (teacher).[30,32,33] In CYL, supervision was provided by a trained coach.[42] One article specified that users received therapist support, but it did not define the manner in which it was provided.[60]

Peer-to-Peer Support

Internet-based social groups (ISG) support offers the prospect of enhancing curricular-based interventions by one of several mechanisms: (1) increasing use of the curricular-based prevention; (2) providing opportunities to discuss contents and increase sociocultural relevance; and (3) directing action of social support.[66] The experience of ReachOut in Australia suggests that sites that incorporate peer-based social support have considerable appeal to the public and may perhaps increase use of other more traditional learning venues.[67] Online groups often sustain individual membership for as long as 12 months (72.6% retention) and some participants experience resolution of depression symptoms after 1 year of participation (33.8%).[68] Likewise, in a study of 5 online one-on-one male-to-female or female-to-female chat sessions, Shaw and Gant[69] found some evidence that participation in Internet-based peer support groups may reduce depressed mood. However, Takahashi and colleagues[70] suggested that ISGs could have negative effects on a person's depressive tendencies, due to the influence of participants with depressive symptoms. With regard to enhancing social support, factors such as subjective view of a social support system, belongingness, and self-esteem may improve with ISG participation.[69]

Adherence

Completion rates, and even the definition of completion, varied across interventions. Overall, half of the guided study participants completed about half of the modules, whereas only about one-fifth to one-tenth of those who had unguided interventions met this mark. Participation in intervention conditions, particularly those including psychotherapy, increased attrition. For example, during the CYL trial, participants completed a mean of only 3.7 of 9 sessions.[42] In a Swedish study, psychotherapy-armed participants experienced more withdrawals than the control group (psychotherapy = 37%, control = 18%).[37] When MoodGYM (self-directed psychotherapy) and BluePages (psychoeducation) were compared, drop rates were greater for the psychotherapy group (MoodGYM: 25.27%, BluePages: 15.15%).[39,43] A structured setting with phone follow-up may reduce dropouts. Phone calls can be for motivation, safety assessments, or education purposes.[34] For example, in the primary care CATCH-IT study, only 7% dropped out at 3 months when phone follow-up was added,[34] whereas 43% dropped out in an earlier study without phone follow-up.[61] Similarly, in the CYL trial, the investigators reported receiving numerous contacts from their participants and provided regular guidance, and reported only a 5% dropout rate. Further, at the 2- and 3-month follow-ups, the investigators reported 95% participation in the intervention group and 91% at the 6-month follow-up.[42] In terms of intervention adherence (modules completed, time on site), baseline factors (younger age, higher education, higher illness severity, favorable attitudes toward the intervention), implementation factors (any structured setting), and intentional use of motivational approaches (referral by mental health specialist, use of brochures, or motivational interview by their primary care physician) may influence the degree of participation in Internet interventions.[32,33,71–73]

IMPLEMENTATION STRUCTURE

A proper behavioral vaccine requires a well thought-out implementation structure, which includes Web site design, varied teaching methods, and effective training.

Delivery Mechanisms

Behavior change sites must balance education, behavior change, and entertainment functions in order to retain the audience, using approaches such as instructional design.[74] Most of the sites providing information primarily in text format were adult intervention studies,[37,39,41,42,45,50,51,60] and most were tested on individuals with moderate to high levels of education.[37,39,41,42,45,50,51,60] Supplying fewer interactive exercises and more textual information could possibly yield lower participation rates because of decreased participation, which could cause lower effect sizes.[40] Conversely, the use of a range of media experiences including, games, music, video, stories, photography, virtual reality, and in-the-moment cell-phone interactions may substantially enhance the intrinsic appeal of sites (eg, ReachOut[67] and YooMagazine[75]). However, we must consider the technical infrastructure available in developing countries, which may not support broadband applications.

Delivery Context

The depression interventions and Internet sites were provided at several locations, depending on the study. Three of the interventions, all MoodGYM, were offered in a school setting[30,32,33] whereas the other interventions were accessed at the users' homes,[31,34–38,41–46,49–51,61] which required home Internet access to participate in the research. However, the main form of variation between most of these studies existed in the form and location of the initial interview and assessment. Five studies conducted the first interview and assessment within a primary care facility,[34,35,42,50,51,61] 3 in a school environment,[30,32,33] 3 by Internet and email,[37,49,60] and 3 by brochures.[31,41] Two assessment strategies producing the best participation were Internet and primary care. In a study of a CBT intervention program with an initial Internet assessment, all participants reached 4 of the 5 modules.[36,37] In the Clarke HMO studies,[36,41] recruitment via search of medical records was used, which may herald future integrative technologies. Integrative technologies such as rule-based algorithms or even artificial intelligence may be able to link interventions to medical records as well as various delivery platforms such as cell phones.

Safety

One challenge to Internet-based depression prevention is the risk of self-harm or progression to major depression among those who are at risk by virtue of subthreshold depressed mood.[34,76] Specifically, the participant may not be observed for an extended period or have meaningful interaction with an experienced care provider. Under these circumstances, the underlying depressive illness as well as self-harm intent can progress. Three studies reported that after becoming aware of such depression scores, the participants were recommended to consult their physician.[31,49–51] Increased monitoring was another method used, including "checking up" on their participants via email, phone, or direct contact to discuss progress and/or concerns.[31,34,35,39,45,49] However, most articles either did not assess self-harm risk and/or did not report additional safety precautions. A comprehensive, standard approach to safety management approaches does not appear to have been developed.

SUMMARY

Considerable progress has been made in developing prototype "behavioral vaccines" for depressive disorders across the life course that include effective components, frameworks for motivation, and a structured implementation strategy. The greatest number of interventions has been developed for middle-aged adults and, to a lesser extent, for adolescents and emerging adults, while no interventions have been developed and published for children or postpartum depression. With regard to effective intervention components, there is substantial evidence that CBT-based interventions can achieve comparable results to face-to-face interventions, with benefits sustained 1 year following treatment. However, the vast majority of studies were not formal prevention studies, so we cannot fully know if components deployed in "treatment" studies would be as effective in prevention. Also, most studies enrolled primarily educated populations of "European ethnic decent"; there is a dearth of research on Internet interventions with ethnically diverse populations. Internet support or peer-to-peer contact offers the promise of providing a "draw" to the interventions while also potentiating the effects of curricular program elements. As with vaccines, schools and primary care may be auspicious environments to implement these interventions, and such settings may engender higher levels of uptake of behavioral vaccines. In the future, artificial intelligence-driven risk monitoring in schools, workplaces, and primary care could deploy personalized behavioral vaccines to alter illness trajectories and consequently reduce morbidity while enhancing positive development.

Future Directions

Interventions over the life course

To determine whether current interventions are effective in the prevention of depression, formal study designs are needed with structured psychiatric interviews, and longitudinal data analysis to examine survival curves (dichotomous outcomes).[15,16] Appropriate comparison groups need to be determined with reference to research ethics and the de facto mental health care system.[77] Behavioral vaccines need to be compared with effective face-to-face preventive strategies that are often unavailable, too complex, and too expensive for general distribution. We need to broaden assessed outcomes to include achievement of developmental milestones in youth and measures of wellbeing, resiliency, productivity, and functional status in adults to enhance relevance to policy makers. Furthermore, the cost effectiveness of such programs needs to be addressed, and the optimal schedule for each intervention, and booster sessions within each intervention, needs to be defined.

Effective intervention components

For behavioral vaccines to develop, we need to identify the key effective content and delivery mechanisms. In addition to dismantling studies, formal moderator and mediator analyses and factorial study designs could facilitate this goal. Methods to inexpensively adapt standard interventions to specific cultural settings worldwide need to be determined. Specifically, we must determine which elements can be shared across large cultural areas and which must be adapted locally. Combining interventions with other modalities, with differing mechanisms of action such as nutritional supplements (eg, essential fatty acids) and exercise, could increase the efficacy of interventions.[78,79]

Framework for motivation

Current interventions may lack sufficient appeal to attain their public health value because relatively few people are "ready" and willing to participate in such self-directed curricular programs.[17] Combinations of education, behavior change, and entertainment need to be created (ReachOut[67] and *YooMagazine*[75]), and/or social media experiences need to be developed, such as peer-to-peer Internet support groups.[37,68–70]

Implementation structure

It is essential that implementation models be developed that allow these interventions to be effectively delivered to defined populations, whereby full public health impact can be assessed.[80] More engaging delivery mechanisms would integrate multiple elements, including peer-to-peer support, games, music, video, advanced technology platforms (eg, virtual reality experiences), cell-phone–based guidance and feedback, and integrative technologies (eg, rule-based programs and true artificial intelligence).

REFERENCES

1. World Health Organization - Regional office for South-East Asia. Conquering depression. New Dehli (India): World Health Organization; 2001.
2. Kessler RC, Berglund P, Demler O, et al. Lifetime prevalence and age-of-onset distributions of DSM-IV disorders in the national comorbidity survey replication. Arch Gen Psychiatry 2005;62(6):593–602.

3. Hankin BL. Adolescent depression: description, causes, and interventions. Epilepsy Behav 2006;8(1):102–14.
4. Kessler RC, Berglund P, Demler O, et al. The epidemiology of major depressive disorder: results from the National Comorbidity Survey Replication (NCS-R). JAMA 2003;289(23):3095–105.
5. DeRubeis RJ, Hollon SD, Amsterdam JD, et al. Cognitive therapy vs medications in the treatment of moderate to severe depression. Arch Gen Psychiatry 2005; 62(4):409–16.
6. Warden D, Rush AJ, Trivedi MH, et al. The STAR*D Project results: a comprehensive review of findings. Curr Psychiatry Rep 2007;9(6):449–59.
7. Lewinsohn PM, Rohde P, Seeley JR, et al. The consequences of adolescent major depressive disorder on young adults. In: Joiner TE, Brown JS, Kistner J, editors. The interpersonal, cognitive and social nature of depression. Mahwah (NJ): Lawrence Erlbaum Associates; 2006. p. 43–68.
8. Weissman MM, Wolk S, Goldstein RB, et al. Depressed adolescents grown up. JAMA 1999;17:7–13.
9. Greenberg PE, Kessler RC, Birnbaum HG, et al. The economic burden of depression in the United States: how did it change between 1990 and 2000? J Clin Psychiatry 2003;64(12):1465–75.
10. Munoz RF, Cuijpers P, Smit F, et al. Prevention of major depression. Annu Rev Clin Psychol 2010;6:181–212.
11. Jaycox LH, Miranda J, Meredith LS, et al. Impact of a primary care quality improvement intervention on use of psychotherapy for depression. Ment Health Serv Res 2003;5(2):109–20.
12. Van Voorhees BW, Walters AE, Prochaska M, et al. Reducing health disparities in depressive disorders outcomes between non-Hispanic whites and ethnic minorities: a call for pragmatic strategies over the life course. Med Care Res Rev 2007; 64(Suppl 5):157S–94S.
13. Cuijpers P, van Straten A, Smit F, et al. Preventing the onset of depressive disorders: a meta-analytic review of psychological interventions. Am J Psychiatry 2008;165(10):1272.
14. Cuijpers P, Muñoz RF, Clarke GN, et al. Psychoeducational treatment and prevention of depression: the "coping with depression" course thirty years later. Clin Psychol Rev 2009;29(5):449–58.
15. Mrazek PB, Haggerty RJ. Reducing risks for mental disorders: frontiers for preventive intervention research. Washington, DC: National Academy Press; 1994.
16. National Research Council and Institute of Medicine. Preventing mental, emotional, and behavioral disorders among young people: progress and possibilities. Washington, DC: The National Academies Press; 2009.
17. Van Voorhees BW, Watson N, Bridges JF. Development and pilot study of a marketing strategy for primary care/internet-based depression prevention intervention for adolescents (The CATCH-IT Intervention). Prim Care Companion J Clin Psychiatry 2010;12(3). pii: PCC.09m00791.
18. Crutzen R, de Nooijer J, Brouwer W, et al. A conceptual framework for understanding and improving adolescents' exposure to Internet-delivered interventions. Health Promot Int 2009;24(3):277–84.
19. De Los Reyes A, Kazdin AE. Conceptualizing changes in behavior in intervention research: the range of possible changes model. Psychol Rev 2006;113(3):554–83.
20. Ritterband LM, Thorndike FP, Cox DJ, et al. A behavior change model for internet interventions. Ann Behav Med 2009;38(1):18–27.

21. Van Voorhees B, Fogel J, Pomper B, et al. Adolescent dose and ratings of an internet-based depression prevention program: a randomized trial of primary care physician brief advice versus a motivational interview. J Cogn Behav Psychother 2009;9(1):1–19.

22. Gray NJ, Klein JD, Cantrill JA, et al. Adolescent girls' use of the internet for health information: issues beyond access. J Med Syst 2002;26(6):545–53.

23. Nation M, Crusto C, Wandersman A, et al. What works in prevention. Principles of effective prevention programs. Am Psychol 2003;58(6–7):449–56.

24. Wandersman A. Community science: bridging the gap between science and practice with community-centered models. Am J Community Psychol 2003;31(3–4):227–42.

25. Landback J, Prochaska M, Ellis J, et al. From prototype to product: development of a primary care/internet based depression prevention intervention for adolescents (CATCH-IT). Community Ment Health J 2009;45(5):349–54.

26. Van Voorhees BW, Ellis JM, Gollan JK, et al. Development and process evaluation of a primary care internet-based intervention to prevent depression in emerging adults. Prim Care Companion J Clin Psychiatry 2007;9(5):346–55.

27. Muñoz R, Barrera A. A worldwide Internet-based CBT intervention for postpartum depression prevention: adaptation, trial and challenges. New York (NY): Association for Behavioral and Cognitive Therapies; 2010.

28. Fung D. Legend of the snow orchid. 2010. Available at: http://www.roc-n-ash.com/imheportal/welcome/2010. Accessed July 15, 2010.

29. Gillham JE, Reivich KJ. Prevention of depressive symptoms in school children: a research update. Psychol Sci 1999;10(5):461–2.

30. Calear AL, Christensen H, Mackinnon A, et al. The Youthmood project: a cluster randomized controlled trial of an online cognitive behavioral program with adolescents. J Consult Clin Psychol 2009;77(6):1021–32.

31. Hoek W, Schuurmans J, Koot HM, et al. Prevention of depression and anxiety in adolescents: a randomized controlled trial testing the efficacy and mechanisms of Internet-based self-help problem-solving therapy. Trials 2009;10:93.

32. O'Kearney R, Gibson M, Christensen H, et al. Effects of a cognitive-behavioural internet program on depression, vulnerability to depression and stigma in adolescent males: a school-based controlled trial. Cogn Behav Ther 2006;35(1):43–54.

33. O'Kearney R, Kang K, Christensen H, et al. A controlled trial of a school-based Internet program for reducing depressive symptoms in adolescent girls. Depress Anxiety 2009;26(1):65–72.

34. Van Voorhees BW, Fogel J, Reinecke MA, et al. Randomized clinical trial of an Internet-based depression prevention program for adolescents (Project CATCH-IT) in primary care: 12-week outcomes. J Dev Behav Pediatr 2009; 30(1):23–37.

35. Van Voorhees BW, Vanderplough-Booth K, Fogel J, et al. Integrative internet-based depression prevention for adolescents: a randomized clinical trial in primary care for vulnerability and protective factors. J Can Acad Child Adolesc Psychiatry 2008;17(4):184–96.

36. Clarke G, Kelleher C, Hornbrook M, et al. Randomized effectiveness trial of an Internet, pure self-help, cognitive behavioral intervention for depressive symptoms in young adults. Cogn Behav Ther 2009;38(4):222–34.

37. Andersson G, Bergstrom J, Hollandare F, et al. Internet-based self-help for depression: randomised controlled trial. Br J Psychiatry 2005;187:456–61.

38. Cavanagh K, Shapiro DA, Van Den Berg S, et al. The effectiveness of computerized cognitive behavioural therapy in routine care. Br J Clin Psychol 2006;45(Pt 4): 499–514.

39. Christensen H, Griffiths KM, Jorm AF. Delivering interventions for depression by using the internet: randomised controlled trial. BMJ 2004;328(7434):265.
40. Christensen H, Griffiths KM, Korten A. Web-based cognitive behavior therapy: analysis of site usage and changes in depression and anxiety scores. J Med Internet Res 2002;4(1):e3.
41. Clarke G, Reid E, Eubanks D, et al. Overcoming depression on the Internet (ODIN): a randomized controlled trial of an Internet depression skills intervention program. J Med Internet Res 2002;4(3):E14.
42. de Graaf LE, Gerhards SA, Arntz A, et al. Clinical effectiveness of online computerised cognitive-behavioural therapy without support for depression in primary care: randomised trial. Br J Psychiatry 2009;195(1):73–80.
43. Mackinnon A, Griffiths KM, Christensen H. Comparative randomised trial of online cognitive-behavioural therapy and an information website for depression: 12-month outcomes. Br J Psychiatry 2008;192(2):130–4.
44. Meyer B, Berger T, Caspar F, et al. Effectiveness of a novel integrative online treatment for depression (Deprexis): randomized controlled trial. J Med Internet Res 2009;11(2):e15.
45. Patten SB. Prevention of depressive symptoms through the use of distance technologies. Psychiatr Serv 2003;54(3):396–8.
46. Proudfoot J, Goldberg D, Mann A, et al. Computerized, interactive, multimedia cognitive-behavioural program for anxiety and depression in general practice. Psychol Med 2003;33(2):217–27.
47. Lewinsohn PM, Antonuccio DO, Breckenridge JS, et al. The 'Coping with Depression' course. Eugene (Oregon): Castalia Publishing Company; 1984.
48. Cavanagh J, Geisler MW. Mood effects on the ERP processing of emotional intensity in faces: a P3 investigation with depressed students. Int J Psychophysiol 2006;60(1):27–33.
49. Warmerdam L, van Straten A, Cuijpers P. Internet-based treatment for adults with depressive symptoms: the protocol of a randomized controlled trial. BMC Psychiatry 2007;7:72.
50. Spek V, Nyklicek I, Smits N, et al. Internet-based cognitive behavioural therapy for subthreshold depression in people over 50 years old: a randomized controlled clinical trial. Psychol Med 2007;37(12):1797–806.
51. Spek V, Cuijpers P, Nyklicek I, et al. One-year follow-up results of a randomized controlled clinical trial on internet-based cognitive behavioural therapy for subthreshold depression in people over 50 years. Psychol Med 2008;38(5):635–9.
52. Clarke GN, Hornbrook M, Lynch F, et al. A randomized trial of a group cognitive intervention for preventing depression in adolescent offspring of depressed parents. Arch Gen Psychiatry 2001;58(12):1127–34.
53. Garber J, Clarke GN, Weersing VR, et al. Prevention of depression in at-risk adolescents: a randomized controlled trial. JAMA 2009;301(21):2215–24.
54. Elliott SA, Leverton TJ, Sanjack M, et al. Promoting mental health after childbirth: a controlled trial of primary prevention of postnatal depression. Br J Clin Psychol 2000;39(Pt 3):223–41.
55. Zlotnick C, Miller IW, Pearlstein T, et al. A preventive intervention for pregnant women on public assistance at risk for postpartum depression. Am J Psychiatry 2006;163(8):1443–5.
56. Lara MA, Navarro C, Navarrete L. Outcome results of a psycho-educational intervention in pregnancy to prevent PPD: a randomized control trial. J Affect Disord 2010;122(1–2):109–17.

57. Clarke GN, Hawkins W, Murphy M, et al. Targeted prevention of unipolar depressive disorder in an at-risk sample of high school adolescents: a randomized trial of a group cognitive intervention. J Am Acad Child Adolesc Psychiatry 1995;34(3):312–21.

58. Christensen H, Griffiths K, Groves C, et al. Free range users and one hit wonders: community users of an Internet-based cognitive behaviour therapy program. Aust N Z J Psychiatry 2006;40(1):59–62.

59. Gellatly J, Bower P, Hennessy S, et al. What makes self-help interventions effective in the management of depressive symptoms? Meta-analysis and meta-regression. Psychol Med 2007;37(9):1217–28.

60. Andersson G, Bergstrom J, Hollandare F, et al. Delivering cognitive behavioural therapy for mild to moderate depression via the Internet: predicting outcome at 6-month follow-up. Verhaltenstherapie 2004;14(3):185–9.

61. Van Voorhees BW, Ellis J, Stuart S, et al. Pilot study of a primary care internet-based depression prevention intervention for late adolescents. Can Child Adolesc Psychiatr Rev 2005;14(2):40–3.

62. Landback J, Prochaska M, Ellis J, et al. From prototype to product: development of a primary care/internet based depression prevention intervention for adolescents (CATCH-IT). Community Ment Health J 2009;45(5):349–54.

63. Resnicow K, Davis RE, Zhang G, et al. Tailoring a fruit and vegetable intervention on novel motivational constructs: results of a randomized study. Ann Behav Med 2008;35(2):159–69.

64. Matthews AK, Sanchez-Johnsen L, King A. Development of a culturally targeted smoking cessation intervention for African American smokers. J Community Health 2009;34(6):480–92.

65. John R, Buschman P, Chaszar M, et al. Development and evaluation of a PDA-based decision support system for pediatric depression screening. Stud Health Technol Inform 2007;129(Pt 2):1382–6.

66. Griffiths KM, Crisp D, Christensen H, et al. The ANU WellBeing study: a protocol for a quasi-factorial randomised controlled trial of the effectiveness of an Internet support group and an automated Internet intervention for depression. BMC Psychiatry 2010;10:20.

67. Coyle D, Doherty G, Sharry J. An evaluation of a solution focused computer game in adolescent interventions. Clin Child Psychol Psychiatry 2009;14(3):345–60.

68. Houston TK, Cooper LA, Ford DE. Internet support groups for depression: a 1-year prospective cohort study. Am J Psychiatry 2002;159(12):2062–8.

69. Shaw LH, Gant LM. In defense of the internet: the relationship between Internet communication and depression, loneliness, self-esteem, and perceived social support. Cyberpsychol Behav 2002;5(2):157–71.

70. Takahashi Y, Uchida C, Miyaki K, et al. Potential benefits and harms of a peer support social network service on the internet for people with depressive tendencies: qualitative content analysis and social network analysis. J Med Internet Res 2009;11(3):e29.

71. Batterham PJ, Neil AL, Bennett K, et al. Predictors of adherence among community users of a cognitive behavior therapy website. Patient Prefer Adherence 2008;2:97–105.

72. Marko M, Fogel J, Mykerezi K, et al. Adolescent internet depression prevention: preferences for intervention and predictors of intentions and adherence. Journal of Cyber Therapy and Rehabilitation Spring 2010;3(1):9–30.

73. Neil AL, Batterham P, Christensen H, et al. Predictors of adherence by adolescents to a cognitive behavior therapy website in school and community-based settings. J Med Internet Res 2009;11(1):e6.

74. Gagne RM, Briggs L, Wager WW. Principles of instructional design. Fort Worth (TX): Harcourt Brace Jovanovich College Publishers; 1992.

75. Santor DA, Poulin C, LeBlanc JC, et al. Online health promotion, early identification of difficulties, and help seeking in young people. J Am Acad Child Adolesc Psychiatry 2007;46(1):50–9.

76. de Graaf LE, Huibers MJ, Cuijpers P, et al. Minor and major depression in the general population: does dysfunctional thinking play a role? Compr Psychiatry 2010;51(3):266–74.

77. Regier DA, Narrow WE, Rae DS, et al. The de facto US mental and addictive disorders service system. Epidemiologic catchment area prospective 1-year prevalence rates of disorders and services. Arch Gen Psychiatry 1993;50(2): 85–94.

78. Cuijpers P. Review: exercise may moderately improve depressive symptoms. Evid Based Ment Health 2009;12(3):76–7.

79. Lakhan SE, Vieira KF. Nutritional therapies for mental disorders. Nutr J 2008;7:2.

80. Glasgow RE, Vogt TM, Boles SM. Evaluating the public health impact of health promotion interventions: the RE-AIM framework. Am J Public Health 1999;89(9): 1322–7.

Infusing Protective Factors for Children in Foster Care

Gene Griffin, JD, PhD[a],*, Erwin McEwen, AM[b],
Bryan H. Samuels, MPP[c], Hayward Suggs, MS, MBA[d],
Juanita L. Redd, MPA, MBA[d], Gary M. McClelland, PhD[e]

KEYWORDS

• Protective factors • Children • Foster care • Trauma

Risk factors are not predictive factors because of protective factors.
Carl Bell

In its report to Congress, the Fourth National Incidence Study of Child Abuse and Neglect[1] found that, during the study year of 2005 to 2006, approximately one child in every 58 in the United States was harmed by child abuse and neglect, whereas an estimated one in every 25 was endangered. The good news is that these statistics represent an improvement from the previous study.[2] The bad news is that during that year 1,256,600 children were harmed and 2,905,800 endangered.

A separate body of research, including the Adverse Childhood Experiences Study, reported how being abused or neglected as a child can lead to an increased risk of developing physical, emotional, cognitive, behavioral, and social problems. This situation makes it more likely that the child will suffer an early death.[3,4] The risks extend beyond the home, because exposure to violence in the schools and communities also increases the risk of trauma.[5]

Is the damage irrecoverable? Do these statistics mean that there is no hope for the millions of youth who are abused or neglected? The answer to those questions seems

[a] Mental Health Services and Policy Program, Northwestern University Feinberg School of Medicine, Suite 1220, 710 North Lakeshore Drive, Chicago, IL 60611-3072, USA
[b] Illinois Department of Children and Family Services, 100 West Randolph Street 6-100, Chicago, IL 60601, USA
[c] Administration on Children, Youth, and Families, 1250 Maryland Avenue, SW, Eighth Floor, Washington, DC 20024, USA
[d] Community Mental Health Council, 8704 South Constance Avenue, Chicago, IL 60617, USA
[e] Mental Health Services and Policy Program, Northwestern University Feinberg School of Medicine, 710 North Lakeshore Drive, Chicago, IL 60611-3072, USA
* Corresponding author.
E-mail address: e-griffin@northwestern.edu

Psychiatr Clin N Am 34 (2011) 185–203
doi:10.1016/j.psc.2010.11.014
0193-953X/11/$ – see front matter © 2011 Elsevier Inc. All rights reserved.
psych.theclinics.com

to be "No." Although the studies on risk factors indicate that it is not sufficient to remove a child from an abusive setting, other research suggests that there are ways to actively intervene with abused or neglected youth that prevent the increased risks they face from becoming reality.

Youth can be helped to overcome early abuse and neglect and can be assisted in building coping skills to confront future adverse experiences.[6] Although some youth naturally have more protective factors, abused and neglected youth can be assisted in becoming more resilient.[7] Risk factors do not become predictive factors if youth develop protective factors.[8,9]

The National Research Council and Institute of Medicine, in their 2009 report, *Preventing mental, emotional, and behavioral disorders among young people: progress and possibilities*,[10] conclude that focusing on early interventions with young people offers the greatest promise for preventing mental, emotional, and behavioral disorders and that these early interventions show potential lifetime benefits. The interventions need to take a child's developmental stage into account. Some of these interventions can be designed to focus on children who have been abused and neglected[11,12] and can incorporate both risk and protective factors.[13,14]

Implementing research findings into direct care can be difficult. Practitioners need to take successful clinical research and apply it to communities in ways that are culturally sensitive[15] and maintain fidelity to the model.[16,17] Real-world applications of research can prove valuable, not only to the children in the community but also as feedback to researchers.[18,19]

Applying interventions to a specific child welfare system requires coordination of federal, state, and local programs.[20] This article looks at an example of infusing protective factors into a child welfare system. Focusing on Illinois and its state child welfare agency, the article reviews some of the research on the relationship between risk behaviors and protective factors of traumatized youth in its child welfare system. Next, it looks at adapting treatment and evidence-based early intervention practices to local child welfare settings. These interventions are then placed in the wider context of a state plan to enhance protective factors. The article also reviews how the state and local plans have been influenced by federal policies and how the Illinois experience might help refine future policy.

THE RESEARCH LINK BETWEEN TRAUMA, RISK BEHAVIORS, AND PROTECTIVE FACTORS IN ILLINOIS CHILD WELFARE

In 2005, the Illinois Department of Children and Family Services (DCFS) began taking a trauma-informed approach in dealing with the youth in its custody. The US Department of Health and Human Services, Administration of Child and Family Services (HHS ACF)[21] had previously conducted its Child and Families Services Review (CFSR) of state and local child welfare programs, noting which areas needed to be improved to avoid loss of federal funding. Illinois had been told, among other things, that it needed to improve the mental health programming for youth in its care. As part of its Performance Improvement Plan (PIP), Illinois integrated child trauma theory into its mental health programming. A full explanation of child trauma, its effect on brain development, and its relationship to mental illness is beyond the scope of this article.[22–24] Suffice to say that a child's mental health and trauma symptoms are closely related and both are affected by risk factors and protective factors.

At DCFS, the new trauma-informed paradigm introduced trauma into 3 phases of mental health programs: training, assessment, and treatment. The 3 phases overlapped. This section focuses on research results from the trauma assessment. The next section looks at the training and treatment.

As part of its integrated assessment program, DCFS began conducting an assessment on every youth coming into its custody through the court system. The assessment included multiple components, one of which was a behavioral health assessment. The behavioral health instrument is the Child and Adolescent Needs and Strengths (CANS) tool,[25] with the DCFS version including sections on trauma experiences and on trauma symptoms.

The CANS is a functional assessment of children that can be used for treatment planning, outcome monitoring, quality improvement, and system design. The DCFS CANS had 105 items, with each item having anchored definitions, allowing it to be ranked from 0 to 3. The definitions translated into action levels (separate for needs and strengths):

For needs:

0. No evidence: no need for action
1. Watchful waiting/prevention
2. Action required (need is interfering with child's individual, family, or community functioning in a notable way)
3. Immediate/intensive action (need is dangerous or disabling).

For strengths:

0. Centerpiece strength (it can be the focus of a strength-based plan)
1. Useful strength (it can be included in a strength-based plan)
2. Strength has been identified (must be developed before being useful)
3. No strength identified (no evidence of a strength).

For purposes of this discussion, strengths are assumed to be equivalent to protective factors. (Specific items in the strengths section of the CANS include estimates of a youth's talents/interests, education, vocation, optimism, interpersonal skills, well-being, spiritual/religious life, family, community life, and relationship permanence.) Also relevant to this discussion, analysis can be based on multiple standardized CANS scales, including traumatic experiences (13 items), traumatic symptoms (5 items), risk behaviors (11 items), and strengths (10 items). Higher scores indicate greater needs or fewer strengths.

Before the use of the CANS, DCFS had not measured trauma or strengths. Children had received diagnoses of mental illness based on the Diagnostic and Statistical Manual (DSM) over the years. Adding measures of trauma and strengths showed immediate benefits. In 2006, after 1 year of administering the CANS to youth entering the DCFS system, the adjustment to trauma item became the most frequently endorsed clinical needs item. Approximately one-quarter of the youth (25.4% of 1375 youth) were assessed to have trauma adjustment at an actionable level (rated a 2 or 3), although more traditional clinical issues of attachment (17.9%), anger (17.7%), or depression (16.7%) were still present. Five years later, in 2010, a recent summary of integrated assessment data (N = 12,938) showed that adjustment to trauma is still running at 24.8%, indicating a stable estimate.

Initial analysis of strengths suggested they might serve as a counterbalance to the trauma. First-year results indicated that approximately 75% of youth showed strengths in multiple categories, including optimism, interpersonal skills, and well-being. The prevalence of these strengths decreased as staff assessed the youth in

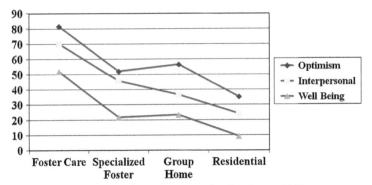

Fig. 1. Illinois DCFS CANS. Level of care by strengths, fiscal year, 2006.

increasing levels of care. That is, as **Fig. 1** shows, when the assessments shifted focus from youth at admission to youth in foster care, specialized foster care, group homes, or residential treatments, estimates of children's strengths declined.

These initial estimates were of different youth at a single point in time and could not distinguish whether children who had fewer strengths at admission required higher levels of care or whether children lost strengths over time while in DCFS custody. Later, more detailed studies have returned to the issue of strengths as well as their relationship to trauma.

In a 2009 study,[26] DCFS looked at trauma experiences and strengths. More than 85% of the youth (N = 8131) had at least one type of significant traumatic experience and nearly 30% had 4 or more types of actionable traumatic experiences. The research found a linear relationship between the number of these types of traumatic experiences and the number of risk behaviors that the child showed, as seen in **Fig. 2**.

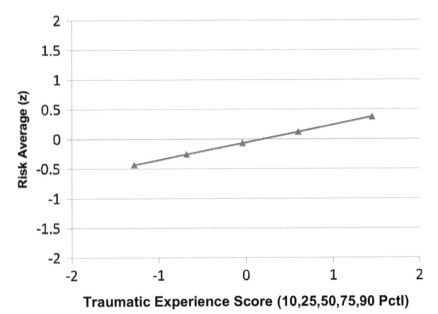

Fig. 2. The relationship between types of traumatic experiences and youth risk behaviors (N = 8131).

Initially, this finding suggested that a risk factor, such as traumatic experiences, is a predictive factor of risk behaviors. However, the picture changes when protective factors are included. The study found that strengths of the child moderated the relationship between trauma experiences and risk behaviors, as shown in **Fig. 3**. High-strength children showed few risk behaviors, regardless of the number of traumatic experiences. Low-strength children proved reactive, with more risk behaviors to begin with and increasing at an accelerating rate.

Like the 2006 study, this research suggests a relationship between trauma and strengths. One study looked at trauma experiences, whereas the other looked at trauma symptoms. Assuming that children are in higher levels of care because of their risk behaviors, both studies suggest an additional relationship between trauma, strengths, and risk behaviors. Neither study looked at change in children over time.

A third, recent study did look at DCFS youth over time, including their trauma symptoms, strengths, and risk behaviors. This study allows for an exploration of change scores and a chance to view the relationship over time between trauma, strengths, and risk behaviors within the same child. The focus of the third study was on DCFS youth who went into residential treatment facilities. The first part of the study examined youth who initially went into community treatment but later were placed in residential care. The results were surprising (**Fig. 4**).

Fig. 4 shows that DCFS staff ratings did not show any significant change in either trauma symptoms or risk behaviors of the youth between the youth's CANS at integrated assessment and the later CANS assessment at admission to residential placement. One might have expected at least the estimate of risk behaviors to have increased to justify taking the youth out of the community and putting them in a more restrictive environment. The one variable that did show a significant change was the estimate of the youth's strengths, with that estimate declining. One possible interpretation is that the youth started with high-risk behaviors (1.8 standard deviations more than the average DCFS youth) but they were offset by higher estimates

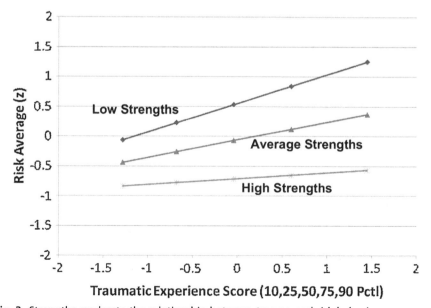

Fig. 3. Strengths moderate the relationship between trauma and risk behaviors.

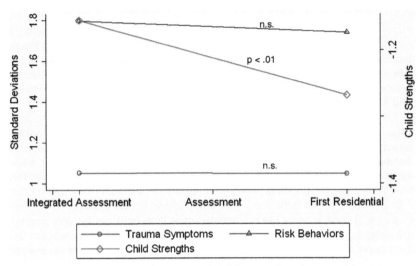

Fig. 4. Trauma symptoms, risk behaviors, and child strengths prior to residential treatment (2010, n = 549).

of the youth's strengths (though still more than a standard deviation below average). Thus, the DCFS workers might have had hope that the youth would improve by foster placement in the community. However, staff saw over time that neither the youth's behavior nor their trauma symptoms improved. The estimate of high risk did not change. Instead, the staff lowered their estimate of the youth's strengths and decided that the youth needed to move from the community to residential placement. In effect, the estimate of strengths may have served as a proxy for the amount of hope that staff had in a youth.

As a follow-up, the study looked at DCFS youth over time while in residential treatment (**Fig. 5**). This second analysis involved a slightly different group of youth than the first analysis because it includes some youth who went directly into residential care, and therefore did not have two CANS assessment before residential care. Also, the second analysis includes only those DCFS youth who were in residential care long enough to have two CANS assessments.

This second analysis, seen in **Fig. 5**, shows that, while in residential care, youth's trauma symptoms and their risk behaviors both improve, as do estimates of the youth's strengths. These results are important, not only because they show improvement while in residential care but also because the results are consistent with the interpretation of the previous analysis (**Fig. 6**).

Fig. 6 combines the previous 2 figures. The prior analysis posited that DCFS staff lost hope when the youth's trauma symptoms and risk behaviors did not improve, resulting in the staff lowering their estimate of a youth's strengths. However, in this second analysis, the youth's trauma symptoms and risk behaviors did improve. The staff also increased their assessment of the youth's strengths. Once again, staff have hope for the youth.

These various studies start to paint a consistent picture of youth in child welfare. First, these youth have experienced multiple traumatic exposures. Approximately one-quarter of youth in child welfare develop significant trauma symptoms, whereas three-quarters show significant strengths. The trauma variables have an effect on a youth's risk behaviors but this effect can be moderated by protective factors. Risk

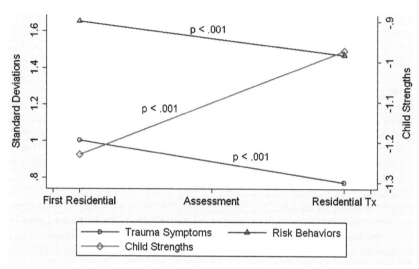

Fig. 5. Trauma symptoms, risk behaviors, and child strengths during residential treatment (2010, n = 603). Tx, treatment.

behaviors and strengths seem to be opposite sides of the trauma coin. Staff estimates of strengths change over time in relation to the youth's improved trauma and risk behaviors. They may serve as a proxy estimate of the hope that staff have for the youth. The next step is to determine how to make practical use of this information.

ADAPTING EVIDENCE-BASED TREATMENTS AND EARLY INTERVENTION PRACTICE TO THE LOCAL CHILD WELFARE SETTING

Although there is no legal finding until after a series of court hearings, there is a high probability that youth who are court ordered into the custody of child welfare have

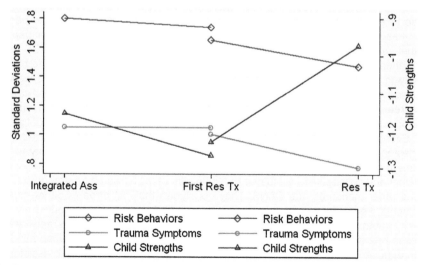

Fig. 6. Trauma symptoms, risk behaviors, and child strengths prior to and during residential treatment. Tx, treatment.

been subject to some form of abuse or neglect. Given that being abused or neglected as a child can lead to an increased risk of developing physical, emotional, cognitive, behavioral, and social problems, DCFS recognized the need for treatment and early intervention. When a youth is given to the custody of DCFS, it is too late for initial prevention. Some damage has already been done, some risk factors put in place. Nor does placement in state custody end the adverse experiences of a child. As the experiences in Illinois show, a child welfare agency removing a youth from their family may save that child's life but can also be considered an additional adverse event. Multiple moves of a child in DCFS custody might also be extremely disruptive to that child and have a negative effect on their development and well-being. The issue becomes one of early intervention and how quickly the department can respond to minimize all these risk factors and put more protective factors in place.

DCFS began by training all caseworkers and foster parents on a basic understanding of trauma, its causes, and its effect on children. To develop the curriculum, DCFS consulted Carl Bell, Bruce Perry,[27] and experts from the National Child Traumatic Stress Network (NCTSN), such as Frank Putnam.[28] Once caseworkers and foster parents had this introduction to trauma theory, DCFS educated staff on how to refer the children for trauma therapy.

There is a growing list of evidence-based practices that therapists can use to treat traumatized children. NCTSN identifies "empirically supported treatments and promising practices."[29] With the rollout of its trauma program, DCFS brought in the designers of 3 of the promising practices to train clinicians treating traumatized youth. DCFS chose child parent psychotherapy (CPP) for 0- to 6-year-olds,[30] trauma-focused cognitive-behavioral therapy (TF-CBT) for 6- to 12-year-old children,[31] and structured psychotherapy for adolescents responding to chronic stress (SPARCS) for teenagers.[32]

Each therapy needed to be adapted to the child welfare culture. For example, with CPP, the classic treatment involved helping a mother interact with her child. However, children in DCFS custody are not living with their mothers. Therefore, depending on the plan regarding reunification with the family, the therapists worked with the foster parent, with another family member, or with both the mother and foster parent. With TF-CBT, the classic model involved teaching a youth to reveal the details of their abuse to a supportive parent. This model needed to be modified when the parent was already involved in the abuse. Other caring adults, such as the foster parent, another relative, or even the caseworker were used as surrogates. SPARCS uses group therapy with adolescents, which avoids the limitations of including the parent directly in the treatment but creates other logistical problems for the child welfare system. The model worked well in an urban setting but was difficult to coordinate in rural areas where group members had to be transported long distances from multiple locations. Workers struggled to minimize disruptions to school and afterschool activities. Eventually, some groups were run for fewer weeks than originally intended, with the designers deciding that the local therapists were able to maintain fidelity to the treatment model.

Weiner and colleagues[33] evaluated the 2006 pilot of the 3 trauma treatments, using, among other measures, the CANS. They concluded that "all three evidence-based treatments were effective in reducing symptoms and improving functioning among minority youth." In addition, the evaluation stated, "analyses revealed no racial differences in retention in the program and no differences in outcomes between minority youth exposed to the intervention and other participants." Thus, with the assistance of experts, DCFS was able to adapt these evidence-based treatments in a culturally appropriate way for its children.

This success in adapting effective treatment of traumatized youth in child welfare gave DCFS an important resource. However, there were still gaps in a child's trauma-informed care. Caseworkers were trained to understand trauma and how to refer a child to trauma therapy. However, these therapies were not available throughout the state. Further, outpatient evidence-based treatment is limited, usually to 1-hour weekly meetings and to certain duration, such as 12 group sessions. In addition, knowing how to refer a youth to professional therapists does not inform the caseworker or foster parent of how they should interact with the traumatized youth. Caseworkers and foster parents have more contact with the mistreated youth than the therapist and have the potential to have a significant effect on a child's life. Also, the caseworkers and foster parents are involved from the beginning of DCFS custody. Evidence-based treatment might not start for some time after the child is in care. Therefore, DCFS needed to come up with some guidelines for its caseworkers and foster parents to use in working with traumatized youth on a daily basis.

The department turned to the NCTSN's guidelines on psychological first aid (PFA).[34] The PFA intervention strategies are intended for use with children, parents, and families exposed to disaster or terrorism. They were originally designed to be used by mental health and direct response providers at disaster settings such as shelters, triage areas, and hospital emergency rooms. It seemed a natural progression for DCFS to apply these principles to help children and families when there is abuse or neglect and the state has just intervened in the crisis by taking custody of the children. DCFS relied on an experienced community provider, the Community Mental Health Council's Institute for Managerial and Clinical Consultation (IMACC), to adapt the material in a culturally appropriate way, maintaining fidelity to the basic PFA model.

IMACC changed the context of PFA from disaster response to child welfare. This change required working with the current standard DCFS training for caseworkers and foster parents, adopting some of the DCFS language and terminology, and writing child welfare specific case scenarios and practice examples. The interventions needed to cover both urban and rural settings and acknowledge the culturally diverse communities. The child welfare PFA needed to fit into the current DCFS policies and procedures as well as union agreements regarding staff roles. The community provider was able to develop a 1-day (7.5-hour) training program, using the DCFS cotrainer and train-the-trainer models.

Whereas the NCTSN intervention was designed to address a crisis, the DCFS training went beyond the immediate crisis and helped staff understand how to interact with DCFS youth at any time. IMACC emphasized to DCFS caseworkers and foster parents that most people have what it takes to be supportive of someone in crisis. The trainers pointed out that the children in custody were normal youth who were responding to an abnormal event. For example, for a child who witnesses community violence and then is unable to concentrate at school or does not remember instructions that were just given, staff should view this behavior as a normal reaction to an extreme circumstance. This child should not be considered defiant or oppositional. Understanding this situation allows caseworkers to see people (both the adults and their children) as injured rather than bad. The child welfare version of PFA avoids pathologizing, or viewing people as mentally ill, because of their response to an event. Instead, it focuses on helping caseworkers and foster parents to recognize that many children's reactions are normal considering their situations. The goal for the caseworkers and foster parents is to help youth build protective factors to return children to their normal precrisis level of functioning.

The NCTSN general steps of PFA for workers, such as engagement, safety and comfort, stabilization, connection with social supports, and linkage with collaborative services are relevant any time that a child welfare worker has contact with the youth or is updating the youth's service plan. Similarly, the PFA handouts, such as those offering *Tips to parents* based on the developmental stage of the youth (infants and toddlers, preschool age, school age, adolescents, and adults), with slight modifications became invaluable resources for caseworkers and foster parents.

IMACC produced several tools, including the *Psychological first aid: child and adolescent care* (PFACAC) instructor manual, learner workbook, school-based instructor manual, school-based learner workbook, community instructor manual, and a series of training vignettes. Using these tools, IMACC certified 50 DCFS-PFA trainers, who went on to train more than 4600 DCFS staff, ranging from receptionists to caseworkers to supervisors to senior level management. IMACC continues to follow up with onsite observations, quality assurance monitoring, coaching meetings, and feedback sessions.

Whereas the evidence-based trauma treatments were implemented to help those youth who were assessed as having trauma symptoms (previously estimated at roughly 25% of the youth), PFACAC applied to all youth in DCFS care. Thus, DCFS moved from its initial focus on assessment and treatment to a larger focus on early intervention.

INCORPORATING PROTECTIVE FACTORS INTO PREVENTION WITH A STATE CHILD WELFARE AGENCY

Incorporating protective factors into a child welfare plan requires more than taking on trauma and risk factors. The Illinois DCFS child trauma approach of training, assessment, and treatment addressed the behavioral health of youth as proposed in its PIP. The department's initial focus on risk factors, through research and practice, led naturally to protective factors. Protective factors have benefits beyond being an antidote to traumatic risk factors. They are relevant to a child's overall well-being, including the well-being of children who never become traumatized. Protective factors, in their own right, need to be incorporated into child welfare.

Rather than being limited to early trauma intervention, protective factors can be part of a plan for prevention. The Center for the Study of Social Policy (CSSP) in Washington, DC[35] has developed a Strengthening Families approach that is intended to reduce the incidence of abuse and neglect. It is an approach that can be integrated into the work of child welfare, education, and early childhood programs. Strengthening Families provides parents with the skills to parent effectively, particularly when the parents are under stress. This focus on the family, rather than the child, allows for prevention, rather than amelioration, of the abuse. The approach focuses on building 6 protective factors: parental resilience; social connections; knowledge of parenting and child development; concrete support in times of need; children's social and emotional development; and parent and child relationships. This Strengthening Families approach is currently being applied in 36 states, including Illinois.

Illinois was one of 7 states selected in 2004 to pilot CSSP's Strengthening Families Through Early Care and Education strategy.[36] DCFS convened more than 20 organizations and state agencies from the child welfare, child abuse prevention, family support, and early childhood fields as well as parents and community leaders to promote the protective factors across systems.

This collaborative partnership, Strengthening Families Illinois (SFI),[37] adopted the basic logic model of the CSSP program shown in **Fig. 7**.

Within the framework of SFI, the starting point is constructing a new normal by which all child-and-family-serving organizations and systems work toward building

HOW POLICIES, PROGRAMS AND PRACTICE CAN PREVENT CHILD ABUSE AND NEGLECT AND PROMOTE OPTIMAL DEVELOPMENT

| a new normal
all child- and family-serving organizations and systems build protective factors | multisystem leadership around levers of change | Program strategies and worker practice that: | protective factors | child abuse & neglect prevention
optimal child development |
|---|---|---|---|---|
| | Parent Partnership | Facilitate friendships and mutual support | Parental Resilience | |
| | Policy/Systems | Strengthen Parenting | Social Connections | |
| | Professional Development | Respond to Family Crises | Knowledge of Parenting & Child Development | |
| | | Link Families to Services and Opportunities | Concrete Supports in Times of Need | |
| | | Value and Support Parents | Social & Emotional Competence | |
| | | Facilitate Children's Social and Emotional Development | Parent Child Relationships | |
| | | Observe and respond to early warning signs of abuse or neglect | | |

Fig. 7. Strengthening families logic model. (*From* Center for the Study of Social Policy (CSSP), 2009. Available at: http://strengtheningfamilies.net/images/uploads/pdf_uploads/%282.3%29_Expanded_Logic_Model_.pdf. Accessed December 28, 2010; with permission.)

protective factors in families. It requires the multisystem leadership to embed a family support approach in its delivery of human services. Each organization, through its program strategies, helps build the protective factors that not only prevent child abuse but also optimize child development, thus achieving the new normal.

DCFS continues to convene SFI, which has now grown to include more than 40 state and local organizations. They include the Illinois Department of Human Services, Voices for Illinois Children, Illinois Federation of Families, Chicago Safe Start, and the Ounce of Prevention Fund.

In order to integrate the Strengthening Families approach with its trauma work, DCFS developed its trauma logic model (**Fig. 8**).

The logic model in **Fig. 8** shows that violence in the home and community results in trauma that affects young children's brain development, youth school performance,

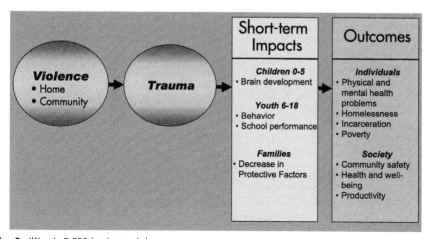

Fig. 8. Illinois DCFS logic model.

and family strengths. In this model, the trauma is seen to decrease the protective factors. The model reflects that there are long-term negative consequences to trauma for individuals and for society. As with SFI, DCFS collaborates with many other state and local organizations in attempting to address the trauma. Trauma-focused collaborators include the Illinois Violence Prevention Authority, Illinois Children's Mental Health Partnership, and the Illinois Childhood Trauma Coalition.

The vision for DCFS is to integrate the protective factors present in the Strengthening Families program model with its own trauma-informed practices. By building the protective factors into the child welfare system as a whole, the objective is to support quality practice and promote children's healing. This integrated and holistic service model required a paradigm shift for the department. It is not enough for DCFS to remove abused children to prevent further harm. DCFS needs to be proactive. However, DCFS did not want to be in the business of taking and raising children. Instead, under this new paradigm, DCFS seeks to be in the business of strengthening families.

The next phase of development in integrating the protective factors with the trauma-informed practices, shown in **Fig. 9**, involved 3 steps: (1) identifying specific problems in treating trauma that arises while a child is in DCFS custody, (2) addressing these problems through DCFS programs, and (3) examining how these programs reflect the relevant protective factors.

Identification of trauma-relevant problems is relatively straightforward. Under this trauma model, DCFS needs to actively address 6 problems: (1) a child's separation from their family, school, and community; (2) lack of resources to serve the child's needs; (3) lack of understanding trauma on the part of adults, which results in misattribution of the child's needs; (4) lack of focus on child and family's strengths and protective capacity; (5) the failure of the department to coordinate care with other

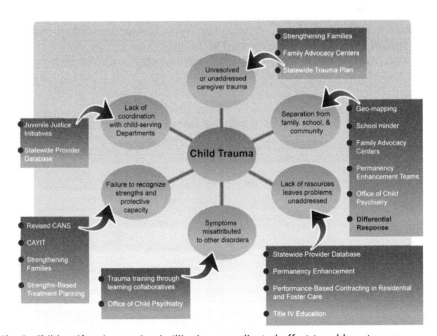

Fig. 9. Child welfare innovation in Illinois: a coordinated effort to address trauma.

child-serving agencies; and (6) lack of understanding of intergenerational trauma and the corresponding failure to address caregiver trauma.

Currently, each of these problems is being addressed by multiple DCFS programs. Some of these programs involve collaboration with SFI members and child advocacy groups. Other programs require the coordination of care with different mandated agencies, such as those dealing with education or juvenile justice. Still other programs involve internal DCFS processes, such as the treatment planning process and a new program, Differential Response. These internal programs are the least obvious, more cutting edge, and require some explanation.

As noted earlier in this article, all youth who come into DCFS custody are given an integrated assessment, which includes the use of the CANS instrument. Based on this assessment, the child's caseworker gathers the relevant parties (including the child, the family, and the foster family) and develops a strength-based treatment plan. DCFS has developed a sophisticated system that integrates CANS data with provider information. When the caseworker enters the child's CANS scores into a Web-based reporting system, that system automatically generates treatment recommendations based on those scores. The system can then use the DCFS statewide provider database to generate a list of relevant service providers, including therapists who offer evidence-based trauma therapies and service providers who offer positive, strength-based programs. Further, the system can use its geomapping function to identify which of the relevant treatment and service providers are closest to the child's residence. The caseworker is not bound by these recommendations but they provide a solid basis for starting the strength-based treatment planning. A child's treatment plan is reexamined (including the addition of updated CANS) every 6 months as part of an administrative case review. Should a youth need to move to another level of care (eg, residential placement, transitional living), the caseworker can also convene a child and youth investment team meeting. This meeting brings together all the providers as well as the youth and family and uses tools in the same manner as the initial planning. The DCFS administration can also combine data from the CANS, statewide provider database, and geomapping tools to perform system level analysis. This analysis can determine the major needs and strengths of youth in its care, where those needs and strengths are most pronounced, and whether there are adequate service providers to meet the demands. This information can drive resources and policy development.

All of this treatment planning is carried out for children in DCFS custody. However, as noted in the Strengthening Families model and as required by HHS ACF,[38] the department is working to reduce the need to take children into custody by strengthening the families before major abuse occurs. The Differential Response program is a new attempt by DCFS to identify and strengthen at-risk families. It is a 5-year demonstration project started in 2010, which requires DCFS initial investigators (who are responding to allegations of abuse or neglect) to identify families who, although problematic, are at low risk of causing a child additional major harm. With these families DCFS then embeds evidence-based practices into its intact family services plan to strengthen the family rather than taking custody of the child. Practices being offered include home visiting and recovery coaches as well as positive, strength-building services, such as learning networks and parent cafés, where groups of parents come together to discuss common problems and effective solutions. The demonstration project uses the CANS, statewide provider database, and geomapping tools in its rollout of Differential Response.

The final DCFS logic model, seen in **Fig. 10**, identifies the relevant protective factors.

Just as the CANS research at the beginning of this article suggested that risk behaviors and strengths were opposite sides of the trauma coin, this logic model also

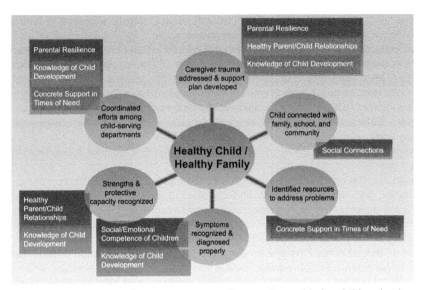

Fig. 10. Building protective factors supports quality practice and helps children heal.

converts the previous trauma problems into protective factors. When DCFS works with families in the appropriate, previously identified ways, the focus can shift from trauma to healthy children and families. The problems get resolved so that: (1) the child is reconnected with their family, school, and community; (2) resources are identified to serve the child's needs; (3) symptoms are recognized and properly diagnosed; (4) the child's and family's strengths and protective capacities are recognized; (5) the department coordinates care with other child-serving agencies; and (6) intergenerational trauma is understood and the caregiver's trauma is addressed. Each of these resolutions integrates some of the Strengthening Families' 6 protective factors of parental resilience; social connections; knowledge of parenting and child development; concrete support in times of need; children's social and emotional development; and parent and child relationships. Achieving this model would represent a true paradigm shift on the part of child welfare and would prove a tremendous benefit to children and families.

APPLYING THE LESSONS LEARNED AND THE LIMITATIONS REGARDING PROTECTIVE FACTORS

Some of the Illinois DCFS work regarding protective factors was in response to the HHS Child and Family Services Reviews, and lessons learned might be of value to national child welfare policies. However, policy discussions of protective factors need not be limited to child welfare. Lessons learned might also benefit other child policy areas such as homeless and runaway youth, children exposed to violence, juvenile justice, substance abuse, mental health, or education.

Lessons Learned

Research with children in the DCFS system supports the proposition that protective factors mediate the effect of adverse experiences. Protective factors can both prevent disruption of a child's normal development and help a child recover from an earlier disruption.

Illinois DCFS has trained staff to incorporate protective factors into early intervention and prevention. In its 5-year demonstration project, DCFS offers community-based services to at-risk families, hoping to build more protective factors and reduce the known risks. In focusing on prevention, DCFS has joined the national Strengthening Families movement and is working with other child-serving agencies to build protective factors in parents as well as children, thereby producing healthier families. In doing so, Illinois DCFS has moved from a traditional symptom/risk child focus to a healthy/protective factor child and family focus. This shift offers a model to other child welfare providers and child-serving agencies.

Limitations

Illinois DCFS faces the usual limitations of inadequate funding and resources to serve all the needs of the children in its custody. By moving to a focus on protective factors and including more early intervention and prevention work, the department hopes that fewer youth will be abused, and harmed youth will recover more completely. In the long run, these changes might result in fewer resources being needed for child welfare.

Although not unique to DCFS, there are some limitations to the research model of protective factors mediating the effect of risk factors. Researchers have not fully defined the model. For example, there is no comprehensive list of adverse experiences. Researchers generally agree that life-threatening events and child abuse can disrupt a child's normal development. However, there is still debate as to what constitutes an adverse experience and whether it should be defined by objective or subjective criteria.

Protective factors are also not well defined. Terms that seem to address the same construct as protective factors include a child's strengths or resilience. Researchers give many different labels to items they include under such terms. Protective factors, by their nature, should be defined in relation to the adverse experiences or risk factors from which these factors are supposed to protect a child. Also, protective factors seem better defined by process variables (eg, a person's ability to cope or self-regulate) rather than static characteristics (eg, a person's age, sex, or race), because protective factors involve adjusting or changing to the environment. Whichever terms are chosen, reaching consensus is essential to moving the research forward.

The research model also relies heavily on the concept of normal development. There is an assumption that a child progresses through normal development if these adverse experiences are absent. The protective factors help a youth maintain the course of normal development. Interventions help a youth achieve a new normal. As with adverse experiences and protective factors, there are not generally accepted standards of normal either.

Yet, this concept of normality is central to the whole discussion of child development. A definition or standard of normal child development could provide a common measure for all agencies working with children (child welfare, juvenile justice, education, mental health), regardless of their particular focus. The goals of all agencies could include maintaining or returning a youth to the normal range of development. Protective factors could be measured by their ability to keep youth in this range. Normal developmental measures would form the center point from which risk factors and protective factors could be studied.

Future Directions

Although no single, formal measure of normal child and adolescent development is currently in use, several of the sources mentioned in this article use a similar approach.

The National Research Council and Institute of Medicine's 2009 report on *Preventing mental, emotional, and behavioral disorders among young people*[10] uses a developmental framework in guiding its prevention recommendations and incorporates some of the latest findings in developmental neuroscience. Perry,[23] in his trauma work, also incorporates developmental neuroscience and proposes functional brain mapping to compare normal neurological development with disruptions caused by trauma. NCTSN, in its PFA, includes a checklist of physical, emotional, cognitive, and behavioral symptoms as well as social problems in its developmental framework.

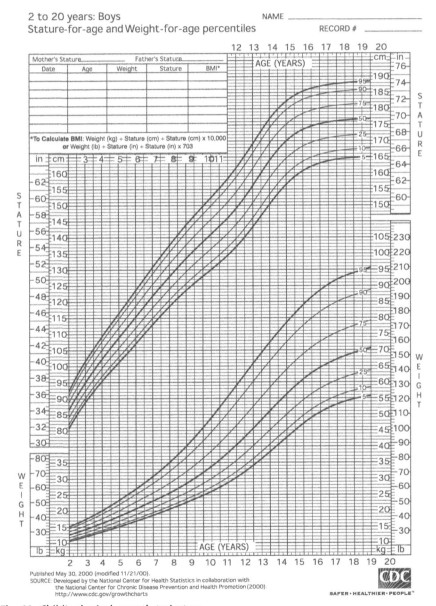

Fig. 11. Child's physical growth trajectory.

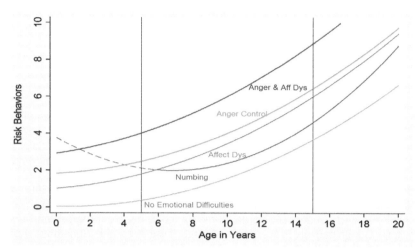

Fig. 12. Trajectory of risk behaviors based on age and emotional functioning. Aff dys, affective dysregulation.

Although they are not currently available, it is theoretically possible to develop a set of measures that would reflect normal child development comprehensively along physical, emotional, cognitive, behavioral, and social dimensions. Each dimension could plot a normal trajectory. For example, every pediatrician can already show new parents a growth chart, similar to **Fig. 11**, placing a newborn within the appropriate percentile for height and weight and projecting that child's future growth.

Illinois DCFS researchers can already use current CANS data to plot the trajectory of risk behaviors based on emotional issues for children in its care, as seen in **Fig. 12**.

Imagine if a trajectory of normal youth could be developed for comparison purposes. The CFSR measure of child well-being could then focus on whether the children in the care of the local child welfare agencies are in the normal range of development. Treatment could focus on bringing youth back into range. All child-serving agencies could collaborate using this common set of measures. Both risk and protective factors could be assessed in their effect against true anchor points. In the process, the focus of working with children could change from measuring symptoms and risk behaviors to measuring positive healthy developments. That would be a true paradigmatic shift toward strengthening families.

REFERENCES

1. Sedlak AJ, Mettenburg J, Basena M, et al. Fourth National Incidence Study of Child Abuse and Neglect (NIS–4): report to Congress. Washington, DC: US Department of Health and Human Services, Administration for Children and Families; 2010.
2. Sedlak AJ, Broadhurst DD. Third National Incidence Study of Child Abuse and Neglect: final report. Washington, DC: US Department of Health and Human Services; 1996.
3. Felitti VJ, Anda RF, Nordenberg D, et al. The relationship of adult health status to childhood abuse and household dysfunction. Am J Prev Med 1998;14:245–58.
4. Nemeroff CB. Commentary: fostering foster care outcomes: quality of intervention matters in overcoming early adversity. Arch Gen Psychiatry 2008;65:625–33.

5. Jenkins EJ, Bell CC. Exposure and response to community violence among children and adolescents. In: Osofsky J, editor. Children in a violent society. New York: Guilford Press; 1997. p. 9–31.
6. Racusin R, Maerlender A, Sengupta A, et al. Psychosocial treatment of children in foster care: a review. Community Ment Health J 2005;4:199–221.
7. Rutter M. Genetic influences on risk and protection: implications for understanding resilience. In: Luthar SS, editor. Resilience and vulnerability: adaptation in the context of childhood adversities. New York: Cambridge University Press; 2003. p. 498–509.
8. Jessor RJ, Van Den Bos J, Vanderryn J, et al. Protective factors in adolescent problem behavior: moderator effects and developmental change. Dev Psychol 1995;31:923–33.
9. Bell C. Editorial: prevention is the future. Clin Psychiatry News 2007;35(1):14.
10. National Research Council and Institute of Medicine. Preventing mental, emotional, and behavioral disorders among young people: progress and possibilities. Committee on Prevention of Mental Disorders and Substance Abuse Among Children, Youth and Young Adults: Research Advances and Promising Interventions. O'Connell ME, Boat T, Warner KE, editors. Board on Children, Youth, and Families, Division of Behavioral and Social Sciences and Education. Washington, DC: The National Academies Press; 2009.
11. Landsverk JA, Burns BJ, Stambaugh LF, et al. Psychosocial interventions for children and adolescents in foster care: review of research literature. Child Welfare 2009;88:49–69.
12. Kessler RC, Pecora PJ, Williams J, et al. The effects of enhanced foster care on the long-term physical and mental health of foster care alumni. Arch Gen Psychiatry 2008;65(6):625–33.
13. Lederman CS, Osofsky JD, Katz L. When the bough breaks the cradle will fall: promoting the health and well being of infants and toddlers in juvenile court. Infant Ment Health J 2007;2:440–8.
14. Hawkins JD, Catalano RF, Miller JY. Risk and protective factors for alcohol and other drug problems in adolescence and early adulthood: implications for substance abuse prevention. Psychol Bull 1992;112:64–105.
15. Bell CC, Bhana A, Petersen I, et al. Building protective factors to offset sexually risky behaviors among black youths: a randomized control trial. J Natl Med Assoc 2008;100:936–44.
16. Kolko DJ, Herschell AD, Costello AH, et al. Child welfare recommendations to improve mental health services for children who have experienced abuse and neglect: a national perspective. Adm Policy Ment Health 2009;36:50–62.
17. Kumpfer KL, Alvarado R, Smith P, et al. Cultural sensitivity and adaptation in family-based prevention interventions. Prev Sci 2002;3:241–6.
18. Chamberlain P, Price J, Leve LD, et al. Prevention of behavior problems for children in foster care: outcomes and mediation effects. Prev Sci 2008;9:17–27.
19. Bell CC. The sanity of survival: reflections on community mental health and wellness. Chicago: Third World Press; 2004.
20. Webb MB, Harden BJ. Beyond child protection: promoting mental health for children and families in the child welfare system. J Emot Behav Disord 2003;11:49–58.
21. US Department of Health and Human Services. Administration for Children and Families, Administration on Children, Youth and Families, Children's Bureau. The Children's Bureau: training and technical assistance network 2010 directory. 2010. Available at: www.acf.hhs.gov/programs/cb/tta/index.htm. Accessed December 28, 2010.

22. Pynoos RS, Steinberg AM, Ornitz EM, et al. Issues in the developmental neurobiology of traumatic stress. Ann N Y Acad Sci 1997;821:176–93.
23. Perry BD. Examining child maltreatment through a neurodevelopmental lens: clinical applications of the neurosequential model of therapeutics. J Loss Trauma 2009;14:240–55.
24. Kazdin A. President's column–trauma in children: how can we communicate what we know? Mon Psychol 2008;39:5.
25. Lyons J. Redressing the emperor: improving our children's public mental health system. Westport (CT), Connecticut: Praeger; 2004.
26. Griffin G, Martinovich Z, Gawron T, et al. Strengths moderate the impact of trauma on risk behaviors in child welfare. Resid Treat Child Youth 2009;26:1–14.
27. Perry BD, Szalavitz M. The boy who was raised as a dog. New York: Basic Books; 2006.
28. Putnam F. The impact of trauma on child development. Juv Fam Court J 2006;57: 1–11.
29. National Child Traumatic Stress Network. National Child Traumatic Stress Network empirically supported treatments and promising practices. 2010. Available at: www.nctsn.org/nccts/nav.do?pid=ctr_top_trmnt_prom. Accessed December 28, 2010.
30. Lieberman A, Van Horn P, Ghosh I. Toward evidence based treatment: child-parent psychotherapy with preschoolers exposed to marital violence. J Am Acad Child Adolesc Psychiatry 2005;44:12.
31. Cohen JA, Deblinger E, Mannarino A, et al. A multisite, randomized controlled trial for children with sexual abuse-related PTSD symptoms. J Am Acad Child Adolesc Psychiatry 2004;43:4.
32. DeRosa R, Pelcovitz. Treating traumatized adolescent mothers: a structured approach. In: Webb N, editor. Working with traumatized youth in child welfare. New York: Guilford Press; 2006. p. 219–45.
33. Weiner D, Schneider A, Lyons J. Evidence-based treatments for trauma among culturally diverse foster care youth: treatment retention and outcomes. Child Youth Serv Rev 2009;31:1199–205.
34. National Child Traumatic Stress Network and National Center for PTSD. Psychological first aid: field operations guide. 2nd edition. 2006. Available at: www. nctsn.org. Accessed December 28, 2010.
35. Center for the Study of Social Policy. 2010. Available at: http://www. strengtheningfamilies.net. Accessed December 28, 2010.
36. Illinois: strengthening families national network partner. Available at: http:// strengtheningfamilies.net/images/uploads/pdf_uploads/Illinois.pdf. Accessed on December 28, 2010.
37. Strengthening Families Illinois. 2010. Available at: http://www.strengthening familiesillinois.org. Accessed December 28, 2010.
38. See, for example, Preventive Services described in US Department of Health and Human Services, Administration for Children and Families, Administration on Children, Youth and Families, Children's Bureau. Child Maltreatment 2008. 2010. Available at: http://www.acf.hhs.gov/programs/cb/stats_research/index.htm#can. Accessed December 28, 2010.

Youth Homicide Prevention

Kobie Douglas, MD[a], Carl C. Bell, MD, DLAPA, FACPsych[a,b],*

KEYWORDS

- Youth • Violence • Prevention

From a societal, public health, and emotional perspective, homicide has long had a devastating effect on individuals, families, and communities. Law enforcement agencies, social scientists, and community leaders have long struggled to find solutions to such a seemingly intractable problem.[1,2] More recently, with the 24-hour news cycle streaming repeated stories of homicide throughout apparently every community, concern about homicide and violence seems to be at a zenith. However, review of existing data shows that there are many different solutions at our disposal, and these interventions are already being used and have proved to be effective.[3,4]

This article reviews homicide and violence data and discusses the developmental dynamics of violence and homicide, noting the different tracks youth take toward violence. The risk factors that lead youth toward a violent lifestyle are compared with the protective factors that shield them from it. The necessary principles involved in the prevention of violent behavior such as homicide are also discussed.

HOMICIDE DATA

Official law enforcement agency reports of criminal behavior and violent crimes such as homicide are typically the most direct and reliable means of obtaining the pertinent epidemiologic data. However, confidential youth surveys can prove useful in obtaining data on violent behavior that may go unreported to such agencies. Although the public perception is that African Americans are more violent than European Americans, there is robust scientific evidence of equal rates of self-report violence between African Americans and European Americans.[5] Analysis of official crime statistics reveals a sharp increase in the arrest rates for homicide in the decade between 1983 and 1993, especially amongst youth.[5] In response to increased numbers of homicide arrests, policies to get tough on youth crime were enacted; gun control laws were passed, boot camps were established, and children were waived from the juvenile justice system into adult

[a] Community Mental Health Council, Inc, 8704 South Constance, Chicago, IL 60617, USA
[b] Institute for Juvenile Research, Department of Psychiatry, College of Medicine, University of Illinois at Chicago, 1747 West Roosevelt Road, Room 155, Chicago, IL 60608-1264, USA
* Corresponding author. Community Mental Health Council, Inc, 8704 South Constance, Chicago, IL 60617.
E-mail address: carlcbell@pol.net

Psychiatr Clin N Am 34 (2011) 205–216
doi:10.1016/j.psc.2010.11.013
0193-953X/11/$ – see front matter © 2011 Elsevier Inc. All rights reserved.

criminal courts.[5] From the authors' perspective, these policies were grave errors because they did not take into account the understanding of youth development, and took a wrong-headed, reactionary, criminal justice approach to youth violence, instead of a scientific, public health approach. The reality is that most youth who perpetrate violent crimes are not arrested. Although arrests for violent crimes decreased in the mid-1990s, self-reports of violence did not reflect a corroborative decrease in violent behavior.[5] Thus, the notion that high arrest rates were decreasing violence was in error. Despite this, in the mid-1990s, overall homicide rates began to decline; however, this punitive approach to youth did not change as readily.[5]

OFFICIAL STATISTICS

Since 1929, when the Federal Bureau of Investigation (FBI) began the Uniform Crime Reporting (UCR) Program, homicide has been one of the leading causes of death in youth in the United States.[6] For decades, this cause of death has occurred disproportionately in the black and Latino populations, and has been the leading cause of death in African American adolescents and young adults.[7–9] Similar to previous years, from 1991 to 2005, homicide rates were consistently higher for non-Hispanic black people than for all other race/ethnicity groups (**Fig. 1**).[10]

Despite the recent media excitement about the new homicide epidemic, homicide rates among all persons aged 10 to 24 years decreased from 15.6 deaths per 100,000 persons in 1991 to 9.0 deaths per 100,000 in 2005 (**Fig. 2**). Homicide rates for non-Hispanic black people declined from 62.6 per 100,000 in 1991 to 32.8 per 100,000 in 2005 (see **Fig. 1**). Consistent with previous years, the most recent statistics, from 2003 to 2005, show that firearms were the leading mechanism for homicide among boys and men aged 10 to 24 years. During these years, the firearm homicide rate among boys and men aged 10 to 24 years was highest for non-Hispanic black people, with 51.4 deaths per 100,000, and was lowest for non-Hispanic white people with 2.4 deaths per 100,000. In 2005, among boys and men aged 10 to 24 years, the homicide rate was highest for non-Hispanic black people, with 58.3 deaths per

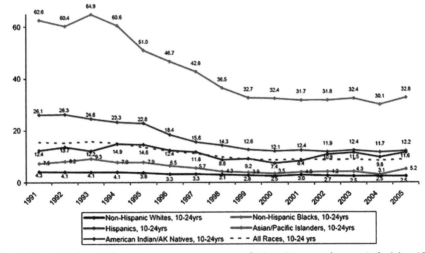

Fig. 1. Trends in homicide rates among persons aged 10 to 24 years, by race/ethnicity, 1991 to 2005. (*From* Centers for Disease Control and Prevention, National Center for Injury Prevention and Control, Division of Violence Prevention. Available at: http://www.cdc.gov/ViolencePrevention/youthviolence/stats_at-a_glance/homicide.html.)

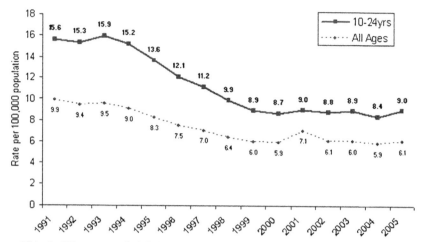

* Rates for All Ages are age-adjusted to the standard 2000 population; rates for the 10-24 yrs age group are age-specific.

Fig. 2. Trends in homicide rates, United States, 1991 to 2005. (*From* Centers for Disease Control and Prevention, National Center for Injury Prevention and Control, Division of Violence Prevention. Available at: http://www.cdc.gov/ViolencePrevention/youthviolence/stats_at-a_glance/homicide.html.)

100,000. Among girls and women aged 10 to 24 years, the homicide rate also was highest for non-Hispanic black people, with 6.6 deaths per 100,000. For comparison, the homicide for non-Hispanic white boys and men was 3.3 per 100,000 and the homicide rate for non-Hispanic white girls and women was 1.5 per 100,000.[10] From a research perspective, although homicide is a leading cause of death in African American men and women, at rates of 58.3/100,000 and 6.6/100,000, homicide is rare, making the scientific study of this phenomenon difficult to accomplish (see Ref.[11] for a discussion of the problem of statistical power for rare events such as suicide).

DEVELOPMENTAL DYNAMICS

Based on decades of youth violence research, it is apparent that youth tend to follow different paths to violent behavior, depending on the age of onset of the behavior in question.[5] Youths who are violent before the age of 13 years tend to show different characteristics than those who become violent afterward. Thus, youths who become violent can be categorized into either an early-onset trajectory or a late-onset trajectory. Violent youths considered with an early-onset trajectory have an onset of violence before puberty. They tend to commit more crimes, and tend to commit more serious crimes. They also tend to commit crimes for a longer period of their lives than do their late-onset counterparts. Such youths exhibit a pattern of escalating violence through childhood and adolescence, and frequently into adulthood. Chronic violent offenders are responsible for most serious violent crime. This finding is in contrast with most violent youths, who exhibit a violent pattern consistent with a late-onset trajectory. Such youths do not exhibit severe violent behavior until they reach adolescence. Their violent behavior tends to peak at about 16 years of age, and then declines greatly by the age of 20 years. They tend to show few signs of violence in either early childhood or adulthood.[5] The problem is that there is no way to accurately identify either the early-onset or late-onset offenders who are going to continue to offend in adulthood. Most of both types do not continue their violent behavior when they mature. Thus, the truism: "Risk factors are not predictive factors due to protective factors."

In addition to these patterns of youth violence, another dynamic of youth violence that must be considered is the prevalence of psychiatric disorders in delinquents. At least one-third of juvenile delinquents have an impairing mental disorder, not including conduct disorder, which often has not been adequately treated.[12] Two of the more common disorders included in this group, attention deficit hyperactivity disorder and major depressive disorder, are treatable. Many of these children also have a comorbid substance abuse diagnosis. These considerations are important as violence prevention efforts in juvenile justice programs in which many of the potentially violent youth are literally a captive audience that can benefit from protective factor approaches to preventing their violent behavior.

NEURODEVELOPMENT

In confidential youth surveys, 30% to 40% of male youth and 15% to 30% of female youth report having committed a serious violent offense at some point in their lives. This cumulative prevalence is consistent amongst African American and European American male youth.[5] Despite the dynamics of youth violence discussed earlier, the violent youth's transition into adulthood is usually marked by an abrupt discontinuation of serious violent behavior. Only roughly 20% of surveyed violent youth continued violent behavior into their 20s. The authors propose that the cause of this shift in behavior is the development of affect regulation.[13] Modern developmental neuroscience indicates, given the development of the brain, that youth are at a high risk for lacking affect regulation. The central nervous system develops from bottom to top and from inside to out.[14] The first part of the brain to develop is the limbic system, which regulates the survival systems of the brain and engages the flight, fight, or freeze behaviors in youth. The frontal lobes (the seat of judgment, deductive reasoning, discernment, and wisdom in the brain) do not fully develop until about 26 years of age.[14] To use a metaphor, children, adolescents, and young adults are neuro-developmentally predisposed to being all gasoline and no brakes. As a car with no brakes will inevitably crash, the lack of emotional brakes often leads to injurious accidents, such as violence.[13] Whatever the reason, the abrupt discontinuation of violence by youth when they enter adulthood, in general, is significant in that there were no observed differences between boys and girls. However, there was a disparity in the findings regarding race. Surveyed African American youths were twice as likely to continue to be arrested for violent behavior into adulthood.[15] Several reasons for this difference are possible, and are discussed later in relation to risk and protective factors for different cultural, racial, and ethnic groups.

RISK FACTORS

A key component of the public health perspective in determining the cause of violence is to track factors that correlate with violence, and determine whether an element is a risk factor or a protective factor. In the context of violent behavior such as homicide, a risk factor is anything that increases the probability than an individual will become engaged in violent behavior. A protective factor is any factor that buffers any harmful risk factors to which an individual may be exposed. The influence a risk factor has on an individual depends on many variables. There is variation in the influence of a single risk factor based on the time it occurs in an individual's life, on the social context in which it occurs, and depending on what protective factors are present.[5] The result is a dynamic interplay between risk and protective factors throughout one's life, rendering such concepts as causation and, more importantly, blame moot in the public health perspective of homicide prevention. Much more useful is the identification of risk and protective factors, determining how they interact, and then designing interventions to incorporate that information into an effective homicide prevention program.

Biological risk factors for youth who exhibit violence, regardless of an early- or late-onset trajectory, include being male, having a low intelligence quotient (IQ), having a psychiatric diagnosis (eg, attention deficit hyperactivity disorder), and having any other general medical condition. Behavioral risk factors include committing general offenses, substance use, aggressive behavior, and problem behavior. Additional individual risk factors include antisocial attitudes and extensive exposure to television violence. Family-related risk factors for violence include low socioeconomic status, having antisocial parents, poor parent-child relations, being from a broken home, and having abusive parents.[5]

Other risk factors include poor school performance, having antisocial peers, and having weak social ties. For youths with a late-onset trajectory pattern for violent behavior such as homicide, other specific risk factors are found. These factors include gang membership, and community-derived risk factors such as neighborhood crime, neighborhood drug usage, and community disorganization.[5]

Closer observation of these risk factors reveals that not all risk factors for violent behavior are equal; they vary in strength and concerning early- or late-onset trajectory. A common way of measuring the strength of a risk factor is with effect size. The larger the effect size, the more predictive value it has. For early-onset trajectory violence, more powerful predictors of future violent behavior are committing general offenses and substance use.[5] Moderate effect size factors for early-onset trajectory violence include being male, family of low socioeconomic status, having antisocial parents, and aggression.[5] Other risk factors (psychological conditions; hyperactivity; poor parent-child relations; harsh, lax, or inconsistent discipline; weak social ties; antisocial behavior; exposure to television violence; poor attitude toward performance in school; medical, physical deficits; low IQ; broken home; separation from parents; antisocial attitudes and beliefs; dishonesty [boys only]; abusive parents; neglect; and antisocial peers) for early-onset trajectory violence were found to have a small effect size (<0.20).[5] For late-onset violence, the risk factors found to have a moderate effect size were weak social ties, having delinquent or antisocial peers (0.37), and gang membership (0.31).[5] The risk factor of committing general offenses was found to have a moderate effect size (0.26).[5] All other risk factors (psychological conditions; restlessness; difficulty concentrating [boys only]; risk taking; aggression [boys only]; being male; poor parent-child relations; harsh or lax discipline; poor monitoring/supervision; low parental involvement; poor attitude toward performance in school; academic failure; physical violence; neighborhood crime, drugs in the neighborhood; neighborhood disorganization; antisocial parents; antisocial attitudes and beliefs; crimes against persons; antisocial behavior; low IQ; broken home; low family socioeconomic status or poverty; abusive parents; family conflict [boys only]; and substance use) were found to have a small effect size (<0.20) for late-onset violent behavior.[5] However, because the public is beset with media epidemiology (ie, bombarded with repeated images and stories about violence and the causes of violence), the public tends to demonize youth from disadvantaged backgrounds without any consideration of the protective factors in these youth's lives. Thus, despite the robust scientific evidence of equal rates of self-report violence between African Americans and European Americans,[5] race is another variable mistakenly assumed to be a risk factor for violent behavior. Race is a risk marker, rather than a risk factor. Race is a proxy for other known risk factors such as poverty, single-parent families, poor educational performance, and exposure to gangs, violence, and crime.[5]

PROTECTIVE FACTORS

Protective factors tend to be consistent in buffering the effects of risk factors for both early- and late-onset trajectories of violence. Individual protective factors include being female, having an intolerant attitude toward deviance, high IQ, having a positive social orientation, and perceiving sanctions for transgressions. There is also some evidence that having sufficient amounts of ω3 in the diet is a protective factor that prevents deficiencies in neurodevelopment and decreases the likelihood of aggression and autonomic dysregulation, all of which affect the social and emotional skill of affect regulation.[16] Family protective factors include having warm supportive relationships with parents or other adults, parents having a positive evaluation of a youth's peers, and having sufficient parental monitoring. School-oriented protective factors include commitment to school and recognition for involvement in conventional activities (eg, organized sports, youth clubs). Having friends who engage in conventional activities is also a protective factor.[5]

EVIDENCE-BASED VIOLENCE PREVENTION PROGRAMS

The Center for the Study and Prevention of Violence suggests that the Olweus Bullying Prevention Program and Greenberg's Promoting Alternative Thinking Strategies (PATHS) program meets the center's standards of evidence provided by experimental design, effect size, replication capacity, and sustainability.[17,18] In addition, the center recommends the Good Behavior Game, FAST Track, Seattle Social Development Project, I Can Problem Solve, and LIFT as promising programs.[19]

In addition, Dr Satcher's report[5] outlined the myths of youth violence as: (1) most future offenders can be identified in early childhood; (2) child abuse and neglect inevitably lead to violent behavior later in life; (3) African American and Hispanic youth are more likely to become involved in violence than any other racial or ethnic group; (4) a new, violent breed of young superpredators threatens the United States; (5) getting tough with juvenile offenders by trying them in adult criminal courts reduces the likelihood that they will commit more crimes; (6) most violent youths will end up being arrested for a violent crime; and, most importantly, (7) nothing works with respect to treating or preventing violent behavior.

More recently, Hahn and colleagues[20] reviewed the current state of violence prevention and found 53 studies of universal school-based programs that met their inclusion criteria. The sample sizes in the 53 studies reviewed ranged from 21 to 39,168 students (median sample size = 563).[20] Slightly more than three-fourths of the studies reviewed measured violence or aggression using direct measures. The rest used outcome measures that served as proxies for violence and aggression.[20] As distal violence prevention outcomes were a consideration in the review, intervention follow-up measures ranged from being performed immediately following the intervention to as far as 6 years (median follow-up time was 6 months).[20]

Studies classified as having the greatest design suitability were characterized by an experimental design with intervention and control subjects with the data being collected prospectively. Of the 53 studies reviewed, 7 were of greatest design suitability and good execution.[21–27] Thirty-two were of greatest design suitability and fair execution. Studies classified as having moderate design suitability were those studies in which data were collected retrospectively or there were multiple before or after measurements without a control condition. Five were of moderate design suitability and fair execution.[28–32] Studies that were classified as having the least suitable designs were studies that lacked a control condition and which had only 1 before and after measure used to determine the outcome of the intervention. Hahn and colleagues[20] conducted a sensitivity analysis, and studies with least suitable designs were excluded from the review. Interventions were identified as desirable when the experimental condition showed a decrease in violent behavior compared with the control condition. Interventions were also classified as effective if they were tested in diverse settings, populations, and circumstances.

PRINCIPLES OF PREVENTION

Establishing a program geared toward homicide prevention should follow certain principles that have proved effective in public health. Complex behavior such as homicide is multidetermined and prevention strategies must be equally complex. The principles of a successful homicide prevention program are those that address the risk factors associated with homicide and accentuate the protective factors linked to violent behavior. As discussed earlier, those risk and protective factors have individual, family, social, and community components. An effective homicide prevention program must navigate them all with some degree of success. Because the Aban Aya violence prevention research project is characterized as greatest design suitability and good execution,[20] and because Aban Aya informed the naturalistic, large-scale, public health research on preventing violence in Chicago Public Schools (CPS),[14,33] we highlight the prevention field principles in this initiative. The public health field principles that decrease risky and violent behavior are: (1) rebuilding the village, (2) access to modern and ancient technology, (3) increasing connectedness, (4) providing activities to improve self-esteem (a sense of power, models, uniqueness, and connectedness), (5) increasing social and emotional skills, (6) reestablishing the adult protective shield, and (7) minimizing the effects of trauma.[34] These principles are interdependent, because each needs the others for success. Because there are multiple ways to actualize these public health field principles, only a few concrete examples are given here.

REBUILDING THE VILLAGE

Since the early 1900s, the hypothesized cause for delinquency was a lack of social fabric surrounding youth.[35] Specifically, they proposed the social disorganization theory of deviance, suggesting that few job opportunities, poverty, single-headed households, isolation from neighbors, and weakened community friendship networks and community institutions lead to reduced informal and formal social control. As mentioned earlier, because of their neurodevelopment, young adults can be conceptualized as being all gasoline and no brakes,[13] and thus at risk for losing control and perpetrating violence. Ergo, young adults need grown adults to provide them with brakes, and this can only be accomplished if social fabric or village surrounds the youth. More recently, Sampson and colleagues[36] showed that, of the 49 equally poor neighborhoods in Chicago, only 6 had high rates of violence, but the other 43 communities with social fabric have less deviant behavior as a result of the prevention of this behavior.

Rebuilding the village refers to the idea that institutions, organizations, businesses, families, and individuals within a given community work together in a way that uses their individual strengths, perspectives, and resources in a way that is beneficial to the community as a whole. Any individual entity can initiate the collaborative process and need not wait for another entity to begin working toward an aim. In this model, every entity contributes toward building a healthier community. Dysfunctional communities are those in which each entity has different goals, has no common language, is activity driven and overly guards resources instead of allowing for their exchange. A functional community can share common, evidence-based goals, communicates effectively, is outcome driven, and collectively maximizes its resources. An example of rebuilding the village is a church or police district helping to organize block clubs and encourage neighbors to monitor each other's children's behavior.[33]

ACCESS TO ANCIENT AND MODERN TECHNOLOGY

As previously noted, a disproportionate number of youth involved with the juvenile justice system have psychiatric disorders.[12] One hypothesis is that, if these youths were provided modern treatment or prevention interventions,[14] their subsequent violence could be prevented. More recently, in an effort to infuse modern biotechnical violence-prevention technology into the CPS system, the CEO of Chicago Public Schools made sure that ω3 was in the CPS diet of all youth (Ron Hubberman, CEO, CPS, Chicago, IL, personal communication, June 23, 2010).

CONNECTEDNESS

According to attachment theory,[37] a young child needs to develop a relationship with at least 1 primary caregiver in order for normal social and emotional development to occur (eg, affect regulation). The Nurse-Family Partnership[38] is an effective intervention that targets the mother-infant bond, which directly affects later affect regulation of the offspring. This intervention improved pregnancy outcomes, maternal caregiving, and the maternal life course, preventing antisocial behavior. A meta-analysis of 60 home visiting programs revealed benefits for children in 3 of 5 areas of children's cognitive and social emotional functioning compared with controls.[39] Using attachment theory as a theoretical model, CPS implemented Cradles to Classroom.[33] This collaborative initiative with Chicago Department of Public Health, 6 hospitals, and other agencies for pregnant and parenting teens trains teens in the development of parenting skills and accessing community resources and provides counseling to new mothers around issues of domestic violence. In addition, it provides teens with access to prenatal, nutritional, medical, social, and childcare services. Some 2000 teenagers in 54 Chicago schools that offer this program had babies in 2002. All 495 seniors graduated, and 78% of them enrolled in 2- or 4-year college programs. Only 5 of the women had a repeat pregnancy while still in school; 4 were graduating seniors, and the other, a junior, stayed in school. Eighty-five teen fathers also participated in the program, learning parenting skills under the supervision of a male mentor at each school.[40]

IMPROVING SELF-ESTEEM

Much research has been done linking low self-esteem with violent behavior such as bullying and domestic abuse.[25] Conversely, improving self-esteem may provide additional protection in buffering the negative effects of risk factors.[25] Self-esteem is operationally defined as (1) a sense of power, (2) a sense of uniqueness, (3) a sense of models, and (4) a sense of connectedness.[41] A sense of power refers to the perception that an individual has the ability to do what they must. One of the key features of building a sense of power is transforming learned helplessness into learned helpfulness, also known as mastery or self-efficacy. A sense of uniqueness comes from acknowledging and respecting the qualities and characteristics about oneself that are special and different. A sense of models comes from observing individuals who have developed effective strategies for success in the world. A sense of connected-ness results in a feeling of satisfaction from being connected to people, places, or things. Thus, the CPS intervention intentionally provided youth with various opportu-nities to increase their self-esteem. These opportunities included improving academic performance, providing youth with opportunities to find their unique gifts and talents, helping assist youth in developing values, and providing them with character educa-tion and conflict resolution skills.[33]

INCREASING SOCIAL AND EMOTIONAL SKILLS

The enhancement of an individual's social and emotional skills creates the opportunity to develop the life skills necessary to prevent and intervene in violence (eg, affect regulation).[13] The development of such skills is crucial not only to the enhancement of intracommunity relations but also within families or school systems. In the CPS intervention, extracurricular activities were used to provide such skills. Such activities provide youth with opportunities to serve their community, resolve disputes peace-fully, and develop leadership skills that will enable them to model and promote healthy alternatives to violence. Some activities particularly suited to the enhancement of social and emotional skills include peer leader programs, teen court, mentoring programs, young negotiators, and service-based clubs.

In the classroom, programs may provide direct teaching of peer mediation, conflict resolution, and anger management skills.[25,33] Programs can support schools, staff, and parents in improving their ability to teach children appropriate social and emotional skills and to use positive interventions to decrease disruptive student behavior.

REESTABLISHING THE ADULT PROTECTIVE SHIELD

Consistent with attachment theory[37] is the idea that young children, in learning to explore the world and beginning to attempt to master it, must at first feel safe and comfortable with a primary caregiver. A child must feel confident that the caregiver can keep them safe. In homicide prevention, the same is true for a community's responsibility toward its youth. Youths need protection not only within their communi-ties but also in their schools and in their homes.

In the CPS intervention, we developed safety and security programs designed to maximize school safety. For example, CPS initiated parent patrols to decrease before-and after-school violence, enhanced training and expansion of security personnel, and rapid response teams.[33] CPS strictly enforce disciplinary rules and provide a safety net of school-based educational opportunities for youth who have been expelled, violated probation, or committed first-time, nonviolent, serious offenses.

MINIMIZING THE EFFECTS OF TRAUMA

One way of describing the phenomenon of anger is as a sense of being hurt. Often attached to that hurt is the fear of being hurt again. Traumatic stress is also associated with a lack of affect regulation.[13] One way of minimizing the effects of trauma is to turn learned helplessness into learned helpfulness. Thus, CPS developed service-learning requirements to enhance the ability of youth to transform their helplessness into help-ful community activities.[33]

SUMMARY

Although homicide continues to be a problematic public health concern, homicide rates have dropped considerably since the mid-1980s, and remain nowhere near their record highs at that point. The authors propose that the decrease in violence was caused by a large number of national and local violence prevention initiatives that are outlined in this article. The science of violence prevention is clear but the political will to disseminate, adapt, and implement these programs waxes and wanes. It is hoped that the science of violence prevention will become so strong that to not provide such programs ubiquitously throughout the United States will become unethical.

REFERENCES

1. Jenkins EJ, Bell CC. Adolescent violence: can it be curbed? Adolesc Med 1992; 3(1):71–86.
2. The role of the pediatrician in youth violence prevention in clinical practice and at the community level. American Academy of Pediatrics Task Force on Violence. Pediatrics 1999;103(1):173–81.
3. Bell CC, Fink P. Prevention of violence. In: Bell CC, editor. Psychiatric aspects on violence: understanding causes and issues in prevention and treatment. San Francisco (CA): Jossey-Bass; 2000. p. 37–47.
4. Bell CC. School-based violence prevention can work – perspective. Clin Psych News 2007;35(10):30.
5. Department of Health and Human Services. Youth violence: a report of the Surgeon General. Rockville (MD): Department of Health and Human Services; 2001.
6. Bell CC, Jenkins E. Prevention of black homicide. In: Dewart J, editor. The state of Black America - 1990. New York: National Urban League; 1990. p. 143–55.
7. Bell CC. Preventive strategies for dealing with violence among blacks. Community Ment Health J 1987;23(3):217–28.
8. Griffith E, Bell CC. Recent trends in suicide and homicide among blacks. JAMA 1989;262(16):2265–9.
9. Hollinger PC, Offer D, Barter JT, et al. Suicide and homicide among adolescents. New York: Guilford Press; 1994.
10. Centers for Disease Control and Prevention, National Center for Injury Prevention and Control, Division of Violence Prevention. Available at: http://www.cdc.gov/ViolencePrevention/youthviolence/stats_at-a_glance/homicide.html. Accessed November 29, 2010.
11. National Research Council, Institute of Medicine Goldsmith SK, Pellmar TC, Kleinman AM, et al. Reducing suicide: a national imperative. Washington, DC: National Academy Press; 2002.
12. Teplin LA, Abram KM, McClelland GM, et al. Psychiatric disorders in youth in juvenile detention. Arch Gen Psychiatry 2002;59(12):1133–43.
13. Bell CC, McBride DF. Affect regulation and prevention of risky behaviors. JAMA 2010;304(5):565–6.
14. National Research Council, Institute of Medicine. Preventing mental, emotional, and behavioral disorders among young people: progress and possibilities. In: O'Connell ME, Boat T, Warner KE, editors. Washington, DC: The National Academies Press; 2009. Available at: http://www.iom.edu/CMS/12552/45572/64120.aspx. Accessed November 29, 2010.
15. Elliott DS. Serious violent offenders: onset, developmental course, and termination. The American Society of Criminology 1993 presidential address. Criminology 1994;32:1–21.
16. Hibbeln JR, Ferguson TA, Blasbalg TL. Omega-3 fatty acid deficiencies in neurodevelopment, aggression and autonomic dysregulation: opportunities for intervention. Int Rev Psychiatry 2006;18(2):107–18.

17. Olweus D, Limber S, Mihalic SF. Bullying prevention program. Boulder (CO): Center for the Study and Prevention of Violence; 1999.
18. Greenberg MT, Kusche CA, Cook ET, et al. Promoting emotional competence in school-aged children: the effects of the PATHS curriculum. Dev Psychopathol 1995;7:117–36.
19. Center for the Study and Prevention of Violence. Blueprints promising programs overview. Boulder (CO): Center for the Study and Prevention of Violence; 2002. Available at: http://www.colorado.edu/cspv/blueprints/promisingprograms.html. Accessed November 29, 2010.
20. Hahn R, Fuqua-Whitley D, Wethington H, et al. Effectiveness of Universal School-Based Programs to prevent violent and aggressive behavior: a systematic review. Am J Prev Med 2007;33(2S):S114–29.
21. Ialongo N, Werthamer L, Kellam SG. Proximal impact of two first-grade preventive interventions on the early risk behaviors for later substance abuse, depression and antisocial behavior. Am J Community Psychol 1999;27:599–641.
22. Conduct Problems Prevention Research Group. Evaluation of the first 3 years of the Fast Track prevention trial with children at high risk for adolescent conduct problems. J Abnorm Child Psychol 2002;30:19–35.
23. Esbensen FA, Osgood DW, Taylor TJ, et al. How great is G.R.E.A.T.? Results from a longitudinal quasi-experimental design. Criminol Public Policy 2001;1: 87–118.
24. Farrell AD, Valois RF, Meyer AL, et al. Impact of the RIPP violence prevention program on rural middle school students. J Prim Prev 2003;24:143–67.
25. Flay BR, Graumlich S, Segawa E, et al. The ABAN AYA Youth Project: effects of comprehensive prevention programs on high-risk behaviors among inner city African American youth: a randomized trial. Arch Pediatr Adolesc Med 2004; 158(4):377–84.
26. O'Donnell L, Stueve A, Doval AS, et al. Violence prevention and young adolescents' participation in community youth service. J Adolesc Health 1999; 24:28–37.
27. Sawyer MG, MacMullin C, Graetz B, et al. Social skills training for primary school children: a one-year follow-up study. J Paediatr Child Health 1997;33: 378–83.
28. Flay BR, Allred C. Long-term effects of the Positive Action program. Am J Health Behav 2003;27(Suppl 1):S6–21.
29. Olweus D. Bully/victim problems in school: facts and intervention. Eur J Psychol Educ 1997;12:495–510.
30. Elias MJ, Gara MA, Schuyler T, et al. The promotion of social competence: longitudinal study of a preventive school-based program. Am J Orthopsychiatry 1991; 61:409–17.
31. Pepler DJ, Craig WM, Ziegler S, et al. An evaluation of an anti-bullying intervention in Toronto schools. Can J Commun Ment Health 1994;13:95–110.
32. Taylor CA, Liang B, Tracy AJ, et al. Gender differences in middle school adjustment, physical fighting, and social skills: evaluation of a social competency program. J Prim Prev 2002;23:261–73.
33. Bell CC, Gamm S, Vallas P, et al. Strategies for the prevention of youth violence in Chicago Public Schools. In: Shafii M, Shafii S, editors. School violence: contributing factors, management, and prevention. Washington, DC: American Psychiatric Press; 2001. p. 251–72.
34. Bell CC, Bhana A, Petersen I, et al. Building protective factors to offset sexually risky behaviors among black South African youth: a randomized control trial.

J Natl Med Assoc 2008;100(8):936–44. Available at: http://www.nmanet.org/images/uploads/Publications/OC936.pdf. Accessed November 29, 2010.

35. Shaw CR, McKay H. Juvenile delinquency and urban areas. Chicago: University of Chicago Press; 1942.

36. Sampson RJ, Raudenbush SW, Earls F. Neighborhoods and violent crime: a multi-level study of collective efficacy. Science 1997;277:918–24.

37. Bowlby J. Attachment and loss, vol. 2, Separation. New York: Basic Books; 1973.

38. Olds DL, Sadler L, Kitzman H. Programs for parents of infants and toddlers: recent evidence from randomized trials. J Child Psychol Psychiatry 2007; 48(3/4):355–91.

39. Sweet MA, Appelbaum ML. Is home visiting an effective strategy? A metaanalytic review of home visiting programs for families with young children. Child Dev 2004;75(5):1435–56.

40. Lamberg L. Programs target youth violence prevention. JAMA 2003;290(5): 585–6.

41. Bean R. The four conditions of self-esteem: A new approach for elementary and middle schools. 2nd edition. Santa Cruz (CA): ETR Associates; 1992.

Human Immunodeficiency Virus Prevention with Youth

Dominica F. McBride, PhD[a], Carl C. Bell, MD, DLAPA, FACPsych[b,c],*

KEYWORDS

• HIV • Prevention • Programs • Youth

The drama of AIDS threatens not just some nations or societies, but the whole of humanity. It knows no frontiers of geography, race, age or social condition... (calling) for a supreme effort of international cooperation on the part of government, the world medical and scientific community and all those who exercise influence in developing a sense of more responsibility in society.

Pope John Paul II (1990)

Pope John Paul (1990) was accurate in his assessment about the extent to which HIV/AIDS has ravaged the world. In January 1981, the first person infected with HIV was discovered in the United States, and by the mid-1980s, the prevalence of those who had contracted the virus doubled each year. By 1985, it was reported that 148 countries worldwide were dealing with an acceleration of HIV infection and AIDS, reaching the level of a pandemic. By 1990, there were more than 1 million people worldwide diagnosed with HIV.[1] Today, that number has reached more than 49 million worldwide.[2] Within the United States alone, 447.8 of 100,000 persons (an estimated 1.1 million adults and adolescents) were living with HIV infection at the end of 2006.[3] People of color comprised most of those cases (65.4%), with the prevalence rate of African Americans reaching 1715.1 per 100,000 persons and Hispanics reaching 585.3 per 100,000. These rates are 7.6 and 2.6 times higher than their European American counterparts.[3]

Although contraction of this virus can be preempted, people have and continue to die prematurely as a result of the progression of this virus to AIDS. This unfortunate

The authors have nothing to disclose.

[a] The HELP Institute, Inc, 2820 Broadview Drive NW, Huntsville, AL 35810, USA

[b] Community Mental Health Council, Inc, 8704 South Constance, Chicago, IL 60616, USA

[c] Institute for Juvenile Research, Department of Psychiatry, University of Illinois, Chicago, 1747 West Roosevelt Road # 155, Chicago, IL 60608-1264, USA

* Corresponding author. Community Mental Health Council (CMHC), Inc, 8704 South Constance, Chicago, IL 60616.

E-mail address: carlcbell@pol.net

reality is rooted in a lack of knowledge on prevention,[4,5] a dearth of motivation, and a paucity of protective factors,[6] especially in youth. Adolescence is the ideal time to provide the proper infrastructure for prevention of risky behaviors. Therefore, the focus of this article is on prevention of HIV in youth. Specifically, the present article delineates: (1) the risk factors that are conducive to risky behaviors, (2) the protective factors that can prevent risky behaviors, and (3) various prevention programs that have been found effective in preempting these behaviors in youth.

RISK FACTORS

Various risk factors have been found to be connected with risky HIV-related behaviors in youth. The reasons for behavior are complex and multidetermined. The most notable and influential factors are those that simultaneously have the power to curb these behaviors and transform them into health behaviors: the individual's personal characteristics, family, and community.[7]

Individual

Resilience in people has been defined as including intrapsychic strengths of trust, self-regulation, autonomy, self-esteem, empathy, altruism, an internal locus of control, flexibility, optimism, invulnerability, aspects of health or social competence,[8] and being stress-resistant.[9] Intrapsychic protective factors, for example, include the manner in which individuals perceive themselves (eg, perceptions of self-reliance, resilience, and invulnerability or vulnerability). Self-perceptions may also be positively shaped by living through trauma, which can create a sense of competence or stress inoculation.[10]

Family

The family is not only the environment in which a child grows but is also the source of potential models and impressive experiences (whether positive or negative). Negative experiences (also known as adverse childhood experiences [ACEs]) are often the root of risky behaviors in youth.[11] ACEs have been linked to numerous behavior problems and mental and emotional disorders, including violence, premature sexual intercourse, and substance abuse.[11] A finding relative to HIV prevention is the evidence that compared with an individual who was not exposed to any of the 7 ACEs (psychological abuse, physical abuse, sexual abuse, violence against mother, living with household members who were substance abusers, living with household members who were mentally ill or suicidal, or living with ex-offender household members), an individual exposed to 4 or more ACEs is 3.2-fold more likely to have 50 or more sexual intercourse partners and 2.5-fold more likely to have a sexually transmitted disease.[11] Maladaptive family functioning clusters (including parental mental illness, substance abuse disorder, and criminality; family violence; physical and sexual abuse; and neglect) have been found to be conducive to various mental health disorders, explaining 32.4% of all disorders, 41.2% of disruptive behavior disorders, 32.4% of anxiety disorders, 26.2% of mood disorders, and 21.0% of substance use disorders.[12,13] These findings demonstrate the acute and indelible effect that family has on behavior and global functioning.

Community and Context

Brown and colleagues[14] provide a detailed and comprehensive review of how various parts of the community affect HIV-related behaviors. As they and many others assert, the community can be constructive or destructive. Community comprises the social resources (eg, people, service organizations) and processes (eg, social interactions including violence and block parties) and physical appearance and structure. If a community is close-knit, collaborative, clean, and kempt, the residents are more likely to be socially secure and behave in a healthy way.[15] However, the opposite is also true; if a community is violent and dilapidated, its members are more likely to be fearful and behave in unhealthy ways. Gladwell[16] writes eloquently on this topic, conveying that context can mold and alter character and behaviors. He provides the example of the 1980s and 1990s in New York City. During this time, the city subway system was littered with graffiti, symbolizing the social disorder that plagued the city at that time. Gladwell[16] poignantly explicated that this contextual predicament was conducive to the social disarray. Hence, when the physical appearance was changed (among other things, such as reinforcing that people pay for entry with both leading to a greater air of social order), the behavior within the subway system also changed; it became safer.

Pertinent to HIV-related behaviors, the socioeconomic conditions of a community have been found to predict risky sexual behaviors in youth, with characteristics including single parenthood, poverty, and instability increasing these behaviors.[14] In 2001, Baumer and South[17] found that living in a disadvantaged community was the strongest predictor of risky sexual behavior among youth, compared with race, owning a home, and gender. Compared with youth who lived in more advantaged communities, Baumer and South found that youth in disadvantaged communities were 39% more likely to have sexual intercourse with various persons and more than twice as likely to have unprotected sex.

The social cohesion within a community also has implications and influences the behavior of youth. The work of the Community Mental Health Council in the child welfare system in Illinois[18] suggests that communities with a lack of social cohesion may result in higher rates of contact with child protective services indicating a higher rate of experiencing ACEs. The Adverse Childhood Study illustrates that children in families that lack support are more at risk for child abuse and neglect resulting in higher numbers of different sexual intercourse partners and rates of sexually transmitted diseases.[11]

With a weak sense of social cohesion, Browning and colleagues[19] found an increase in sexual promiscuity, indicating the possibility that community cohesion has a positive relationship with healthy behaviors in youth. These investigators also found that this relationship strengthened with the age of the youth. As they became older, the likelihood of them having 2 or more partners decreased with the increase of social cohesion.

As stated previously, the physical community environment, including the buildings, layout, and structure of the community, has been shown to also influence health-related behaviors (Brown and colleagues, in press). Semenza and March[20] describe the acute deleterious effects of the way communities are structured. They stated, "These fractured metropolises can stifle physical activity, degrade the environment, and curb spontaneous social interactions."[(p23)] Communities structured in a way that is conducive to physical activity (eg, walking, jogging) have been found to provide an environment ripe for more positive social interaction.[21] The buildings themselves, whether kempt or decrepit, seem to also be associated with HIV and other health-related behaviors.[16,22] Hopfer and colleagues[23] asserted that environmental factors play a significant role in adolescent alcohol use. Berstein and colleagues[24] narrowed the broader category of environmental factors down to physical dilapidation, finding those living in dilapidation to be more likely to drink heavily than those living in more enhanced environments. More direct links have been found concerning community ramshackle and the rate of sexually transmitted diseases. For example, Cohen and colleagues[25] found that there was a positive correlation between the number of broken windows and cases of gonorrhea. This indicator appeared to be more influential than other variables, including unemployment and income.

PROTECTIVE FACTORS

Many researchers have fallen into the trap of focusing on deficiencies and risk factors and have forgotten the more important and potent aspects of development and healing: the protective factors. Protective factors are not only integral but they are also powerful in that they have been shown to prevent risk factors from becoming predictive.[26–29] This section discusses 7 field principles that have been shown to be conducive to the development of empowerment and healthy behaviors. Applied to the prevention of HIV-related risk behaviors, they have also been proved to be effective in reducing this likelihood and even increasing social cohesion and holistic well-being: (1) rebuild the village or create social fabric, (2) provide access to modern technology, (3) facilitate connectedness on various levels, (4) facilitate improvement of self-esteem, (5) develop social and emotional skills and intelligence, (6) reestablish the adult protective shield, and (7) minimize the effects of trauma. Bell and colleagues[30,31] provide detailed and concrete accounts of how to execute these principles.

Rebuild the Village or Create Social Fabric

Creating social fabric (or social cohesion) is an anecdote for the aforementioned risk factor of community dissolution. A village in the old adage is defined as a cohesive social unit in which its members work together and collaborate in caring for one another and their community as a whole. This sentiment is the goal of this principle. The purpose is 3-fold: (1) to build a sense of empowerment and motivation for change and progress within community members, (2) to develop and enhance social and interpersonal processes and partnerships or coalitions, and (3) to establish a strong and unified community. Often, this ambition is accomplished through first examining the social capital currently existing within a community (eg, schools, churches, people, organization); second, bringing these various elements together in partnership and collaboration; and third, moving collectively toward a common vision.[32] These processes help to create a true and holistic collective through uniting community members in work, physical interaction, and mental and emotional motivation and empowerment.

Provide Access to Modern and Ancient Technology

Merriam-Webster's dictionary definition of technology is "the practical application of knowledge especially in a particular area." Thus, technology includes knowledge, adjunctive physical facilities, and action (eg, treatments for drug addiction, prosthetics, heart transplants) and from a public health perspective, technology can be biotechnical or psychosocial. Unfortunately, disadvantaged or historically oppressed communities often do not receive and, therefore, benefit from technology. This discrepancy is the cause of the present health disparities between European Americans and African Americans, for example. Therefore, the provision of technology, particularly health care, is integral in the movement toward social equity.

Providing access to these technologies includes offering and effectively applying health care services such as health insurance, physical and mental health screenings (eg, breast cancer, depression, dental), and medications. A perfect example of a biotechnical technology would be circumcision in men to prevent the spread of HIV. This technology also encompasses evidence-based knowledge and practices including prevention programming (eg, HIV prevention programs, cardiovascular disease prevention education). This list centers on modern technology but ancient technology is also effective in healing, including certain homeopathic remedies and soft martial arts (eg, tai chi).[33] Ancient technology such as meditative practices that formed the development of cognitive behavioral therapy are also useful in developing affect regulation and important social and emotional skills and intelligence that prevents youth from being driven by their limbic system instead of their frontal lobe.[34]

Facilitate Connectedness on Various Levels

Human beings are social creatures, as shown through not only physiological responses to human relationships but also mental and emotional well-being or harm caused by interpersonal interaction.[35] From infancy to adulthood, connectedness with one another is integral to holistic well-being. Bowlby[36] and Meloy[37] (1992) assert that attachment between caregivers and their dependents during infancy acts as a conductor of behaviors, whether healthy or unhealthy. Renken and colleagues[38] demonstrated that those with insecure or unstable attachments in infancy exhibited violent or risky behaviors later in life. Fortunately, the potential damage done in infancy can be attenuated through later intervention, focused on bridging social gaps and bolstering positive and meaningful connectedness between the person and others.

Social connectedness can be manifested on various levels (intrafamilial, peer-to-peer, neighborhood, and school or community) and at various times in the rearing of a person (eg, infancy, adolescence). Caregivers can be taught how to form strong attachments between themselves and their infants.[39] Parents can be trained in how to mend relational breaks through communication, empathy, and acceptance. Teachers and other adult actors in a youth's life can hone their social and emotional skills and become mentors and confidants. Even institutions, such as schools[31] and churches, can be entities to which a young person connects and heals. Therefore, all is not lost if mistakes are made early in a child's life and connectedness is a potent protective factor, both physically and mentally.

Facilitate Improvement of Self-esteem

Self-esteem is a construct defining how people feel about or value themselves. It is associated with health-related behaviors and mental and emotional disorders, from depression to anxiety states.[40] Bell and colleagues[31] purport that "improving the target recipients' self-esteem is a critical component in any successful prevention/intervention strategy to change health behavior."[(pp260-1)] Bean[41] delineates 4 conditions that are conducive to producing self-esteem: (1) a sense of connectedness, (2) a sense of uniqueness, (3) a sense of power, and (4) a sense of models.

Connectedness

This construct relates to the previous discussion on connectedness. However, in Bean's research,[41] this sense was more expansive and encompassed not only people and institutions but also groups, a past or culture, things, or places, a sense of belonging. Similar to the third field principle, in cases of interpersonal relations, there must be a bidirectional relationship in which the child perceives that the object (ie, person or group) of her affection also exhibits a sense of being connected to the child, ergo a sense of belonging. Connectedness, in this regard, also includes feeling connected and trusting in one's body; hence, the child feels connected to himself.

Uniqueness

A sense of uniqueness is a realization and embracing of special qualities. When a child experiences feeling unique, the child identifies and respects characteristics, skills, and/or talents that are specific to him or her. This condition encompasses the child knowing and actualizing their uniqueness as well as others validating and reaffirming the importance of their special traits or skills. Thus, there are 4 components to manifesting this condition: having a space and opportunity to identify unique aspects, the actual identification and respect for these characteristics, enacting or engaging the skills or facets, and the external validation of the features.

Power

A sense of power in this case refers to empowerment and trust of self; children perceive and trust in their own capability to accomplish their ambitions and what they need and want to do. When children have a sense of power, they also view that they can influence circumstances within their life and make a difference in the lives of others. Children perceive their own competence and they are, ideally, given opportunities to apply their skills and build confidence in their competence. From academics to philanthropy, a sense of power can be manifest in various areas. Children should be given ample opportunity to manifest their skills to build their competence and sense of power.

Models

To feel safe and secure, children must be able to make sense of the world. A sense of human, philosophical, and operational models facilitates this process and forms the foundation for the formation of goals, values, personal principles, and ideals. Children who have a strong sense of models are connected with positive role models, have an accurate internal moral compass, feel a sense of purpose and direction, and are able to make sense of and influence their circumstances.

Develop Social and Emotional Skills

Emotional and social skills have been identified as one of the main causes of success in life.[42] Emotional skills are synonymous with affect regulation, which is "a set of processes individuals use to manage emotions and their expression to accomplish goals."[34] Emotional skills can also encompass emotional and mental inclinations such as empathy and compassion.[42] Social skills refer to the way in which an individual can and does interact with others. They include the ability to resolve conflict and facilitate social interactions appropriately. Social and emotional skills can engender healthy interpersonal interactions and relationships. The lack of both these skill sets are conducive to the opposite, including interpersonal conflict, isolation, and even violence.[43] This paucity can even influence HIV-related behaviors, with an individual armed with emotional and social skills being better able to protect and assert themselves in potentially dangerous situations (eg, peer pressure toward drug use, sexual encounters). Thus, the acquisition and use of emotional and social skills can be a potent protective factor.

Reestablish the Adult Protective Shield

The adult protective shield is a synchronized buffer against potential emotional and physical dangers for youth. Adults can include parents, school personnel, and community members who act as mentors. Within this protective factor, adults are active in coordinating efforts to preempt conflict, disorder, and violence (eg, metal detectors in schools, prevention programs). As a result of how the brain develops, with the limbic system developing first and the frontal lobes developing last (by age

26 years), youth are susceptible to reacting without logic, reason, or conscious thought. Metaphorically, the youth are operating as vehicles with no brakes. Therefore, adults must act as their inhibition or brakes; in other words, protect the youth from their lack of forethought and/or reactivity.[34] This biological, social, and emotional predicament constitutes the importance and integrality of the adult protective shield, especially in preventing HIV-related risk behaviors.

Minimize the Effects of Trauma

As conveyed previously, ACEs contribute significantly and are often responsible for later mental and behavioral disorder. The untreated effects of trauma can lead to behaviors that place an individual in grave danger and are conducive to premature death. Therefore, minimizing the effects of trauma is a necessary component, in many cases, to preventing these behaviors. One reason for pernicious and indelible effects is a sense of victimization that never changes into a survivor or conqueror stance. The person victimized perceives a lack of power over the situation and, thus, a sense of helplessness, which often leads to insidious choices and risky behavior. One such way of preempting this behavior and minimizing trauma is transforming a sense of learned helplessness into learned helpfulness or empowerment.[44]

These 7 field principles are effective because of their holism, working on multiple levels. Bronfenbrennor[45] perceived the necessity of a multifaceted and multilayered approach to helping an individual, for each is embedded within and affected by multiple systems. The principles address the individual internally (eg, self-esteem) and interpersonally (eg, social skills), the family system (eg, adult protective shield), and the neighborhood and community (eg, social fabric). Conducive to transformation and empowerment, the intersection and harmony of these components has been shown to effectively prevent risky behaviors,[30,31] improve systems,[30] and enhance communities.[18] To endanger lasting prevention mechanisms for youth, one must work on all these levels.

OVERVIEW OF HIV PREVENTION PROGRAMS

There are prevention programs and initiatives that have applied some of these principles and have been effective in preventing HIV-related risky behaviors in youth. This section delineates various prevention intervention programs targeted at youth and/or the family.

PATH

Parent-Preadolescent Training for HIV Prevention (PATH) is a prevention intervention that targets HIV risk behaviors by focusing on healthy family relations, delay of sexual initiation, accurate information on HIV/AIDS, and how to implement skills to reduce the risk of infection. PATH integrates principles focused on connectedness through targeting family relationships, enhancing the adult protective shield through bolstering parenting skills, and indirectly touches on self-esteem through information and skills implementation. PATH was designed to prevent risky sexual behaviors in youth, particularly those aged 10 to 13 years. It consists of 4 sessions, provided once per week, lasting 3 hours each for the parents. Sessions cover topics including knowledge and skills on preventing risky behaviors related to sex, HIV and drugs, parent-child communication, and child development. Three months after the end of the program, parents meet again with facilitators to discuss their family life after the program.

The trial of this program consisted of 238 families who participated in either the treatment or control condition (materials only). The children of the parents who participated in PATH showed increased HIV knowledge, higher intentions to use condoms,[46] and a greater delay of first intercourse.[47]

The SAAF Project

The Strong African American Families Program (SAAF)[48] incorporates the field principles of connectedness, the adult protective shield, and self-esteem. SAAF consists of 7 consecutive weekly 2-hour meetings. Youth and their caregivers begin with a meal together, divide into separate groups, and come together at the end to focus on family relationships. The content for caregivers focuses on limit setting, monitoring, racial socialization, clear expectations about sexual risk, including sexual initiation, alcohol/substance use, communication, and inductive discipline. The youth content focuses on strengthening protective factors including dealing with experiences of racism, planning for the future, differences between themselves and peers who engage in HIV-related and other risk behaviors. Family modules focus on problem solving, conflict resolution, communication skills, the promotion of positive parent-child affectivity about sex, and the establishment of clear expectations about sexual behavior and substance use.

SAAF was evaluated in a randomized prevention trial with 667 African American 11-year-old students and their caregivers who were recruited from public schools in 8 rural Georgia counties.[48] Of the participating SAAF families, 65% attended 5 or more of the 7 weekly sessions; 44% attended all 7 sessions. Families who participated in SAAF had increased communication and their youth had enhanced protection, including enhanced future orientation, and improved attitudes and self-efficacy about resisting influences to risky behavior. Most importantly, the program reduced young people's HIV-related risk behavior, including early onset of substance use and sexual intercourse.

Keepin' it R.E.A.L.!

Diorio and colleagues[49] developed a prevention program for mothers and adolescents called Keepin' it R.E.A.L.! (Responsible, Empowered, Aware, and Living) to enhance the role of mothers in postponing the sexual debut of their 11- to 14-year-old adolescents. This program also focused on bridging possible gaps between parents and their children through enhancing their communication (or connectedness). The program had 2 versions: one focused on preventing risky sexual behavior and the other focused more broadly on reducing multiple problem behaviors. A randomized trial comparing the 2 versions of the program with a control condition indicated that there were no differences among conditions in delay of sexual intercourse, but the program focused on multiple problems increased condom use.

Diorio and colleagues[50] also developed a version of the program for fathers. The fathers attended 7 weekly sessions, and sons attended the final session. The program included goal setting and take-home activities. A randomized trial showed that fathers who participated in the program reported significantly more conversations about sexuality, greater intentions to have future conversations about sexuality, more confidence discussing sexual issues, and more positive outcomes associated with these conversations with their sons. Their adolescents reported significantly higher rates of sexual abstinence, condom use, and the intent to delay initiation of sexual intercourse.

Familias Unidas

Familias Unidas (United Families) is a multilevel, family-centered, ecodevelopmental, Hispanic-focused, HIV prevention intervention.[51] This program integrates the principles of connectedness through targeting parent-child relationships, the adult protective shield through parental involvement and school bonding, and self-efficacy through adolescent self-regulation and behavior control. It targets Hispanic immigrant parents and their children in an urban community in Miami, Florida. The first study was a 9-month randomized trial that showed that the program increased parental involvement, improved communication and support, and resulted in fewer adolescent behavior problems.[51] Active participation in the group was shown to predict engagement and retention in the intervention, and in turn, engagement and retention facilitated improved outcomes for adolescents and families participating in the intervention.[52]

A second study randomly assigned 266 eighth-grade Hispanic adolescents and their primary caregivers to 1 of 3 conditions: (1) Familias Unidas + Parent-Preadolescent Training for HIV Prevention (PATH); (2) English for speakers of other languages (ESOL) + PATH; and (3) ESOL + HeartPower! For Hispanics (HEART). The results showed that Familias Unidas + PATH was efficacious in preventing and reducing cigarette use relative to both control conditions and more efficacious than ESOL + HEART in reducing illicit drug use. Familias Unidas + PATH was efficacious, relative to ESOL + PATH, in reducing unsafe sexual behavior. Results showed that Familias Unidas + PATH was efficacious in reducing illicit drug use relative to ESOL + HEART. There were 2 surprising results. First, Familias Unidas + PATH was more efficacious in reducing cigarette use than ESOL + HEART, in which HEART directly targeted cigarette use. Second, Familias Unidas + PATH was more efficacious in reducing unsafe sexual behavior at last sexual intercourse than ESOL + PATH.[53]

CHAMP

The Chicago HIV Prevention and Adolescent Mental Health Project (CHAMP) targeted all 7 field principles throughout its development and iterations. CHAMP is a family-based HIV prevention intervention that targets young adolescents (fourth and fifth grades). It includes 10 to 12 manualized, multiple-family group sessions that engage the guardians and their dependants. The sessions educate the participants on HIV and risky behaviors and situations, and promote parental skills (eg, parental connectedness with youth, parenting styles, parental monitoring, and engaging caregiver support from the community and peers). Through skills-building practice, the participants learn to apply and hone prevention skills. The sessions also encourage comfort around family discussion on sensitive topics, connectedness between the caregivers and their youth, and apt monitoring and discipline for parents. All of the CHAMP programs are designed to allow youth the opportunity to practice the social and emotional skills necessary to extricate themselves from risky sexual situations and to avoid being influenced by sexual and drug use peer pressure.[29] The program facilitators are also integral parts of the program and the realization of social fabric. A CHAMP research staff member and a target community member conduct the sessions.[29] The required community partnership is yet another way in which CHAMP interventions are conducive to the actualization of rebuilding the village.[29]

The first CHAMP research study involved more than 300 control and more than 300 experimental families assigned to multiple-family groups, 1 with an attention control and 1 with the manualized CHAMP HIV prevention. Three of 4 families in the experimental condition completed the entire program. In addition, the experimental families showed an increase in family decision making, improved caregiver monitoring, greater comfort in discussing hard to talk about topics with their children, more neighborhood support systems in place, and fewer aggressive and rule-breaking behaviors.[29,54] Based on the findings from the original, CHAMP was adapted to contexts in

New York, Chicago's Westside, Durban, South Africa; and Trinidad and Tobago.[55,56] The adaptations did not change the core family-based HIV prevention principles of this evidence-based intervention, but rather shifted the packaging of the core principles to be welcoming to the target culture as measured by focus group endorsement, not offensive to the target culture, contain issues of relevance to the targeted culture, recognizable to the target culture, familiar to the target culture, and endorsed by the target culture. Accordingly, the basic goals of increasing family connectedness, communication about difficult topics, social skills training and practice, HIV transmission knowledge, and so forth were preserved in each adaptation of the CHAMP intervention.

An analysis of the key elements of all the CHAMP interventions illustrates that a major goal of the intervention was to rebuild the village by guiding families to cultivate social fabric or collective efficacy[15] to assist in child rearing. The principle of providing modern psychological technology was accomplished by using the multiple-family groups to deliver a manualized HIV prevention intervention. This manual had exercises to develop connectedness and social and emotional skills (eg, communication using I messages). Thus, South African caregivers were supported in obtaining a sense of power and models along with reestablishing the adult protective shield so that youth could feel safer. Thus, families were taught how to set family rules, monitor their and other's children's whereabouts, and cooperate with neighbors to watch out for their children. The intervention also aimed at creating a sense of mastery to address the HIV/AIDS epidemic in South Africa and this was achieved by cultivating a sense of learned helpfulness as these families were actively doing something to prevent HIV infections.

In Durban, South Africa, compared with the control group, the caregivers in the experimental arm had increased their monitoring of their youth and had more family rules. These families also had more comfort and frequency in talking to their youth about the epidemic. Caregivers who experienced the CHAMP manualized intervention reported less neighborhood disorganization along with more social control and cohesion where they lived. The youth in the experimental conditions had more knowledge and less stigmatizing attitudes toward people afflicted with HIV/AIDS. Because, like the original CHAMP, indigenous Zulu community residents were hired to recruit, retain, and deliver the intervention, the participation rate was 94%.[29] These outcomes are proximal, therefore it is too early to tell whether they will be sustained; however, it is clearly a step in the right direction.

SUMMARY

For years, the HIV pandemic was seemingly mysterious and uncontrollable. However, it is now known that with technology, this virus can be stopped from becoming fatal, and with prevention further infection can be stopped. With the application of certain principles and knowledge, this pandemic can be turned into something much less nocuous and pervasive. Various researchers and programs have effectively demonstrated this reality, showing the possibilities of ameliorating the propagation of this virus through prevention. Future research and policy should indicate the furtherance of these programs and designate more time and resources for more targeted research on prevention.

REFERENCES

1. Fanning D. Frontline: the age of AIDS [television broadcast]. Washington, DC. New York: Public Broadcasting System; 2006.

2. Tree of Life Gallery. AIDS orphans 2006. Available at: http://treeoflifegallery.org/AidsOrphans.htm. Accessed May 1, 2006.

3. Centers for Disease Control and Prevention. HIV prevalence estimates: United States; 2006. Available at: http://www.cdc.gov/mmwr/preview/mmwrhtml/mm5739a2.htm. Accessed June 15, 2008.

4. Pequegnat W, Stover E. Behavioral prevention is today's AIDS vaccine! AIDS 2000;14:S1–7.

5. Pequegnat W. Family and HIV/AIDS: first line of health promotion and disease prevention. In: Pequegnat W, Bell CC, editors. Families and HIV/AIDS: culture and contextual issues in prevention and treatment. New York: Springer, in press.

6. National Research Council and Institute of Medicine. Preventing mental, emotional, and behavioral disorders among young people: progress and possibilities. Washington, DC: The National Academies Press; 2009.

7. Flay BR, Snyder F, Petraitis J. The theory of triadic influence. In: DiClemente RJ, Kegler MC, Crosby RA, editors. Emerging theories in health promotion practice and research. 2nd edition. New York: Jossey-Bass; 2009. p. 451–510.

8. Zigler E, Trickett PK. IQ, social competence, and evaluation of early childhood intervention programs. Am Psychol 1978;33:789–98.

9. Masten AS. Resilience in development: implications of the study of successful adaptation for developmental psychopathology. In: Cicchetti D, editor, Rochester symposium on developmental psychopathology. The emergence of a discipline, vol. 1. Hillsdale (NJ): Erlbaum; 1989. p. 261–94.

10. Bell CC, Richardson J, Blount MA. Suicide prevention. In: Lutzker JR, editor. Preventing violence: research and evidence-based intervention strategies. Washington, DC: American Psychological Association; 2005. p. 217–37.

11. Felitti VJ, Anda RF, Nordenberg D, et al. Relationship of child abuse and household dysfunction to many of the leading causes of death in adults. The Adverse Childhood Experiences (ACE) Study. Am J Prev Med 1998;14:245–58.

12. Green JG, McLaughlin KA, Berglund PA, et al. Childhood adversities and adult psychiatric disorders in the national comorbity survey replication I. Arch Gen Psychiatry 2010;67:113–23.

13. McLaughlin KA, Green JG, Gruber MJ, et al. Childhood adversities and adult psychiatric disorders in the national comorbity survey replication II. Arch Gen Psychiatry 2010;67:124–32.

14. Brown SC, Flavin K, Kaupert S, et al. The role of settings in family-based prevention of HIV/STDs. In: Pequegnat W, Bell CC, editors. Families and HIV/AIDS: culture and contextual issues in prevention and treatment, vol. 304. New York: Springer; 2010. p. 565–6.

15. Sampson RJ, Raudenbush SW, Earls F. Neighborhoods and violent crime: a multilevel study of collective efficacy. Science 1997;277:918–24.

16. Gladwell M. Tipping point: how little things can make big difference. New York: Little, Brown and Company; 2000.

17. Baumer EP, South SJ. Community effects on youth sexual activity. J Marriage Fam 2001;63:540–54.

18. Redd J, Suggs H, Gibbons R, et al. A plan to strengthen systems and reduce the number of African-American children in child welfare. Illinois Child Welfare 2005;2:34–46.

19. Browning CR, Burrington LA, Leventhal T, et al. Neighborhood structural inequality, collective efficacy, and sexual risk behavior among urban youth. J Health Soc Behav 2008;49:269–85.

20. Semenza JC, March TL. An urban community-based intervention to advance social interactions. Environ Behav 2009;41:22–42.
21. Toit L, Cerin E, Leslie E, et al. Does walking in the neighborhood enhance local sociability? Urban Stud 2007;44:1677–95.
22. Collins RL, Ellickson PL, Orlando M, et al. Isolating the nexus of substance use, violence and sexual risk for HIV infection among young adults in the United States. AIDS Behav 2005;9:73–87.
23. Hopfer CJ, Crowley TJ, Hewitt JK. Review of twin and adoption studies of adolescent substance use. J Am Acad Child Adolesc Psychiatry 2003;42:710–9.
24. Bernstein KT, Galea S, Ahern J, et al. The built environment and alcohol consumption in urban neighborhoods. Drug Alcohol Depend 2007;91:244–52.
25. Cohen D, Spear S, Scribner R, et al. "Broken windows" and the risk of gonorrhea. Am J Public Health 2000;90:230–6.
26. National Institute of Medicine. Reducing suicide: a national imperative. Washington, DC: The National Academies Press; 2002.
27. US Department of Health and Human Services. Youth violence: a report of the surgeon general. Washington, DC: US Department of Health and Human Services; 2001.
28. Bell CC, Bhana A, McKay MM, et al. A commentary on the Triadic Theory of Influence as a guide for adapting HIV prevention programs for new contexts and populations: the CHAMP-South Africa story. Soc Work Men Health 2007;5: 243–67.
29. Bell CC, Bhana A, Petersen I, et al. Building protective factors to offset sexually risky behaviors among black South African youth: a randomized control trial. J Natl Med Assoc 2008;100:936–44.
30. Bell CC, Gamm S, Vallas P, et al. Strategies for the prevention of youth violence in Chicago Public Schools. In: Shafii M, Shafii SF, editors. School violence: assessment, management, prevention. Arlington (VA): American Psychiatric Press; 2001. p. 251–72.
31. Bell CC, Flay B, Paikoff R. Strategies for health behavior change. In: Chunn J, editor. The health behavioral change imperative. New York: Kluwer Academic/ Plenum Publishers; 2002. p. 17–39.
32. Bell CC. Keeping promises: ethics and principles in psychiatric practice. In: The art and science of psychiatry. Boston: Aspatore Books; 2007. p. 7–38.
33. Bell CC. Endurance, strength, and coordination exercises without cardiovascular or respiratory stress. J Natl Med Assoc 1979;71:265–70.
34. Bell CC, McBride DF. Affect regulation and the prevention of risky behaviors. JAMA, in press.
35. Levey J, Levey M. Living in balance: a dynamic approach for creating harmony and wholeness in a chaotic world. Berkeley (CA): Conari Press; 1998.
36. Bowlby J. Separation. Attachment and loss, vol. 2. New York: Basic Books; 1973.
37. Meloy R. Violent attachments. Northvale (NJ): Jason Aronson; 1992.
38. Renken B, Egeland B, Marvinney D, et al. Early childhood antecedents of aggression and passive-withdrawal in early elementary school. J Pers 1989; 57:257–81.
39. Sweet MA, Appelbaum ML. Is home visiting an effective strategy? A meta-analytic review of home visiting programs for families with young children. Child Dev 2004;75:1435–56.
40. Fisher M, Schneider M, Pegler C, et al. Eating attitudes, health-risk behaviors, self-esteem, and anxiety among adolescent females in a suburban high school. J Adolesc Health 1991;12:377–84.

41. Bean R. The four conditions of self-esteem: a new approach for elementary and middle schools. 2nd edition. Santa Cruz (CA): ETR Associates; 1992.
42. Goleman D. Emotional intelligence: why it can matter more than IQ. New York: Batman Books; 1994.
43. Flay BR, Graumlich S, Segawa E, et al. The ABAN AYA youth project: effects of comprehensive prevention programs on high-risk behaviors among inner city African American youth: a randomized trial. Arch Pediatr Adolesc Med 2004; 158:377–84.
44. Bell CC. Cultivating resiliency in youth. J Adolesc Health 2001;29:375–81.
45. Bronfenbrennor U. The ecology of human development: experiments by nature and design. Cambridge (MA): Harvard University Press; 1979.
46. Krauss B, Tiffany J, Goldsamt L. Research notes: parent and pre-adolescent training for HIV prevention in a high seroprevalence neighbourhood. AIDS STD Health Promot Exch 1997;1:10–2.
47. Krauss B, McGinniss S, O'Day J, et al. Delaying tactics: parent HIV education as a protective factor for early sexual debut. Poster presented at NIMH International Conference on the Role of Families in Preventing and Adapting to HIV/AIDS. San Francisco (CA), July 2007.
48. Willis TA, Murry VM, Brody GH, et al. Ethnic pride and self-control related to protective and risk factors: test of the theoretical model for the Strong African American Families Program. Health Psychol 2007;26:50–9.
49. Dilorio C, Resnicow K, Denzmore P, et al. Keepin' It R.E.A.L.! a mother-adolescent HIV prevention program. In: Pequegnat W, Szapocznik J, editors. Working with families in the era of AIDS. Thousand Oaks (CA): Sage; 2000. p. 113–32.
50. Dilorio C, McCarty F, Denzmore P. An exploration of social cognitive theory mediators of father-son communication about sex. J Pediatr Psychol 2006;31:1–11.
51. Pantin H, Coatsworth JD, Feaster DJ, et al. Familias Unidas: the efficacy of an intervention to promote parental investment in Hispanic immigrant families. Prev Sci 2003;4:189–201.
52. Prado G, Pantin H, Schwartz SJ, et al. Predictors of engagement and retention into a parent-centered, ecodevelopmental HIV preventive intervention for Hispanic adolescents and their families. J Pediatr Psychol 2006;31:874–90.
53. Prado G, Pantin H, Briones E, et al, Family-based HIV prevention with African American and Hispanic youth. In: Pequegnat W, Bell CC, editors. Families and HIV/AIDS: culture and contextual issues in prevention and treatment. New York: Springer, in press.
54. McKay MM, Chasse KT, Paikoff R, et al. Family-level impact of the CHAMP family program: a community collaborative effort to support urban families and reduce youth HIV risk exposure. Fam Process 2004;43:79–93.
55. McKay MM, Paikoff RL, editors. Community collaborative partnerships: the foundation for HIV prevention research efforts. Binghamton (NY): Haworth Press; 2007.
56. Bell CC. Family as the model for prevention of mental and physical health problems. In: Pequegnat W, Bell CC, editors. Families and HIV/AIDS: culture and contextual issues in prevention and treatment. New York: Springer, in press.

Psychological Protective Factors Across the Lifespan: Implications for Psychiatry

Ipsit V. Vahia, MD[a,b,c,*], Elizabeth Chattillion, BA[b],
Harish Kavirajan, MD[d], Colin A. Depp, PhD[a,b]

KEYWORDS

- Positive psychology • Aging • Psychological protective factors
- Positive psychological constructs • Resilience • Spirituality
- Wisdom • Self-efficacy

The field of positive psychology has advanced rapidly in the past several years, and a particularly active application of this area of inquiry has been in understanding the determinants of healthy aging and longevity. Two decades ago, in their seminal article published in *Science*, Rowe and Kahn noted that much of the research on aging had focused on the distinction between pathological aging from "usual,"[1,2] and urged the field to embark on rigorous scientific study of the biological, social, and psychological factors that determined "successful aging." Around the same time period, positive psychology began to emerge, which, like successful aging, offered a counterpoint to the field's historical focus on pathological conditions, traits, and experiences.[3,4] Although it remains the case that there is much more known about negative emotions and age-associated diseases, there have been several studies that have enlightened the intersection of positive psychology and lifespan development.

According to Seligman, positive psychology concerns itself with individual traits (resilience, wisdom), subjective experiences (eg, well being, happiness), and attributes of groups (eg, civic-mindedness, altruism).[3] In this review, the authors focus on

[a] Sam and Rose Stein Institute for Research on Aging, University of California, San Diego, 9500 Gilman Drive #0664, La Jolla, CA 92093, USA
[b] Department of Psychiatry, University of California, San Diego, 9500 Gilman Drive #0664, La Jolla, CA 92093, USA
[c] Sun Valley Behavioral Medical Center, 2417 Marshall Avenue #1, Imperial, CA 92251, USA
[d] Department of Psychiatry and Biobehavioral Sciences, University of California, Los Angeles, 950 South Coast Drive, Suite 202, Costa Mesa, CA 92626, USA
* Corresponding author. Sam and Rose Stein Institute for Research on Aging, Division of Geriatric Psychiatry, University of California, San Diego, 9500 Gilman Drive #0664, La Jolla, CA 92093.
E-mail address: ivahia@ucsd.edu

Psychiatr Clin N Am 34 (2011) 231–248
doi:10.1016/j.psc.2010.11.011
0193-953X/11/$ – see front matter © 2011 Elsevier Inc. All rights reserved.

individual psychological traits that may protect against morbidity and mortality in later life. There are several reasons why positive psychological constructs are fertile territory in the study of the determinants of healthy cognitive and emotional development. First, and probably the most significant reason, is that several longitudinal studies suggest that adults who report higher levels of positive psychological traits, such as optimism, positive attitudes toward aging, and purpose in life, appear to live longer and healthier lives. These effects are present when statistically adjusting for other more frequently studied predictors of morbidity and mortality, such as depression and physical illnesses. A second reason for interest in positive psychological traits is that qualitative studies indicate that older people appear to include these traits in how they define successful aging. The components of the definition of successful aging employed in quantitative studies have been most often indicators of higher functional status, physical health, and cognitive status (eg, freedom from cognitive impairment)[5,6]; whereas, qualitative studies indicate that older adults define successful aging in terms of resilience[7,8] and positive outlook toward the future.[9] A third reason why the intersection of positive psychology and aging has intrigued researchers is that in contrast to declining trajectories (or mitigation in declines) in most physical and cognitive phenotypes, aging seems to be associated with higher levels of some positive psychological traits[10] and states.[11] Thus, studying positive constructs in older people may be instructive toward understanding their development throughout the lifespan. A fourth reason why positive psychological constructs offer great promise is that, unlike genes at the present time, these are predictors of outcome in later life that are potentially modifiable through psychosocial interventions, policies, and behavior changes.

Nevertheless, like any new field, there are several challenges to the study of positive psychology and successful aging. The boundaries around the definitions of positive psychological traits are each intensely debated, in part, because there is no clinical mandate to define these boundaries (as would be the case for depression, for instance). Another key concern is whether successful aging and positive psychological constructs represent the opposite of, or freedom from, pathology (ie, that positive psychology is simply psychology).[4,12] In addition, available data are limited by the almost exclusive use of self-report measures[13]; few available data on the psychometric properties relative to pathological measures; and limited understanding about the impact of cohort effects, selective mortality, age differences, and cultural factors.

Notwithstanding the challenges in understanding the psychological predictors of healthy aging, there are clear merits to furthering the understanding of this area from the perspective of psychiatry. The following is a review of the best-studied positive psychological constructs in the context of aging, selected based on the presence of more than one empirical study with physical or mental health status as the dependent variable. For each psychological construct, the authors describe the definition/conceptualization, measurement/operationalization, and associations, and synthesize the findings at the conclusion. As previously noted, positive psychological traits appear to play a greater role in cognitive and emotional functioning as one ages. Therefore, in this review the authors' focus is on the impact of these traits in late adulthood and old age because future research in this area is likely to be of most immediate relevance to older adults.

RESILIENCE
Definition/Conceptualization

Resilience is broadly defined in physiological terms as the ability to return to homeostasis in the presence of stressful experiences that would be expected to bring about negative effects.[14] Resilience can be conceptualized and studied as a general personality trait (eg, hardiness), as a process that entails positive responses to specific and acute stressors, or as a set of physiological responses to stressors. By and large, the study of resilience has primarily focused on childhood development and surviving early childhood trauma, given that some children seem to show no ill effects of difficult, disadvantaged early years. However, there has been a more recent focus on resilience in early and later adulthood. The interest in resilience in regard to aging relates to the consistent observation that older adults, on average, are able to maintain levels of subjective well-being, despite increasing biological vulnerabilities to stressors. To this end, a related concept to resilience is adaptation, which pertains more to the behavioral plasticity that serves to compensate for loss of function. Life-span developmental theories conceptualize adaptation as central to success in the management of physical decline that accompanies aging (Baltes[15] and later Schulz & Heckhausen[16]).

Measurement/Operationalization

The approach to measuring resilience varies according to the characteristics of the stressors. When conceptualized as a general personality trait, resilience is measured with global self-report measures, such as the Connor Davidson Resilience Scale (CD-RISC).[17] The original CD-RISC includes 25 items, with later studies culling the scale to 10 items[18] or even 2 items[19] (the 2-item measure includes "able to adapt to change" and "tend to bounce back after illness or hardship"). The CD-RISC has evidenced sound psychometric properties in normal population samples, clinical samples with anxiety disorders, and older primary care patients.[20] An alternative to the CD-RISC is the Hardy Gill Resilience Scale, which asks the respondent to identify a single major stressor experienced in the past 5 years, with subsequent ratings of experienced positive and negative effects. The Hardy Gill scale thus may tap into resilience as a state rather than a general tendency. In physiologic terms, a deleterious response to chronic stress is called allostatic load.[21] Allostatic load is operationalized as an index of biomarkers of cardiovascular, immune, and hypothalamic-pituitary-adrenal axis overactivation. Resilient individuals may then be evidenced by low levels of allostatic load in the context of chronic stressors. Finally, a concept that is related to resilience, but not the same, is posttraumatic growth. This concept has been operationalized based on the model proposed by Tedeschi and Calhoun[22] as positive changes in self-perception, interpersonal relationships, or philosophy of life after a traumatic experience. A measure, the Post Traumatic Growth Inventory, has been developed based on this model.[22]

Correlates/Associations

In comparison to other positive traits, resilience has been studied with translational methods. There is considerable literature on physiological effects of stress, animal models, and the genetic, cellular, and neural systems involved in resilience. There are several general conclusions about resilience, reviewed in greater depth elsewhere.[23,24] One conclusion is that, during and after adverse circumstances, resilient individuals appear to experience more positive emotions and maintain optimism. Resilient individuals display more active, problem-focused coping, as opposed to avoidant or passive coping. At the physiological level, resilience may be characterized by reduced exposure to stress hormones, such as cortisol. Neuropeptide Y and dehydroepiandrosterone (DHEA) are also thought to reduce autonomic response and therefore protect the brain, thereby possibly increasing resilience. Therefore, a second conclusion regarding resilience is that it appears to be an active physiological process, not simply a function of attenuated stress response, and one that integrates a complex physiological system.[23]

Predictors of residence include higher educational attainment, which appears to relate to reduced allostatic load.[25,26] Greater social support is also implicated in speedier recovery from illness and stressors[27] and reduced inflammatory markers.[28] In examining whether age itself is related to resilience, Lamond and colleagues[20] assessed predictors of resilience in a cross-sectional sample of 1741 older women, measuring resilience with the CD-RISC. In comparison to previously published data from younger healthy controls, scores on the CD-RISC were similar among older women. Among older adults, resilience was associated with higher levels of optimism and more positive attitudes toward aging. The factor structure of the CD-RISC was somewhat different, with greater prominence of more emotion-focused coping strategies (eg, tolerating negative affect) over problem-focused strategies. The investigators theorized that that the shift toward emotion-focused coping may be caused by the changing nature of stressors in the latter half of life; older adults are more likely to face chronic uncontrollable stressors (eg, medical problems) than acute stressors that require active problem solving (eg, losing a job).[29]

OPTIMISM
Definition/Conceptualization

Optimism is among the better-studied positive psychological traits[30] and is generally defined by the tendency to hold positive expectations of the future. *Explanatory* optimism can be defined by the tendency to explain positive events in terms of stable, global, and internal factors, and to attribute negative events to causes that are unstable, specific, and external to the self. A pessimist would view positive and negative events in the converse. *Dispositional* optimism is more focused on orientation toward the future, in particular to expect that more positive than negative events will occur. Hence, the primary distinction is that explanatory optimism rests on the individual's interpretations of past events; whereas, dispositional optimism is more focused on future expectations.

Measurement/Operationalization

The primary measure used to reflect dispositional optimism is the Life Orientation Test (LOT or LOT-R)[31] and the instrument associated with explanatory optimism is the Attributional Styles Questionnaire (ASQ).[32] Although self-report instruments are the primary tools used to measure optimism, a recent article employed an econometric approach to operationalizing optimism, defining it as the discrepancy between predicted life expectancy based on actuarial tables and how long individuals expect to live.[33]

Correlates/Associations

Based on a large volume of available data on optimism, several general conclusions can be drawn. One is that people, on average, tend be more optimistic than pessimistic. Optimism appears to be quite stable over time, with test-retest correlation estimated at approximately 0.70 over 10 years.[34] The heritability of optimism was estimated to be 0.25 in a sample of over 500 twin pairs,[35] which is similar to the heritability of other personality traits. Although generally thought to be on a continuum, optimism and pessimism have also been found to demonstrate independent effects.[36] Although dispositional optimism is nearly universally related to positive mental health, there may both positive and negative physiological outcomes, especially with regard to immune response.[37]

In a recent meta-analysis of 83 studies,[38] the mean effect size for optimism in predicting a range of physical health outcomes (including mortality, cardiovascular health, immune function, cancer, pain, and physical symptoms) was estimated to be small to moderate (mean d = 0.17). These effects persisted after adjustment for other health variables, demographic factors, and other subjective indicators and were larger for subjective outcomes than objective indicators. Giltay and colleagues[39] followed 999 older Dutch men and women for an average of 9 years. Participants who reported higher levels of optimism at baseline had a lower risk of all cause mortality (especially cardiovascular mortality) after adjusting for age, sex, disease, education, and several other health risks at baseline. These effects were stronger in men than in women. Thus, optimism appears to produce a small but substantial protective effect on a range of health-related variables, including mortality.

Much of the research on physiological effects of optimism has focused on individual differences in cardiovascular, immune, and neuroendocrine function. The previously described study by Giltay indicated that optimism may be particularly related to cardiovascular mortality and there is some evidence that optimists have a heightened immune response. In one study of 124 law students, optimism predicted greater cell mediated immunity as measured by skin tests.[40] In behavioral studies, it appears that greater optimism predicts greater participation in health protective behavior,[41] greater persistence in regard to reducing negative health behaviors (eg, alcohol use), and greater resilience in the presence of health-related challenges.

PERSONAL CONTROL/MASTERY/SELF-EFFICACY
Definition/Conceptualization

Personal control broadly refers to an individual's belief in the self as an agent whose actions or behaviors are capable of changing the social or physical environment to obtain a desired outcome.[42,43] Two related but distinct constructs that have received attention in the positive psychology literature are mastery and self-efficacy. Mastery involves a global sense of control over one's future and life circumstances, in contrast to a fatalistic sense of a predetermined future. Individuals with high mastery have a sense of control over events that happen to them and feel confident that they can solve problems that arise in their lives.[44] Self-efficacy[45] is distinguished from mastery in that self-efficacy is most often related to a specific task or domain,[42,45–47] although the term has, on occasion, been used to represent a more universal trait.[47–49]

Measurement/Operationalization

Given that constructs of control represent internal states, existing measures of personal control, mastery, and self-efficacy used in older adults are self-report instruments. The most commonly used measure of mastery in adults is the Pearlin Mastery Scale, consisting of 7 Likert scale items.[44] A wider variety of self-report instruments exist to measure self-efficacy because of the specificity of the construct to particular tasks or domains. Measures of general (ie, non task-specific) self-efficacy include Sherer's General Self-efficacy Scale[49] and the 9-item Rodin and McAvay General Self-efficacy Scale,[48] which are of particular relevance to older adults. There exists a myriad of other domain-specific self-efficacy measures, such as those measuring intellectual self-efficacy or exercise self-efficacy. The varying level of specificity of these self-efficacy measures may make it difficult to accurately aggregate and interpret research findings related to self-efficacy.[47]

Correlates/Associations

Accumulated research findings on these constructs of control and their effects on morbidity and mortality in older adults support the notion that an increased sense of personal control contributes to successful aging. For example, in healthy older adults, a high sense of mastery is associated with fewer anxiety symptoms.[50,51] Low levels of mastery are associated with greater depressive symptoms in healthy older adults[51] and in those with severe arthritis.[52] Furthermore, high mastery has also been shown to be protective against the detrimental impact of economic hardship on increased depressive and anxiety symptoms[51] and the effect of deteriorating health on decreased life satisfaction.[53] A high level of general self-efficacy has been associated with increased quality of life[54]; whereas, high levels of domain-specific self-efficacy have been shown to predict less loneliness and less psychological distress in older adults.[55] Self-efficacy for managing instrumental daily activities has been positively associated with better cognitive functioning (ie, memory and abstraction)[56] as well as greater maintenance of cognitive performance (ie, verbal memory) over time in elderly men.[57]

These findings are further substantiated by longitudinal data, where higher self-efficacy for engaging in physical activity was indirectly associated with a less severe trajectory of physical decline over a 2-year period in older women, independent of chronic health conditions.[58] Furthermore, a longitudinal study of older adults demonstrated that higher mastery was associated with lower overall mortality risk (after controlling for relevant factors, such as chronic diseases)[52] and lower risk for mortality and injury in disabled older women.[59]

In healthy older women, eudaimonic well-being, which includes a sense of environmental mastery, is associated with lower levels of salivary cortisol and proinflammatory cytokines, decreased cardiovascular risk, and longer duration of rapid eye movement (REM) sleep.[60] In a highly stressed population of older caregivers, high levels of mastery have been shown to protect against stress-related decreases in immune function,[61] stress-related increases in sympathetic arousal,[62] and stress-induced depressive symptoms.[63] Of most immediate interest are findings suggesting that greater self-efficacy may promote adherence to healthy behaviors, such as adoption and maintenance of regular exercise.[64–66]

POSITIVE ATTITUDES TOWARD OWN AGING
Definition/Conceptualization

Self-perception of aging includes cultural and personal beliefs about aging,[67,68] age identity,[69,70] as well as physical and other psychological factors.[67,71] Related research has focused on the constructs of "expectations regarding aging"[72] and "attribution to aging" of health problems,[73] both of which assess general beliefs about aging.[69] These constructs focus on younger persons' attitudes toward aging rather than older persons' personal experience of aging.

Measurement/Operationalization

Several approaches have been used to measure positive attitudes toward own aging in the literature. The most common approach is self-report measures, such as the 38-item Expectations Regarding Aging survey (ERA-38)[72] and the shorter 12-item Expectations Regarding Aging survey (ERA-12).[74] Both of these measures assign a score between 0 and 100, with higher scores indicating higher (more positive) expectations from old age. Other studies, including those conducted by the authors' group, have used shorter self-report measures, such as the Attitude Toward Own Aging subscale of the Philadelphia Geriatric Morale scale.[75] To assess intrinsic stereotypes toward aging, Levy[76] has used the Implicit Association Test (IAT).

Correlates/Associations

Evidence from the medical, psychological, sociological, and gerontological literature indicates that older persons who hold more negative views regarding their experience of aging have greater morbidity (eg, more hearing, cognitive, and mood disturbances,[67,71,77–79] poorer function,[71,80] and higher mortality rates)[80–82] than those with more positive views of their aging.

Sarkisian[72] found that better mental and physical health predicted positive aging attitudes, and that advanced age and greater depression predicted negative aging attitudes, but that gender, income, education, religiosity, medical comorbidity, and function are not determinants of aging perceptions. In a separate study, attribution of newly emergent health problems to age was associated only with older age and grip strength; whereas, coefficients for gender, education, social network score, depression, smoking, and various physical health indicators were not significant.[73] Barrett[69] reported that more youthful "age identity" (ie, felt age minus actual age) is associated with being older, female gender, nonwhite race, various self-rated health measures, and having a parent in poor health.[69] Therefore, the existing literature provides consistent support for negative associations between depression and poor physical functioning and positive attitudes toward aging, but discrepant evidence on whether chronological age predicts positive or negative views on aging.

Several reports have identified associations between health and psychosocial measures and attitudes toward aging, but given the vast differences in methodological rigor of such studies, it is difficult to estimate how valid and reliable these associations might be. Prominently associated factors include ethnicity and culture,[67,70,83,84] education,[84] socioeconomic status,[69] and age (with higher age associated with increasingly negative views of aging).[67,72,84] Positive perceptions of own aging is also associated with general health measures, such as self-rated global health,[68] health-related function,[85] and medical comorbidity,[69,83] as well as specific health problems (eg, hearing impairment,[79] cognitive decline,[67,86] incontinence,[87,88] and increased body mass index [BMI]).[82]

SPIRITUALITY
Definition/Conceptualization

In recent years there has been a growing interest in understanding the role of spirituality and religious practices in relation to mental health and well-being, especially among older adults. There is much ongoing debate about the definitions of, and distinctions between, religiosity and spirituality, and no globally accepted definitions exist for either. However, as suggested by Blazer,[89] literature in this area is best studied in the context of definitions and measures used in individual studies, rather than in the context of an overarching global construct. A discussion on the differences between spirituality and religiosity, and a complete appraisal of all literature in this area is beyond the scope of this article, so the authors have restricted the focus to the impact of religiosity/spirituality on physical, psychological, and cognitive functioning in older adults.

Measurement/Operationalization

Reflecting the lack of consensus in definitions of spirituality and religiosity, there have been few measures that comprehensively encompass the multiple domains of spirituality and religiosity. Recently, the Brief Multidimensional Measure of Religiosity and Spirituality[90] has been validated and increasingly used in research. This scale, developed in collaboration between the National Institute of Aging and the Fetzer Corporation, comprises 38 items that measure 11 domains: daily spiritual experience, belief that god is watching, forgiveness, private spiritual experience, religious/spiritual coping, religious support, religious/spiritual history, commitment, organizational religiousness, religious meaning and an overall religious/spiritual ranking.

Correlates/Associations

Crowther[91] has proposed an amendment to Rowe and Kahn's well-established model of successful aging to include the construct of positive spirituality. This theory is an indicator of the prominence attributed to spirituality by some authors. Several studies indicate an association of religious involvement with longevity,[92] better adaptation to medical illness,[93] greater resilience[94] and improved health behaviors such as lower rates of smoking and alcohol use.[95] Some authors have suggested a role for spirituality in health promotion.[91]

Recent studies have focused on the association between religious attendance and cognitive function. van Ness and Kasl[96] and Hill and colleagues[97] demonstrated that people who attend religious services more frequently demonstrated slower rates of age-related cognitive decline, and Reyes-Ortiz and colleagues[98] reported that rates of cognitive decline were faster in individuals who attended religious services less frequently. The latter investigators also found that cognitive decline associated with chronic depressive symptoms was faster in persons who were not religious. Religious support positively impacts emotional health.[99] One limitation of most studies is that they are restricted to specific clinical populations (eg, patients with cancer, patients with chronic pain). In a study of spirituality in a community-dwelling population of older adults, Vahia and colleagues[94] noted that greater spirituality was associated with greater resilience as well as lower income and education levels. Thus, precise correlates of spirituality/religiosity may be dependent to some extent on the nature of the population sample in which such correlates are assessed.

WISDOM
Definition/Conceptualization

Wisdom is a new area of research for psychiatry, though it has been studied by gerontologists, psychologists, and sociologists for almost 3 decades. Understanding of wisdom has evolved considerably. Early work conceptualized wisdom as expert comprehensive knowledge and focused on its use for decision making,[100] with later work broadening the definition to include social and emotional aspects. Meeks and Jeste[101] describe wisdom in terms of pragmatic life knowledge and decision making, emotional homeostasis, value relativism, and management of ambiguity. Ancient and modern definitions tend to be more similar than different. Comparing definitions in the modern scientific literature (based on Western philosophy) to the definition of wisdom in the *Bhagavad Gita*, an ancient Indian text that is at least 2500 years old, Jeste and Vahia[102] noted that the concepts of wisdom in these 2 bodies of literature from different eras and different cultural sources were remarkably similar. Meeks and Jeste[101] provided a conceptual review proposing a possible neurobiological basis for wisdom. Based on their review, the investigators proposed a neurobiological model where the lateral prefrontal cortex (PFC), especially the dorsolateral PFC, works in concert with the dorsal anterior cingulated cortex (ACC), orbitofrontal cortex (OFC) and medial prefrontal cortex (MPFC) to exert an important inhibitory effect on several brain areas associated with emotionality and immediate reward dependence (eg, amygdala, ventral striatum). Thus, a rational/analytical aspect of wisdom possibly operates in synergy with a more emotion-based subcomponent, including prosocial attitudes and behaviors that involve MPFC, PCC, OFC, superior temporal sulcus, and reward neurocircuitry. Likewise, MPFC seems to mediate self-reflection and self-awareness; a certain amount of lateral PFC inhibition of this process may, however, be required to stop this function short of maladaptive self-absorption.

Measurement/Operationalization

Currently, the most commonly operationalized model of wisdom is the 3-dimensional model proposed by Clayton and Birren[103] and refined by Ardelt,[104] which divides wisdom into cognitive, affective, and reflective domains. This model postulates that to be considered wise a person must simultaneously demonstrate cognitive qualities (ie, expert knowledge, reasoning ability, problem solving/decision making), affective qualities (ie, positive emotions, fewer negative emotions, ability to regulate emotion), and a reflective component (ie, ability to overcome subjective perspectives and accept other views, including contradictory ones). The 3-Dimensional Wisdom Scale (3D-WS) is a self-rated quantitative measure of wisdom developed using this model, and has been demonstrated as valid and reliable.[104]

In a study using the Delphi method to characterize wisdom, Jeste and colleagues[105] invited 30 experts on wisdom to rate 53 Likert-style statements related to wisdom, spirituality, and intelligence. After phase 1, the list was narrowed to 12 statements to better characterize wisdom and the experts were invited to rate these 12 items. At the end of the study, there was agreement that wisdom is a uniquely human but rare personal quality, which can be learned and measured, and increases with age through advanced cognitive and emotional development that is experience driven. At the same time, the experts agreed that wisdom was not expected to increase by taking medication. The study also discerned an overlap between wisdom and intelligence, but noted that wisdom and spirituality seemed to be distinct entities.

Correlates/Associations

Although the association of wisdom with age is complex, there is evidence that the process of acquiring wisdom-related traits (eg, intellectual capacity) begins in childhood.[106] It remains unclear whether aging is associated with wisdom. It is likely that acquiring wisdom with age is dependent on opportunities to gather experiences, the nature of those experiences, and the ability to learn from such experiences.[107]

At present, wisdom has limited utility in psychiatry, largely because of deficiencies in the ability to operationalize and measure wisdom. However, because of recent advances in our understanding of wisdom and its underlying mechanisms, as well as the availability of more psychometrically sound measures, such as the 3D-WS,[104] focus on the association of wisdom with psychopathology, physical and emotional functioning, and its utility as a measure of developmental outcomes are all fertile areas for study.

SUMMARY AND DIRECTIONS FOR FUTURE RESEARCH

As is evident from the studies previously reviewed, there are some provocative data supporting a link between positive psychological constructs and the maintenance and promotion of health, especially in older persons. People who are optimistic about the future and about aging itself, who are resilient after stressful events, and who are confident in their abilities to manage day-to-day affairs and hassles seem to experience better cognitive and emotional health into later adulthood. Although the strength of these associations vary across studies and the causal influences among variables is difficult to tease apart, the impact of these constructs seems to be at least somewhat independent from established pathological predictors of morbidity and mortality in longitudinal studies employing statistical controls. These studies also seem to suggest that positive psychological constructs are not simply the converse of risk factors.

It is clear that there are remaining challenges in operationalizing and measuring these protective factors, with some constructs attaining greater consensus than others. In addition to advances in measurement, the next steps are to identify the mechanisms and moderators of the impact of positive psychological traits on health, as well as evaluate whether interventions can modify or amplify their expression. Reconceptualization of positive traits as processes rather than stable qualities may help to guide future work in understanding how positive traits are manifested and what can be done to promote them.

For example, such research would ask how resilient responses to stress are manifested rather than whether resilient people are healthier. To this end, expanding the repertoire of assessment beyond global self-report measures, to include methods, such as ecological momentary assessment and laboratory-based experiments, may help identify how positive psychological traits are expressed in daily life.[108]

Investigation of the mechanisms of positive traits will need to address whether their effects are a result of indirect or direct pathways toward health maintenance,[109] and what physiological systems are involved. As the authors describe in previous sections, positive psychological traits are associated with greater engagement in healthy lifestyle behaviors.[76,110] However, it remains unclear whether they also have a role in reversing physiological and cellular pathways that underlie deleterious effects of stressors. It may be quite possible that there are effects of positive psychological constructs that are unmediated by stress, immune response, or lifestyle behavior.[111] For example, in a study that applied an innovative ambulatory monitoring protocol in which people were asked to rate their mood while their cardiovascular functioning was monitored, periods of happiness were associated with lower heart rate.[112] Among positive traits, stress and resilience appear to be furthest along in regard to mapping psychological constructs onto physiological systems. The deleterious effects of chronic stress on the brain and cardiovascular systems are well established, with chronic overactivation of hypothalamic-pituitary-adrenal axis leading to atrophy of brain structures, such as the hippocampus, and cardiovascular changes.[113] Chronic inflammation associated with stress has been linked with purported markers of accelerated aging, such as the telomere.[1]

Studying the mechanisms of positive psychological constructs at the community/ social level is also of great recent interest. Advances in social network analyses have opened a window into the dynamic spread of negative health behaviors (eg, smoking, obesity)[114] and happiness.[115] Happy people tend to be in the center of large social networks and an individual's level of happiness seems to influence the well-being of other network members over time. Thus, social network analyses could be used to determine how positive psychological constructs are transmitted and reciprocally influence the social environment. Similarly, several investigations have assessed the impact of media and other environmental influences on health behaviors. For example, Levy and Langer[67] showed that television watching predicted worse attitudes toward aging in older people. A separate issue that has received recent attention is the evident between-subjects differences in the strength of associations between positive traits and other measures. For example, the relationship between positive affect and health is less consistent among older people who have chronic medical illnesses compared with healthy older adults.[109] The reasons for this difference are not well understood. In addition, there may be important gender differences, with a stronger effect of optimism on cardiovascular health in older men than women.[39] In a study of self-reported resilience in older women, factor analyses revealed somewhat different factor structure than reported in younger samples,[17] and greater positive associations for emotion-focused items (eg, being able to tolerate distress) than associations with problem-focused items (eg, feeling confident in overcoming problems).[20] There may also be relevant genetic variation that influences the expression of positive traits. Stein and colleagues[116] found that the short allele of the serotonin transporter promoter polymorphism (5HTTLPR) was associated with lower resilience.

Once the mechanisms of protective factors are better elucidated, is may be possible to enhance them toward prevention of morbidity (eg, increase levels of optimism in pessimistic people). At present, positive constructs in intervention research are typically conceptualized as mediators or intervention effects. Many psychological interventions, such as cognitive behavioral therapy (CBT), are presumed to work because they enhance self-efficacy or optimism, thereby reinforcing adaptive beliefs about the self or the future. In addition, there is a small but compelling body of literature suggesting that some of the positive psychological constructs previously described could be modified in older people. Levy and colleagues[78] provide evidence in randomized experiments that altering implicit messages about aging can produce subsequent changes in handwriting or mobility. Older adults who engage in volunteer programs report greater purpose in life.[117]

Based on an understanding of resilience as the ability to achieve positive developmental outcomes despite adversity in early childhood and the ability to achieve/regain sustained well-being in response to adversity in later life, therapeutic techniques have been developed to promote resilience.[118] One such technique, termed *well-being therapy* postulates that by identifying components of well-being (eg, environmental mastery, personal growth, purpose in life, autonomy, self-acceptance, positive relations with others) and maximizing these components in therapy sessions, resilience can be promoted. In a small pilot trial of 20 subjects, well-being therapy was found to be superior to CBT in treating residual affective symptoms in persons with depressive disorders.[119] Other validation studies, although mainly small, nonblinded trials, have documented the efficacy of well-being therapy in prevention of relapse in persons with recurrent depression and a role for well-being therapy as a step in a sequential treatment approach to generalized anxiety disorder (GAD)[118] and remission of active symptoms of posttraumatic stress disorder (PTSD).[120]

Interventions have also been developed to promote posttraumatic growth in persons suffering from psychiatric and medical illnesses. In an exploratory trial of 51 subjects, assessing whether an Internet-based cognitive-behavioral intervention for complicated grief resulted in changes in posttraumatic growth and optimism, Wagner and colleagues[121] noted that in comparison to the waitlist group, the CBT group demonstrated clinically and statistically significant reductions in complicated grief symptoms and concomitant increases in posttraumatic growth, though they did not show changes in their personality. The investigators suggest that although optimism is a stable personality trait, posttraumatic growth may be amenable to interventions.

Of all the positive traits discussed, spirituality/religiosity may be the most extensively used to promote clinical outcomes. Studies assessing the use of spirituality or religiosity as interventions to promote wellness have not been the domain of psychiatrists. Although a comprehensive discussion of these studies is beyond the scope of this review, multiple trials have demonstrated that participating in religious activity[122] and spiritual involvement can serve as a coping mechanism for a variety of stressors, including bereavement,[123] chronic illness,[124] and pain[125] in a range of clinical populations, including patients with cardiac illnesses, patients with cancer, those suffering from chronic pain, and patients with terminal illnesses. Spirituality is the basis for

12-step programs to promote sobriety in persons with alcohol or substance dependence,[126] and is being evaluated as a tool to promote well-being of caregivers of persons with chronic physical and psychiatric illness.[127] It is, however, important to note that the subjective benefits of spiritual or religious engagement appear to be more consistently demonstrable across studies than objective benefits.

SUMMARY

In conclusion, it is clear that several major strides have been made in refining constructs related to positive psychological traits. Perhaps the most striking finding has been the suggestion that these traits may have an independent positive effect on health, especially in older adults. As psychiatry prepares to deal with the impending growth in the older population, a future research agenda in this area should include refining the definitions of these constructs to promote consensus on these domains and broadening our understanding of psychological and biological mechanisms that underlie these constructs. It is also imperative to devise and assess interventions aimed at promoting positive psychological traits. More immediately, psychiatric clinicians should dedicate time and effort to the identification of positive psychological traits in patients, especially older adults, and to incorporating means to reinforce these traits as part of ongoing psychiatric treatment.

REFERENCES

1. Epel ES, Blackburn EH, Lin J, et al. Accelerated telomere shortening in response to life stress. Proc Natl Acad Sci U S A 2004;101:17312–5.
2. Rowe JW, Kahn RL. Human aging: usual and successful. Science 1987;237:143–9.
3. Seligman ME, Csikszentmihalyi M. Positive psychology. An introduction. Am Psychol 2000;55:5–14.
4. Sheldon KM, King L. Why positive psychology is necessary. Am Psychol 2001;56:216–7.
5. Depp CA, Glatt SJ, Jeste DV. Recent advances in research on successful or healthy aging. Curr Psychiatry Rep 2007;9:7–13.
6. Depp CA, Jeste DV. Definitions and predictors of successful aging: a comprehensive review of larger quantitative studies. Am J Geriatr Psychiatry 2006;14:6–20.
7. Knight T, Ricciardelli LA. Successful aging: perceptions of adults aged between 70 and 101 years. Int J Aging Hum Dev 2003;56:223–45.
8. von Faber M, Bootsma-van der Wiel A, van Exel E, et al. Successful aging in the oldest old: who can be characterized as successfully aged? Arch Intern Med 2001;161:2694–700.
9. Reichstadt J, Depp CA, Palinkas LA, et al. Building blocks of successful aging: a focus group study of older adults' perceived contributors to successful aging. Am J Geriatr Psychiatry 2007;15:194–201.
10. Roberts BW, Walton KE, Viechtbauer W. Patterns of mean-level change in personality traits across the life course: a meta-analysis of longitudinal studies. Psychol Bull 2006;132:1–25.
11. Mroczek DK, Kolarz CM. The effect of age on positive and negative affect: a developmental perspective on happiness. J Pers Soc Psychol 1998;75:1333–49.
12. Miller SM, Sherman AC, Christensen AJ. Introduction to special series: the great debate–evaluating the health implications of positive psychology. Ann Behav Med 2010;39:1–3.

13. Coyne JC, Tennen H. Positive psychology in cancer care: bad science, exaggerated claims, and unproven medicine. Ann Behav Med 2010;39:16–26.
14. Rutter M. Implications of resilience concepts for scientific understanding. Ann N Y Acad Sci 2006;1094:1–12.
15. Baltes PB, Staudinger UM, Lindenberger U. Lifespan psychology: theory and application to intellectual functioning. Annu Rev Psychol 1999;50:471–507.
16. Schulz R, Heckhausen J. Aging, culture and control: Setting a new research agenda. J Gerontol B Psychol Sci Soc Sci 1999;54:P139–45.
17. Connor KM, Davidson JR. Development of a new resilience scale: the Connor-Davidson Resilience Scale (CD-RISC). Depress Anxiety 2003;18:76–82.
18. Campbell-Sills L, Stein MB. Psychometric analysis and refinement of the connor-davidson resilience scale (CD-RISC): validation of a 10-item measure of resilience. J Trauma Stress 2010;20:1019–28.
19. Vaishnavi S, Connor K, Davidson JRT. An abbreviated version of the Connor-Davidson Resilience Scale (CD-RISC), the CD-RISC2: psychometric properties and applications in psychopharmacological trials. Psychiatry Res 2007;152:293–7.
20. Lamond AJ, Depp CA, Allison M, et al. Measurement and predictors of resilience among community-dwelling older women. J Psychiatr Res 2008;43:148–54.
21. McEwen BS. Interacting mediators of allostasis and allostatic load: towards an understanding of resilience in aging. Metabolism 2003;52:10–6.
22. Tedeschi RG, Calhoun LG. The posttraumatic growth inventory: measuring the positive legacy of trauma. J Trauma Stress 1996;9:455–71.
23. Charney DS. Psychobiological mechanisms of resilience and vulnerability: implications for successful adaptation to extreme stress. Am J Psychiatry 2004;161:195–216.
24. Feder A, Nestler EJ, Charney DS. Psychobiology and molecular genetics of resilience. Nat Rev Neurosci 2009;10:446–57.
25. Seeman T, Glei D, Goldman N, et al. Social relationships and allostatic load in Taiwanese elderly and near elderly. Soc Sci Med 2004;59:2245–57.
26. Seeman T, Singer B, Ryff C, et al. Social relationships, gender, and allostatic load across two age cohorts. Psychosom Med 2002;64:395–406.
27. Ryff CD, Singer BH. Biopsychosocial challenges of the new millennium. Psychother Psychosom 2000;69:170–7.
28. Loucks EB, Berkman LF, Gruenwald TL, et al. Relation of social integration to inflammatory marker concentrations in men and women 70–79 years. Am J Cardiol 2006;97:1010–6.
29. Karel MJ. Aging and depression: vulnerability and stress across adulthood. Clin Psychol Rev 1997;17:847–79.
30. Carver CS, Scheier MF, Segerstrom SC. Optimism. Clin Psychol Rev 2010. [Epub ahead of print].
31. Scheier MF, Carver CS, Bridges MW. Distinguishing optimism from neuroticism (and trait anxiety, self-mastery, and self-esteem): a reevaluation of the life orientation test. J Pers Soc Psychol 1994;67:1063–78.
32. Schulman P, Castellon C, Seligman ME. Assessing explanatory style: the content analysis of verbatim explanations and the attributional style questionnaire. Behav Res Ther 1989;27:505–12.
33. Puri M, Robinson DT. Optimism and economic choice. J Financ Econ 2007. Available at SSRN: http://ssrn.com/abstract=1010023. Accessed April 30, 2010.
34. Gitlay EJ, Zitman FG, Kromhout D. Dispositional optimism and the risk of depressive symptoms during 15 years of follow-up: the Zutphen Elderly Study. J Affect Disord 2006;91:45–52.

35. Plomin R, Scheier MF, Bergeman CS, et al. Optimism, pessimism and mental health: a twin/adoption analysis. Pers Individ Dif 1992;13:921–30.
36. Chang EC, Maydeu-Olivares A, D'Zurilla TJ. Optimism and pessimism as partially independent constructs: relationship to positive and negative affectivity and psychological well-being. Pers Individ Dif 1997;23(3):433–40, 2010.
37. Segerstrom SC. Optimism and immunity: do positive thoughts always lead to positive effects? Brain Behav Immun 2005;19:195–200.
38. Rasmussen HN, Scheier MF, Greenhouse JB. Optimism and physical health: a meta-analytic review. Ann Behav Med 2009;37:239–56.
39. Giltay EJ, Geleijnse JM, Zitman FG, et al. Dispositional optimism and all-cause and cardiovascular mortality in a prospective cohort of elderly dutch men and women. Arch Gen Psychiatry 2004;61:1126–35.
40. Segerstrom SC, Sephton SE. Optimistic expectancies and cell-mediated immunity: the role of positive affect. Psychol Sci 2010;21:448–55.
41. Giltay EJ, Geleijnse JM, Zitman FG, et al. Lifestyle and dietary correlates of dispositional optimism in men: the Zutphen Elderly Study. J Psychosom Res 2007;63:483–90.
42. Skinner EA. A guide to constructs of control. J Pers Soc Psychol 1996;71: 549–70.
43. Thompson SC. Will it hurt less if i can control it? A complex answer to a simple question. Psychol Bull 1981;90:89–101.
44. Pearlin LI, Schooler C. The structure of coping. J Health Soc Behav 1978;19:2–21.
45. Bandura A. Self-efficacy: the exercise of control. New York: Freeman; 1997.
46. Bandura A. Social foundations of thought and action: a social cognitive theory. Englewood Cliffs (NJ): Prentice-Hall; 1986.
47. Berry JM, West RL. Cognitive self-efficacy in relation to personal mastery and goal setting across the life span. Int J Behav Dev 1993;16:351–79.
48. Rodin J, McAvay G. Determinants of change in perceived health in a longitudinal study of older adults. J Gerontol Psychol Sci 1992;47:P373–84.
49. Sherer M, Maddux JE, Mercadante B, et al. The self-efficacy scale: construction and validation. Psychol Rep 1982;51:663–71.
50. Mehta KM, Simonsick EM, Penninx BW, et al. Prevalence and correlates of anxiety symptoms in well-functioning older adults: findings from the health aging and body composition study. J Am Geriatr Soc 2003;51:499–504.
51. Pudrovska T, Schieman S, Pearlin LI, et al. The sense of mastery as a mediator and moderator in the association between economic hardship and health in late life. J Aging Health 2005;17:634–60.
52. Penninx BW, van Tilburg T, Kriegsman DM, et al. Effects of social support and personal coping resources on mortality in older age: the longitudinal aging study Amsterdam. Am J Epidemiol 1997;146:510–9.
53. Jonker AA, Comijs HC, Knipscheer KC, et al. The role of coping resources on change in well-being during persistent health decline. J Aging Health 2009; 21:1063–82.
54. Kostka T, Jachimowicz V. Relationship of quality of life to dispositional optimism, health locus of control and self-efficacy in older subjects living in different environments. Qual Life Res 2010;19:351–61.
55. Fry PS, Debats DL. Self-efficacy beliefs as predictors of loneliness and psychological distress in older adults. Int J Aging Hum Dev 2002;55:233–69.
56. Seeman T, Rodin J, Albert M. Self-efficacy and cognitive performance in high-functioning older individuals: MacArthur studies of successful aging. J Aging Health 1993;5:455–74.

57. Seeman T, McAvay G, Merrill S, et al. Self-efficacy beliefs and change in cognitive performance: MacArthur studies of successful aging. Psychol Aging 1996; 11:538–51.

58. McAuley E, Hall KS, Motl RW, et al. Trajectory of declines in physical activity in community-dwelling older women: social cognitive influences. J Gerontol B Psychol Sci Soc Sci 2009;64:543–50.

59. Penninx BW, Guralnik JM, Bandeen-Roche K, et al. The protective effect of emotional vitality on adverse health outcomes in disabled older women. J Am Geriatr Soc 2000;48:1359–66.

60. Ryff CD, Singer BH, Dienberg LG. Positive health: connecting well-being with biology. Philos Trans R Soc Lond B Biol Sci 2004;359:1383–94.

61. Mausbach BT, von Kanel R, Patterson TL, et al. The moderating effect of personal mastery and the relations between stress and plasminogen activator inhibitor-1 (PAI-1) antigen. Health Psychol 2008;27:S172–9.

62. Roepke SK, Mausbach BT, Aschbacher K, et al. Personal mastery is associated with reduced sympathetic arousal in stressed Alzheimer caregivers. Am J Geriatr Psychiatry 2008;16:310–7.

63. Mausbach BT, Patterson TL, von Kanel R, et al. The attenuating effect of personal mastery on the relations between stress and Alzheimer caregiver health: a five-year longitudinal analysis. Aging Ment Health 2007;11:637–44.

64. Ayotte BJ, Margrett JA, Hicks-Patrick J. Physical activity in middle-aged and young-old adults: the roles of self-efficacy, barriers, outcome expectancies, self-regulatory behaviors and social support. J Health Psychol 2010;15:173–85.

65. Dunton GF, Atienza AA, Castro CM, et al. Using ecological momentary assessment to examine antecedents and correlates of physical activity bouts in adults age 50+ years: a pilot study. Ann Behav Med 2009;38:249–55.

66. Kirk A, MacMillan F, Webster N. Application of the transtheoretical model to physical activity in older adults with type 2 diabetes and/or cardiovascular disease. Psychol Sport Exerc 2010;11:320–4.

67. Levy B, Langer E. Aging free from negative stereotypes: successful memory in China and among the deaf. J Pers Soc Psychol 1994;66:989–97.

68. Moor C, Zimprich D. Personality, aging self-perceptions, and subjective health: a mediation model. Int J Aging Hum Dev 2006;63:241–57.

69. Barrett A. Socioeconomic status and age identity: the role of dimensions of health in the subjective construction of age. J Gerontol B Psychol Sci Soc Sci 2003;58:S101–9.

70. Westerhof G, Barrett A. Age identity and subjective well-being: a comparison of the United States and Germany. J Gerontol B Psychol Sci Soc Sci 2005;60: S129–36.

71. Barker M, O'Hanlon A, McGee H, et al. Cross-sectional validation of the aging perceptions questionnaire: a multidimensional instrument for assessing self-perceptions of aging. BMC Geriatr 2007;7:9.

72. Sarkisian CA, Hays RD, Mangione CM. Do older adults expect to age successfully? The association between expectations regarding aging and beliefs regarding healthcare seeking among older adults. J Am Geriatr Soc 2002;50:1837–43.

73. Sarkisian C, Liu H, Ensrud K, et al. Correlates of attributing new disability to old age. J Am Geriatr Soc 2001;49:134–41.

74. Sarkisian CA, Steers WN, Hays RD, et al. Development of the 12-item expectations regarding aging survey. Gerontologist 2005;45:240–8.

75. Lawton MP. The Philadelphia geriatric center morale scale: a revision. J Gerontol 1975;30:85–9.

76. Levy BR. Mind matters: cognitive and physical effects of aging self-stereotypes. J Gerontol B Psychol Sci Soc Sci 2003;58:203–11.

77. Levy B. Improving memory in old age through implicit self-stereotyping. J Pers Soc Psychol 1996;71:1092–107.

78. Levy B, Hausdorff J, Hencke R, et al. Reducing cardiovascular stress with positive self-stereotypes of aging. J Gerontol B Psychol Sci 2000;55:205–13.

79. Levy B, Slade M, Gill T. Hearing decline predicted by elders' stereotypes. J Gerontol B Psychol Sci 2006;61:P82–7.

80. Levy B, Slade M, Kunkel S, et al. Longevity increased by positive self perceptions of aging. J Pers Soc Psychol 2002;83:261–70.

81. Uotinen V, Rantanen T, Suutama T. Perceived age as a predictor of old age mortality: a 13-year prospective study. Age Ageing 2005;34:368–72.

82. Rakowski W, Hickey T. Mortality and the attribution of health problems to aging among older adults. Am J Public Health 1992;82:1139–41.

83. Goodwin J, Black S, Satish S. Aging versus disease: the opinions of older black, hispanic, and non-hispanic white Americans about the causes and treatment of common medical conditions. J Am Geriatr Soc 1999;47:973–9.

84. Sarkisian CA, Shunkwiler SM, Aguilar I, et al. Ethnic differences in expectations for aging among older adults. J Am Geriatr Soc 2006;54:1277–82.

85. Harrison T, Blozis S, Stuifbergen A. Longitudinal predictors of attitudes toward own aging among women with multiple sclerosis. Psychol Aging 2008;23: 823–32.

86. Best D, Hamlett K, Davis S. Memory complaint and memory performance in the elderly: the effects of memory-skills training and expectancy. Appl Cogn Psychol 1992;6:405–16.

87. Gjorup T, Hendriksen C, Lund E, et al. Is growing old a disease? A study of the attitudes of elderly people to physical symptoms. J Chronic Dis 1987;40: 1095–8.

88. Locher JL, Burgio KL, Goode PS, et al. Effects of age and causal attribution to aging on health-related behaviors associated with urinary incontinence in older women. Gerontologist 2002;42:515–21.

89. Blazer DG. Religious beliefs, practices and mental health outcomes: what is the research question? Am J Geriatr Psychiatry 2007;15:269–72.

90. Fetzer Institute. Multidimensional measurement of religiousness/spirituality for use in health research. Bethesda (MD): Fetzer Institute, National Institute of Aging; 1999. p. 1–95.

91. Crowther M, Parker M, Achnebaum W, et al. Rowe and kahn's model of successful aging revisited: positive spirituality–the forgotten factor. Gerontologist 2002; 42:613–20.

92. Glass TA, de Leon CM, Marottoli RA, et al. Population based study of social and productive activities as predictors of survival among elderly Americans. BMJ 1999;319:478–83.

93. Ell K, Nishimoto R, Morvay T, et al. A longitudinal analysis of psychological adaptation among survivors of cancer. Cancer 1989;63:406–13.

94. Vahia IV, Depp CA, Palmer BW, et al: Correlates of spirituality in older women. Aging Ment Health 2010;Oct:1–6.

95. Koenig HG, George LK, Cohen HJ, et al. The relationship between religious activities and cigarette smoking in older adults. J Gerontol A Biol Sci Med Sci 1998;53:M426–34.

96. Van Ness PH, Kasl SV. Religion and cognitive dysfunction in an elderly cohort. J Gerontol B Psychol Sci Soc Sci 2003;58:S21–9.

97. Hill TD, Burdette AM, Angel JL, et al. Religious attendance and cognitive functioning among older Mexican Americans. J Gerontol B Psychol Sci Soc Sci 2006;61:3–9.
98. Reyes-Ortiz CA, Berges IM, Raji MA, et al. Church attendance mediates depressive symptoms and cognitive functioning among older Mexican Americans. J Gerontol A Biol Sci Med Sci 2008;63:480–6.
99. Blazer DG. Psychiatry and the oldest old. Am J Psychiatry 2000;157:1915–24.
100. Baltes PB, Smith J. The psychology of wisdom and its ontogenesis. In: Sternberg RJ, editor. Wisdom: its nature, origins and development. New York: Cambridge University Press; 1990.
101. Meeks TW, Jeste DV. Neurobiology of wisdom: a literature overview. Arch Gen Psychiatry 2009;66:355–65.
102. Jeste DV, Vahia I. Comparison of the conceptualization of wisdom in ancient Indian literature with modern views: focus on the Bhagavad Gita. Psychiatry 2008;71:197–209.
103. Clayton VP, Birren JE. The development of wisdom across the life-span: a reexamination of an ancient topic. In: Baltes PB, Brim OG, editors. Life-span development and behavior, vol. 3. New York: Academic Press; 1980. p. 103–35.
104. Ardelt M. Empirical assessment of a three-dimensional wisdom scale. Res Aging 2003;25:275–324.
105. Jeste DV, Ardelt M, Blazer D, et al. Expert consensus on the characteristics of wisdom: a Delphi method study. Gerontologist 2010;50(5):668–8.
106. Sternberg RJ, Jordan J. A handbook of wisdom: psychological perspectives. New York: Cambridge University Press; 2005.
107. Webster JD. An exploratory analysis of a self-assessed wisdom scale. J Adult Dev 2003;10:13–22.
108. Lai JC, Evans PD, Ng SH, et al. Optimism, positive affectivity, and salivary cortisol. Br J Health Psychol 2005;10:467–84.
109. Pressman SD, Cohen S. Does positive affect influence health? Psychol Bull 2005;131:925–71.
110. Steptoe A, Wright C, Kunz-Ebrecht SR, et al. Dispositional optimism and health behaviour in community-dwelling older people: associations with healthy ageing. Br J Health Psychol 2006;11:71–84.
111. Steptoe A, Wardle J. Positive affect and biological function in everyday life. Neurobiol Aging 2005;26(Suppl 1):108–12.
112. Steptoe A, Wardle J, Marmot M. Positive affect and health-related neuroendocrine, cardiovascular, and inflammatory processes. Proc Natl Acad Sci U S A 2005;102:6508–12.
113. Lupien SJ, Wan N. Successful aging: from cell to self. Phil Trans R Soc Lond 2004;359:1413–26.
114. Christakis NA, Fowler JH. The spread of obesity in a large social network over 32 years. N Engl J Med 2007;357:370–9.
115. Fowler JH, Christakis NA. Dynamic spread of happiness in a large social network: longitudinal analysis over 20 years in the Framingham Heart Study. BMJ 2008;337:a2338.
116. Stein MB, Campbell-Sills L, Gelernter J. Genetic variation in 5HTTLPR is associated with emotional resilience. Am J Med Genet B Neuropsychiatr Genet 2009;150:900–6.
117. Greenfield EA, Marks NF. Formal volunteering as a protective factor for older adults' psychological well-being. J Gerontol B Psychol Sci Soc Sci 2004;59:S258–64.

118. Fava GA, Tomba E. Increasing psychological well-being and resilience by psychotherapeutic methods. J Pers 2009;77:1903–34.
119. Fava GA, Rafanelli C, Cazzaro M, et al. Well-being therapy. A novel psychotherapeutic approach for residual symptoms of affective disorders. Psychol Med 1998;28:475–80.
120. Belaise C, Fava GA, Marks IM. Alternatives to debriefing and modifications to cognitive behavior therapy for posttraumatic stress disorder. Psychother Psychosom 2005;74:217.
121. Wagner B, Knaevelsrud C, Maercker A. Post-traumatic growth and optimism as outcomes of an internet-based intervention for complicated grief. Cogn Behav Ther 2007;36:156–61.
122. Koenig HG, Larson DB, Larson SS. Religion and coping with serious medical illness. Ann Pharmacother 2001;35:352–9.
123. Michael ST, Crowther MR, Schmid B, et al. Widowhood and spirituality: coping responses to bereavement. J Women Aging 2003;15:145–65.
124. Greenstreet W. From spirituality to coping strategy: making sense of chronic illness. Br J Nurs 2006;15:938–42.
125. Wachholtz AB, Pearce MJ, Koenig H. Exploring the relationship between spirituality, coping, and pain. J Behav Med 2007;30:311–8.
126. Brown AE, Pavlik VN, Shegog R, et al. Association of spirituality and sobriety during a behavioral spirituality intervention for Twelve Step (TS) recovery. Am J Drug Alcohol Abuse 2007;33:611–7.
127. Hebert RS, Weinstein E, Martire LM, et al. Religion, spirituality and the well-being of informal caregivers: a review, critique, and research prospectus. Aging Ment Health 2006;10:497–520.

Prevention in Psychiatry: Effects of Healthy Lifestyle on Cognition

David A. Merrill, MD, PhD*, Gary W. Small, MD

KEYWORDS

• Healthy lifestyle • Cognition • Longevity

People are living longer than ever. With greater longevity, a critical question becomes whether or not our memories endure across the life span. This article reviews the common forms of age-related memory change and the emerging evidence related to putative risk and protective factors for brain aging. With increasing awareness of Alzheimer disease (AD) and related dementias, patients, families, and clinicians are eager for concise and accurate information about the effects and limitations of preventative strategies related to lifestyle choices that may improve cognitive health.

DEMOGRAPHICS AND OVERVIEW OF AGING AND COGNITIVE HEALTH

We are living in an increasingly older world; the estimated 76 million Baby Boomers, born in the United States between 1946 and 1964, will begin entering the 65-years-plus age bracket in 2011. The increasing numbers of such Golden Boomers will soon result in people more than age 65 years outnumbering children less than age 5 years.[1] In addition to this generational dynamic, the past 150 years have seen a remarkably linear increase in life expectancy at birth, at a rate of roughly 3 months per year, every year, since 1840. During this time, life expectancy has increased from 45 years to 80 years. This increase was initially a result of decreases in infant mortality, better sanitation, and improved treatment of infectious diseases with antibiotics. More recently, we have seen a 50-year-long, worldwide trend of increased life expectancy after age 65 years.[1] Those reaching 65 years today can expect to live 16 to 20 years more, with women generally living 3 to 6 years longer than men. Overall, the number of people living beyond age 80 years will be higher than at any time in

Department of Psychiatry and Biobehavioral Sciences, Division of Geriatric Psychiatry, Memory & Aging Research Center, Semel Institute for Neuroscience & Human Behavior, David Geffen School of Medicine at the University of California, Los Angeles, 760 Westwood Plaza, Suite 38-231, Los Angeles, CA 90024-1759, USA
* Corresponding author.
E-mail address: dmerrill@mednet.ucla.edu

Psychiatr Clin N Am 34 (2011) 249–261
doi:10.1016/j.psc.2010.11.009
0193-953X/11/$ – see front matter © 2011 Elsevier Inc. All rights reserved.

recorded history. If the 160-year-long life expectancy trend continues, it will be only 6 decades until the average life span is 100 years.

Aging is associated with memory decline, with the degree of decline varying considerably among individuals. We know that some cognitive changes occur with normal aging. For example, beginning in midlife, processing speed declines and many people develop difficulty with spontaneous recall of facts and events, including names, although their recognition abilities remain intact.[2] Such mild objective changes and subjective reports of memory change have been classified as age-associated memory impairment, which affects approximately 40% of people aged 65 years or older but does not increase the risk of developing AD.[3] More prominent memory loss, as shown by significantly poor performance on one or more standardized cognitive tests (generally defined as scoring greater than one standard deviation less than average on age-controlled scales), but without functional impairment, affects approximately 10% of individuals aged 65 years or older and defines the diagnosis of mild cognitive impairment (MCI).[4] MCI can further be classified as primarily involving memory (amnestic), other cognitive domains (nonamnestic), or both (multiple domain). A diagnosis of MCI is considered a risk factor for AD, with approximately 15% of patients with MCI developing AD each subsequent year.

Once memory and other cognitive declines reach the threshold of causing significant impairment in daily function, a diagnosis of dementia is warranted.[5] Dementia is a syndrome of memory loss plus decline in one or more additional cognitive domains (including speech and language production or comprehension, object naming or recognition, execution of motor activities, abstraction, planning of complex tasks, and judgment). Declines must interfere with daily life, commonly causing difficulty initially with complex tasks, such as driving or managing finances, and later difficulties with more basic activities, such as bathing or dressing. AD is the most common cause of dementia, currently affecting 5.3 million people in the United States.[6] Less common causes of dementia include vascular dementia (VD), frontotemporal dementia (FTD), dementia with Lewy bodies, and Parkinson disease dementia. AD is currently the seventh leading cause of death, and the number of AD cases is expected to increase 50% over the next 2 decades to 7.7 million.[6] With a current annual cost of $172 billion, and the potential looming effect of a sharp increase in AD cases, it is remarkable that for every $25,000 on spent clinical care of patients with AD, only $100 is allocated for AD-related research. Thus, preventative strategies related to healthy lifestyle and cognition in aging offer the potential for a major public health effect.

A small number of early-onset (<65 years of age) familial AD cases (<5% of total AD cases) have been linked to specific genetic mutations involving increased production of pathological forms of β-amyloid protein, including mutations of presenilin 1, presenilin 2, and the amyloid precursor protein.[7] Although neither necessary nor sufficient to cause AD, the major known genetic risk factor for AD is the apolipoprotein E4 allele, which also may increase risk for VD.[8,9] Despite these known genetic associations with AD, the landmark MacArthur Study of Successful Aging found that for most people, genetics accounts for only about one-third of what contributes to successful aging, defined as both cognitive and physical health.[10] Thus, an entire range of environmental nongenetic factors, including lifestyle choices, combine and interact with an individual's genetics to determine how well that individual ages.

CLINICAL ASSESSMENT OF COGNITION IN AGING

Patients who come to clinicians requesting a memory evaluation can expect to start with a complete history and physical examination. A simple screening question asking about the patient's memory ability is often informative, as are queries regarding family history of dementia and personal history of medical illnesses that increase risk for dementia (eg, diabetes, Parkinson disease, stroke). A thorough inventory of prescription medications and over-the-counter medicines and supplements should be completed to eliminate the possibility of drug toxicity as a cause of memory loss. Brief cognitive screens, such as the Mini-Mental Status Examination or Montreal Cognitive Assessment, can be used initially to decide whether or not to order complete neuropsychological testing.[11,12] Laboratory studies (such as metabolic tests, complete blood counts, thyroid function tests, and vitamin B_{12} levels) can also reveal potentially reversible contributors to cognitive decline. A structural brain imaging study (computed tomography or magnetic resonance imaging [MRI]) is used to rule out occult mass lesions and may yield additional information about the extent of vascular damage and/or cerebral atrophy of memory-critical brain regions, such as the medial temporal lobe.[13] In diagnostically challenging cases, fluorodeoxyglucose (FDG)-positron emission tomography (PET) can differentiate between AD and FTD patterns of metabolism.[14] More recently developed PET ligands, such as 2-(1-{6-[(2-[^{18}F]fluoroethyl)(methyl)amino]-2-naphthyl}ethylidene)malononitrile, measure the load of plaque and tangle neuropathology in the living brain.[15] Such information has classically been used at autopsy to yield a definitive diagnosis of AD. Peripheral and cerebrospinal fluid biomarkers are also in development for clinical use, such as levels of amyloid-β protein or phosphorylated-τ protein.[16]

LIFESTYLE CHOICES AND BRAIN AGING

The National Institutes of Health recently funded an exhaustive review by the Agency for Healthcare Research and Quality, performed through its Evidence-Based Practice Centers, of the existent clinical literature on potential risk and protective factors related to the development of AD and cognitive decline.[17] The review included 25 systematic reviews and 250 primary research studies on various factors, subdivided into the following categories: nutritional factors, medical conditions and prescription and nonprescription medications, social/economic/behavioral factors, toxic environmental factors, and genetics. Only a few factors showed a consistent association with AD or cognitive decline across multiple observational studies and the available randomized controlled trials (RCTs). Factors associated with increased risk of AD and cognitive decline were diabetes, ε4 allele of the apolipoprotein E gene (APOE4), smoking, and depression. Factors consistently associated with a decreased risk of AD and cognitive decline were cognitive engagement and physical activity. The modification of risk for reported associations was typically small to moderate, and the currently available data were believed to be limited and generally of low strength. The overall conclusion of the review was that further research is necessary before definitive recommendations can be made regarding behavioral, lifestyle, and pharmaceutical interventions/modifications.

However, patients facing the possibility of age-related memory loss continue to request recommendations from clinicians regarding lifestyle choices and brain aging, leaving clinicians in the potentially difficult position of giving advice without a definitive evidence base. In general, patients can be educated about the current state of the field (ie, that the definitive studies are yet to be completed regarding the various putative risk and/or protective factors).

A challenge to the field is in confirming causal relationships. Although the epidemiological association studies are helpful in elucidating potential risks for and protections from dementia, prospective, RCTs are needed to verify whether a particular lifestyle choice truly has an effect on future brain health. Patients should be cautioned about spending large amounts of money on any commercial products claiming to preserve or improve memory function with aging. However, as reviewed later, this strategy should not prevent clinicians from communicating that several generally healthy lifestyle modifications can be adopted immediately; these changes often improve physical health, pose little to no risk or harm, and may end up significantly improving or preserving memory function with aging.

SMOKING

Cigarette smoking has been identified as the most important source of preventable morbidity and premature mortality in the United States, with smoking-related diseases causing an estimated 440,000 American deaths each year.[18] Meta-analysis of 10 prospective cohort studies on the potential link between smoking and dementia found an increased risk of dementia with continued smoking (summary relative risk 1.79; 95% confidence interval [CI] 1.43–2.23), whereas quitting smoking appeared to lessen risk toward the level of risk seen in those who had never smoked.[19] Although there is insufficient evidence to conclude how much smoking over what time period is necessary to increase risk of dementia, it seems that smoking increases risk for development of AD and cognitive decline.[17] The physical and psychological aspects of nicotine addiction curtail the initial success rates of smoking cessation efforts. Greater success is found with a combination of nicotine replacement, smoking cessation medications (bupropion or varenicline), and use of psychological treatments, such as cognitive behavioral therapy or government-sponsored quit programs (1-800-QUIT-NOW). Even with active intervention, initial quit rates are less than 50%, with increasing success observed with repeated attempts to quit.

DRINKING

The French Paradox of regular red wine consumption leading to low rates of heart disease, despite a high intake of dietary cholesterol and saturated fats, may hold true for brain health. Light to moderate alcohol consumption (defined as <3 to 4 drinks per night) has been associated with a decreased risk of dementia.[20,21] It is unclear whether this reflects selection effects in cohort studies commencing in late life, a protective effect of alcohol consumption throughout adulthood, or a specific benefit of alcohol in late life. It would be premature to recommend that all older adults drink wine regularly to prevent dementia. Nutritional deficits associated with severe alcoholism lead to dementia, and acute alcohol intoxication can lead to increased confusion and disinhibition, especially in persons already experiencing memory loss.

Midlife Vascular Conditions

What is good for heart health is likely good for brain health, with conditions such as hypertension, hyperlipidemia, diabetes, and obesity being implicated in studies examining risk of dementia.[22–25] The relationships may be complex, with health conditions present during earlier stages of midlife having a larger effect on brain function in old age. For example, whereas studies of obesity in late life have not found a consistent relationship to dementia, and have at times found that obesity in late life decreases relative risk of dementia, midlife obesity has been more consistently linked to an increased risk of dementia in old age.[26] This reversal in direction of the association of obesity with dementia risk in late life may relate to the physical changes seen in older adults headed toward disability.

Head Trauma

People with a history of head trauma with loss of consciousness for an hour or more have double the risk for developing AD later in life.[27] Further, a study comparing amateur soccer players with runners and swimmers (who were less likely to have had concussive head injuries) in their mid-20s found that more than 30% of soccer players had memory impairments, compared with less than 10% of the runners and swimmers.[28] Results of studies examining head injury and risk of dementia have been mixed; however, meta-analysis of 15 case-control studies found an excess history of head injury in those with AD.[29] Thus, avoiding head trauma seems to be a prudent strategy to maintain brain health throughout life. Clinicians can promote brain health by recommending use of seat belts while driving, wearing helmets during contact sports, and minimizing fall risks by fall proofing the home (eg, eliminating throw rugs, minimizing clutter, and optimizing lighting).

OCCUPATION

Complex occupations (intellectually demanding jobs or those involving coordinating tasks and working with people) have been associated with decreased risk of dementia, whereas more simple occupations have been implicated with increased risk.[30–32] Similar to the benefits observed with increased educational level, occupational attainment may reduce the risk of AD by enhancing an individual's cognitive reserve, which delays the onset of clinical signs of disease.

ENVIRONMENTAL EXPOSURES

There are limited data on environmental exposures and risk for AD and cognitive decline. One systematic review of case-control and cohort studies on the association between AD and occupational exposures found increased and statistically significant associations with pesticides.[33] For the remaining exposures studied, the evidence of association was less consistent (for solvents and electromagnetic fields) or absent (for lead and aluminum).

LIFESTYLE STRATEGIES FOR MAINTAINING BRAIN HEALTH
Maintaining Social Connections

Findings suggest that maintaining rich social connections may decrease risk of dementia, likely from the intellectual stimulation provided by social interactions. The Kungsholmen Project, a long-term population study in Sweden, showed over 6 years that continuing frequent (daily to weekly) engagement in mental, social, or productive activities during late life was related to a decreased incidence of dementia.[34] Furthermore, poor or limited social networks increased risk of dementia by 60% (95% CI 1.2–2.1) in this same Swedish population.[35] These findings parallel results from a sample of community-dwelling elderly adults in New Haven, Connecticut, which found that global social disengagement was a risk factor for developing cognitive impairment.[36] The MacArthur Study of Successful Aging found that staying in close contact with people and remaining involved in meaningful activities predicted successful aging.[10] Because a large component of the MacArthur Study definition for successful aging was cognitive function, such activities likely promote brain health as well. Level of social engagement has also been related to depression, which may itself be an independent risk factor for dementia.[37,38]

STRESS REDUCTION

Chronic stress negatively affects brain health and memory performance. Animal studies show that prolonged exposure to stress hormones has an adverse effect on the hippocampus, a brain region involved in learning and memory, leading to decreased brain plasticity.[39] Human studies of stress and cognition indicate that several days of exposure to the stress hormone cortisol impairs memory.[40] The deleterious effects of increased stress levels can be mitigated by other protective environmental factors. For example, a study of New York City traffic enforcement agents showed that increased levels of workplace support decrease stress levels, as measured by changes in blood pressure, especially during stressful periods.[41] Chronic stress can also contribute to depression and anxiety disorders, which often interfere with normal memory processing, particularly as people age. Taken together, these findings suggest that minimizing stress may have a beneficial effect on brain health.

Physical Activity

Increasing biological evidence supports the idea that physical activity promotes brain health through changes in brain structure and function. When laboratory animals exercise regularly they develop new neurons in the hippocampus, which then form functional connections with other brain cells.[42] Physical exercise may also increase cerebral blood flow, which in turn promotes nerve cell growth and expression of brain-derived neurotrophic factor, further enhancing brain plasticity.[43] Neuropsychological examinations of healthy adults ages 60 to 75 years found that involvement in an aerobic exercise program improved performance on mental tasks involved in frontal lobe function (monitoring, scheduling, planning, inhibition, and memory) when compared with a control group.[44] Aerobic fitness has also more recently been shown to relate to increased hippocampal volume and superior spatial memory in older adults.[45]

The current literature of cohort studies supports the conclusion that aerobic physical activities, particularly at high levels, are associated with lower risk of developing AD.[17] A meta-analysis of RCTs comparing aerobic physical activity programs with control interventions found that aerobic exercise is protective against loss of cognitive function in healthy older adults.[46] In particular, meta-analysis showed significant effects of physical activity on motor function, cognitive speed, and auditory and visual attention. In one such study, adults with subjective memory impairment but no dementia showed a modest improvement in cognition at 18-month follow-up after a 6-month program of increased physical activity.[47] Although such findings are promising, additional clinical interventional studies are needed to define the optimal preventive and therapeutic strategies for cognitive maintenance in terms of type, duration, and intensity of physical activity.

Healthy Diet

Greater adherence to a Mediterranean diet, especially when combined with higher levels of physical activity, has been shown to decrease risk of developing AD.[48] Rates of cognitive decline and conversion of patients from MCI to AD have also been shown to be decreased by a higher adherence to a Mediterranean diet.[49,50] Mediterranean diets typically include high amounts of fruits and vegetables, fish or shellfish twice weekly, olive oil or canola oil, nuts such as walnuts or pecans, moderate amounts of red wine, and plentiful herbs and spices as seasonings.

Such diets limit the amounts of added salt and animal fats found in red meats and butter; foods typically associated with increased risk for vascular disease. Furthermore, diets rich in carbohydrates with high glycemic indices (eg, pretzels, French fries) can increase the risk for diabetes and can lead to stroke disease and VD,[51] whereas dietary changes can reverse such effects. For example, the combination of weight loss, eating a healthy diet, and exercising regularly has been shown to reduce the risk of developing type 2 diabetes by more than 50%.[52]

Given the association of midlife obesity with increased risk of dementia,[26] a healthy brain diet should emphasize moderate caloric intake, with total daily amounts ranging from 2000 to 2500 kcal/d depending on total body mass and gender. Taken one step further, caloric restriction of roughly 30% has been shown repeatedly across species to increase longevity substantially, apparently through a reduction in both inflammation and oxidative stress.[53] Even without frank caloric restriction, dietary choices can be informed by the antioxidant potency of various foods as measured by nutrition scientists, with high antioxidant capacity foods potentially protecting brain health.[54] Examples of such foods include blueberries, strawberries, and green vegetables (eg, broccoli, spinach).

Omega-3 fatty acids figure prominently in Mediterranean diets, are found naturally in foods like fish and nuts, and have potential as protective factors for brain health. Currently available observational and clinical trial data support a role of omega-3 fatty acids in slowing cognitive decline in older adults without dementia.[55] Large clinical trials of extended duration with various dosages and formulations of supplements are needed to provide definitive answers regarding the potential of omega-3 fatty acids for the prevention or treatment of AD and related dementias.

Mental Challenge/Cognitive Training

Higher levels of education have been found to decrease the risk for developing AD and related dementias.[56] An increase in cognitive reserve that can postpone the clinical manifestations of dementia is the hypothesized mechanism of this effect.[57] In support of this hypothesis are animal studies showing that environmental enrichment (modeling an increased level of mental challenge) results in hippocampal neurogenesis, synaptogenesis, and enhanced neuronal plasticity within the brain.[58]

Beyond the effects of education, twin studies have found that higher midlife engagement in cognitively stimulating activities decreases dementia risk.[59,60] Prospective studies of late-life cognitive stimulation have also reported slowing of cognitive decline[61] and overall decreased risk of developing cognitive impairment[62] and dementia.[63] When compared with persons who spend time on more intellectually challenging tasks, the undemanding task of watching television has been shown to increase risk of cognitive decline over time.[64]

Observational and initial RCTs of cognitive training in normal aging have found a protective effect of such training on risk of cognitive decline.[17,65] One landmark study, the Advanced Cognitive Training for Independent and Vital Elderly (ACTIVE) study, reported sustained improvements in the cognitive areas trained (speed of processing, verbal memory, and reasoning compared with a no-contact control condition) at 2 years after the intervention.[66] Although the initial study failed to find transfer of skills to everyday function, later 5-year follow-up of the same group has shown that problem-solving training resulted in less functional decline.[67] More recent work has explored the possibility of training older adults individually using computer-based training. Taken together, cognitive training interventions in older adults show promise but, similar to the study of physical activity, the exact form, frequency, duration, and intensity of training interventions necessary for delaying or preventing cognitive decline and development of dementia remain an elusive target requiring further rigorous study.

Despite the lack of definitive proof of brain protection from mental stimulation, many clinicians encourage patients to explore their natural curiosity through cognitively active hobbies such as reading and writing, learning a new language or musical instrument, or completing crossword or Sudoku puzzles. Patients can challenge the brain by using their nondominant hand for otherwise routine daily tasks. Joining a book club or discussing current events with family and friends can help some people to combine the potentially synergistic benefits of cognitive stimulation and enriched social connections. However, it is important for people to realize that the evidence of the brain health benefits of these activities is not definitive. Moreover, patients should find the level of mental stimulation that is comfortably challenging, whether they have normal aging, MCI, or dementia.

For those asking for help with memory, basic principles for improving memory performance can be reviewed, learned from courses, books, or computer programs.[68] For example, we live in a distracting world. Teaching patients to stop multitasking while learning new things (ie, paying full undivided attention with all senses) can bolster the likelihood of retaining new information. We can also ask ourselves about the meaning of the new information and how it makes us feels. Combined use of associations and visual imagery can further enhance the learning process for tasks such as remembering new names. When introduced to a new person with the same name as a familiar person, one may imagine that person shaking hands with the familiar person, mentally linking the two. Patients can also be counseled about the usefulness of practical aids such as written lists or memory places or set locations for keys, wallets, and glasses. Such techniques can reduce frustration levels over otherwise normal memory lapses and help ward off related feelings of anxiety or depression.

Technology

Use of technology in promoting a cognitively healthy lifestyle holds both challenges and opportunities. One can imagine that the progressive invasion of electronic forms of communication into our daily lives, including cell phones, text messaging, and the Internet, could produce negative effects on brain function. However, recent research suggests that common computer tasks such as searching online may activate and strengthen neural networks.[69] Our group compared functional MRI measurements in middle-aged and older adults with previous Internet search experience with those who were naive to Internet searching, while they performed simulated Internet search or book-reading tasks. The reading task activated brain regions controlling language, reading, memory, and visual abilities, and both the magnitude and the extent of brain activation were similar in the Internet-naive and experienced groups. During the Internet search task, the naive group showed an activation pattern similar to that of their text reading task, whereas the experienced group showed significant increases in signal intensity in additional regions controlling decision making, complex reasoning, and vision. Internet searching was associated with a more than 2-fold increase in the extent of activation in the experienced group compared with the naive group, suggesting that previous experience with Internet searching may alter the responsiveness of the brain in neural circuits controlling decision making and complex reasoning.

Another potentially useful avenue for the marriage of technology and cognitive preservation is in brain training for both healthy older adults and those already experiencing MCI.[70] For example, in younger adults, experience with recreational video games has been shown to improve speed and skill of surgeons performing laparoscopic surgery, as measured by shorter surgery times and fewer surgical errors.[71] Personalized data assistance devices can also aid with memory capacity, as a readily accessible and potentially expansive peripheral brain for important dates like birthdays or anniversaries, allowing us greater freedom to pick and choose the items we commit to our biologically based memory systems.

Combining Healthy Lifestyle Strategies

Although the effect size of a particular lifestyle strategy is best determined when compared with a control condition, anecdotal evidence suggests that combining more than one approach may provide a synergy that enhances individual strategies. For example, an individual with anxiety about memory abilities might show greater benefits from memory training classes when combined with stress reduction exercises. Our group studied a 2-week combined healthy lifestyle program (diet plan along with relaxation, physical, and memory training exercises) on cognition and cerebral metabolism in people with mild age-related memory complaints.[72] Volunteers in the intervention group objectively showed greater word fluency, as well as a significant reduction in left dorsolateral prefrontal cortical glucose metabolism (measured with FDG-PET). Reduced resting activity in left dorsolateral prefrontal cortex may reflect greater cognitive efficiency of a brain region involved in working memory.

SUMMARY

Healthy lifestyle choices have numerous potential benefits that may prevent cognitive decline. Although definitive large-scale RCTs represent a major challenge for scientists in the coming years, clinicians in practice need not wait to encourage patients and their family members who come into the office to discuss such healthy lifestyle choices and guide them in practical approaches to integrating them into their daily lives. Considerable data already indicate that many of these factors improve cardiac and general health, in many cases increasing life expectancy significantly and augmenting quality of life. The potential for these same factors to improve and maintain cognitive performance is another reason to promote healthy lifestyle choices with patients who otherwise face a constant barrage of motivators generated by the mass media to remain sedentary, understimulated, and overly indulgent. Although the exact components and amounts of activities necessary to enhance brain health and induce positive cognitive effects remain unanswered questions, healthy lifestyle factors on aggregate hold many potential benefits that outweigh the minimal risks involved in their adoption, especially when applied in combination in an enjoyable and consistent manner.

REFERENCES

1. Kinsella K, He W. US Census Bureau, international population reports, P95/09-1. An aging world: 2008. Washington, DC: USGP Office, 2009.
2. Christensen H. What cognitive changes can be expected with normal ageing? Aust N Z J Psychiatry 2001;35:768.
3. Larrabee GJ, Crook TH 3rd. Estimated prevalence of age-associated memory impairment derived from standardized tests of memory function. Int Psychogeriatr 1994;6:95.
4. Petersen RC, Smith GE, Waring SC, et al. Mild cognitive impairment: clinical characterization and outcome. Arch Neurol 1999;56:303.
5. Small GW, Rabins PV, Barry PP, et al. Diagnosis and treatment of Alzheimer disease and related disorders. Consensus statement of the American Association

for Geriatric Psychiatry, the Alzheimer's Association, and the American Geriatrics Society. JAMA 1997;278:1363.

6. Alzheimer's Association. 2010 Alzheimer's disease facts and figures. Alzheimers Dement 2010;6:158.

7. Hsiung GY, Sadovnick AD. Genetics and dementia: risk factors, diagnosis, and management. Alzheimers Dement 2007;3:418.

8. Li H, Wetten S, Li L, et al. Candidate single-nucleotide polymorphisms from a genomewide association study of Alzheimer disease. Arch Neurol 2008;65:45.

9. Slooter AJ, Cruts M, Hofman A, et al. The impact of APOE on myocardial infarction, stroke, and dementia: the Rotterdam Study. Neurology 2004;62:1196.

10. Kahn RL. Successful aging. New York: Pantheon; 1998.

11. Folstein MF, Folstein SE, McHugh PR. "Mini-mental state". A practical method for grading the cognitive state of patients for the clinician. J Psychiatr Res 1975; 12:189.

12. Nasreddine ZS, Phillips NA, Bedirian V, et al. The Montreal Cognitive Assessment, MoCA: a brief screening tool for mild cognitive impairment. J Am Geriatr Soc 2005;53:695.

13. Frisoni GB, Fox NC, Jack CR Jr, et al. The clinical use of structural MRI in Alzheimer disease. Nat Rev Neurol 2010;6:67.

14. Silverman DH, Small GW, Chang CY, et al. Positron emission tomography in evaluation of dementia: regional brain metabolism and long-term outcome. JAMA 2001;286:2120.

15. Small GW, Kepe V, Ercoli LM, et al. PET of brain amyloid and tau in mild cognitive impairment. N Engl J Med 2006;355:2652.

16. Blennow K, Hampel H, Weiner M, et al. Cerebrospinal fluid and plasma biomarkers in Alzheimer disease. Nat Rev Neurol 2010;6:131.

17. Williams JW, Plassman BL, Burke J, et al. Preventing Alzheimer's Disease and cognitive decline. Evidence Report/Technology Assessment No. 193. (Prepared by the Duke Evidence-based Practice Center under Contract No. HHSA 290-2007-10066-I.) AHRQ Publication No. 10-E005. Rockville (MD): Agency for Healthcare Research and Quality; 2010.

18. National Institutes of Health NCI. Smoking facts and tips for quitting. Bethesda (MD): National Institutes of Health; 2010.

19. Anstey KJ, von Sanden C, Salim A, et al. Smoking as a risk factor for dementia and cognitive decline: a meta-analysis of prospective studies. Am J Epidemiol 2007;166:367.

20. Anstey KJ, Mack HA, Cherbuin N. Alcohol consumption as a risk factor for dementia and cognitive decline: meta-analysis of prospective studies. Am J Geriatr Psychiatry 2009;17:542.

21. Orgogozo JM, Dartigues JF, Lafont S, et al. Wine consumption and dementia in the elderly: a prospective community study in the Bordeaux area. Rev Neurol (Paris) 1997;153:185.

22. Anstey KJ, Lipnicki DM, Low LF. Cholesterol as a risk factor for dementia and cognitive decline: a systematic review of prospective studies with meta-analysis. Am J Geriatr Psychiatry 2008;16:343.

23. Beydoun MA, Beydoun HA, Wang Y. Obesity and central obesity as risk factors for incident dementia and its subtypes: a systematic review and meta-analysis. Obes Rev 2008;9:204.

24. Lu FP, Lin KP, Kuo HK. Diabetes and the risk of multi-system aging phenotypes: a systematic review and meta-analysis. PLoS One 2009;4:e4144.

25. McGuinness B, Todd S, Passmore P, et al. The effects of blood pressure lowering on development of cognitive impairment and dementia in patients without apparent prior cerebrovascular disease. Cochrane Database Syst Rev 2006; 2:CD004034.
26. Fitzpatrick AL, Kuller LH, Lopez OL, et al. Midlife and late-life obesity and the risk of dementia: cardiovascular health study. Arch Neurol 2009;66:336.
27. Mayeux R. Gene-environment interaction in late-onset Alzheimer disease: the role of apolipoprotein-epsilon4. Alzheimer Dis Assoc Disord 1998;12(Suppl 3):S10.
28. Matser EJ, Kessels AG, Lezak MD, et al. Neuropsychological impairment in amateur soccer players. JAMA 1999;282:971.
29. Fleminger S, Oliver DL, Lovestone S, et al. Head injury as a risk factor for Alzheimer's disease: the evidence 10 years on; a partial replication. J Neurol Neurosurg Psychiatr 2003;74:857.
30. Helmer C, Letenneur L, Rouch I, et al. Occupation during life and risk of dementia in French elderly community residents. J Neurol Neurosurg Psychiatr 2001; 71:303.
31. Jorm AF, Rodgers B, Henderson AS, et al. Occupation type as a predictor of cognitive decline and dementia in old age. Age Ageing 1998;27:477.
32. Stern Y, Gurland B, Tatemichi TK, et al. Influence of education and occupation on the incidence of Alzheimer's disease. JAMA 1994;271:1004.
33. Santibanez M, Bolumar F, Garcia AM. Occupational risk factors in Alzheimer's disease: a review assessing the quality of published epidemiological studies. Occup Environ Med 2007;64:723.
34. Wang HX, Karp A, Winblad B, et al. Late-life engagement in social and leisure activities is associated with a decreased risk of dementia: a longitudinal study from the Kungsholmen Project. Am J Epidemiol 2002;155:1081.
35. Fratiglioni L, Wang HX, Ericsson K, et al. Influence of social network on occurrence of dementia: a community-based longitudinal study. Lancet 2000;355: 1315.
36. Bassuk SS, Glass TA, Berkman LF. Social disengagement and incident cognitive decline in community-dwelling elderly persons. Ann Intern Med 1999;131:165.
37. Glass TA, De Leon CF, Bassuk SS, et al. Social engagement and depressive symptoms in late life: longitudinal findings. J Aging Health 2006;18:604.
38. Ownby RL, Crocco E, Acevedo A, et al. Depression and risk for Alzheimer disease: systematic review, meta-analysis, and metaregression analysis. Arch Gen Psychiatry 2006;63:530.
39. Sapolsky RM. Glucocorticoids, stress, and their adverse neurological effects: relevance to aging. Exp Gerontol 1999;34:721.
40. Newcomer JW, Selke G, Melson AK, et al. Decreased memory performance in healthy humans induced by stress-level cortisol treatment. Arch Gen Psychiatry 1999;56:527.
41. Karlin WA, Brondolo E, Schwartz J. Workplace social support and ambulatory cardiovascular activity in New York City traffic agents. Psychosom Med 2003; 65:167.
42. Gage FH. Neurogenesis in the adult brain. J Neurosci 2002;22:612.
43. Rolland Y, Abellan van Kan G, Vellas B. Physical activity and Alzheimer's disease: from prevention to therapeutic perspectives. J Am Med Dir Assoc 2008;9:390.
44. Kramer AF, Hahn S, Cohen NJ, et al. Ageing, fitness and neurocognitive function. Nature 1999;400:418.
45. Erickson KI, Prakash RS, Voss MW, et al. Aerobic fitness is associated with hippocampal volume in elderly humans. Hippocampus 2009;19:1030.

46. Angevaren M, Aufdemkampe G, Verhaar HJ, et al. Physical activity and enhanced fitness to improve cognitive function in older people without known cognitive impairment. Cochrane Database Syst Rev 2008;3:CD005381.
47. Lautenschlager NT, Cox KL, Flicker L, et al. Effect of physical activity on cognitive function in older adults at risk for Alzheimer disease: a randomized trial. JAMA 2008;300:1027.
48. Scarmeas N, Luchsinger JA, Schupf N, et al. Physical activity, diet, and risk of Alzheimer disease. JAMA 2009;302:627.
49. Feart C, Samieri C, Rondeau V, et al. Adherence to a Mediterranean diet, cognitive decline, and risk of dementia. JAMA 2009;302:638.
50. Scarmeas N, Stern Y, Mayeux R, et al. Mediterranean diet and mild cognitive impairment. Arch Neurol 2009;66:216.
51. Brand-Miller J, Volwever TM, Colaguiri S, et al. The glucose revolution. New York: Marlow; 1999.
52. Eriksson J, Lindstrom J, Tuomilehto J. Potential for the prevention of type 2 diabetes. Br Med Bull 2001;60:183.
53. Holloszy JO, Fontana L. Caloric restriction in humans. Exp Gerontol 2007;42:709.
54. Joseph JA. The color code: a revolutionary eating plan for optimal health. New York: Hyperion; 2002.
55. Fotuhi M, Mohassel P, Yaffe K. Fish consumption, long-chain omega-3 fatty acids and risk of cognitive decline or Alzheimer disease: a complex association. Nat Clin Pract Neurol 2009;5:140.
56. Caamano-Isorna F, Corral M, Montes-Martinez A, et al. Education and dementia: a meta-analytic study. Neuroepidemiology 2006;26:226.
57. Ngandu T, von Strauss E, Helkala EL, et al. Education and dementia: what lies behind the association? Neurology 2007;69:1442.
58. van Praag H, Kempermann G, Gage FH. Neural consequences of environmental enrichment. Nat Rev Neurosci 2000;1:191.
59. Carlson MC, Helms MJ, Steffens DC, et al. Midlife activity predicts risk of dementia in older male twin pairs. Alzheimers Dement 2008;4:324.
60. Crowe M, Andel R, Pedersen NL, et al. Does participation in leisure activities lead to reduced risk of Alzheimer's disease? A prospective study of Swedish twins. J Gerontol B Psychol Sci Soc Sci 2003;58:P249.
61. Wilson RS, Bennett DA, Bienias JL, et al. Cognitive activity and cognitive decline in a biracial community population. Neurology 2003;61:812.
62. Verghese J, LeValley A, Derby C, et al. Leisure activities and the risk of amnestic mild cognitive impairment in the elderly. Neurology 2006;66:821.
63. Wilson RS, Scherr PA, Schneider JA, et al. Relation of cognitive activity to risk of developing Alzheimer disease. Neurology 1911;69:2007.
64. Wang JY, Zhou DH, Li J, et al. Leisure activity and risk of cognitive impairment: the Chongqing aging study. Neurology 2006;66:911.
65. Acevedo A, Loewenstein DA. Nonpharmacological cognitive interventions in aging and dementia. J Geriatr Psychiatry Neurol 2007;20:239.
66. Ball K, Berch DB, Helmers KF, et al. Effects of cognitive training interventions with older adults: a randomized controlled trial. JAMA 2002;288:2271.
67. Willis SL, Tennstedt SL, Marsiske M, et al. Long-term effects of cognitive training on everyday functional outcomes in older adults. JAMA 2006;296:2805.
68. Small GW. The memory bible: an innovative strategy for keeping the brain young. London: Penguin Press; 2002.
69. Small GW, Moody TD, Siddarth P, et al. Your brain on Google: patterns of cerebral activation during internet searching. Am J Geriatr Psychiatry 2009;17:116.

70. Faucounau V, Wu YH, Boulay M, et al. Cognitive intervention programmes on patients affected by Mild Cognitive Impairment: a promising intervention tool for MCI? J Nutr Health Aging 2010;14:31.
71. Rosser JC Jr, Lynch PJ, Cuddihy L, et al. The impact of video games on training surgeons in the 21st century. Arch Surg 2007;142:181.
72. Small GW, Silverman DH, Siddarth P, et al. Effects of a 14-day healthy longevity lifestyle program on cognition and brain function. Am J Geriatr Psychiatry 2006; 14:538.

Index

Note: Page numbers of article titles are in **boldface** type.

A

Acetylcholinesterase inhibitors, in AD, 131
Adolescent depression, **35–52**. See also *Youth homicide.*
  epidemiology of, 35–36
  Internet-based behavioral vaccine for, 171–172
  intervention in, timing of, 38–39
  orevention research in, future directions for, 46–47
  prevention, defined in, 39
  prevention research in, conceptual framewok for, 36–37
    for resilience and protective factors, 38
    for risk factors, 37–38
  review of prevention efforts for, indicated programs in, 45–46
    selective programs, 41–45
    universal programs, 39–41
Adolescents. See also *Youth homicide.*
Aging, cognition in, clinical assessment of, 250–251
    demographics and overview of, 249–250
    familial AD and, 250
    memory decline and dementia, 250
  of brain, drinking and, 252
    environmental exposures and, 253
    head trauma and, 253
    lifestyle choices and, 251–252
    midlife vascular conditions and, 252
    occupation and, 253
    risk factors for, 251
    smoking and, 252
Alzheimer disease (AD). See also *Dementia.*
  characterization of, 127
  cognitive impairment in, mild, 128, 130
    vascular, 128
  incidence of, 129
  National Institutes of Health State-of-the-Science conference and report on, 136–137
  prevalence of, 128–129
  prodromal phase, 128
  reduction of risk for, cognitive training and, 134
    intellectual activities in, 133–134
    Mediterranean Diet in, 134–135
    physical activity in, 132–133
    social networks in, 135
Antidepressant medication, for postpartum depression, 55–56

Psychiatr Clin N Am 34 (2011) 263–274
doi:10.1016/S0193-953X(11)00011-6
0193-953X/11/$ – see front matter © 2011 Elsevier Inc. All rights reserved.

psych.theclinics.com

Antipsychotic medications, metabolic syndrome prevention, antipsychotic choice in, 114
   switching antipsychotics in, 115
   weight gain with, in children and youth, 114

B

Behavioral vaccines, for mental, emotional, and behavioral disorders, **1–34**
   nonpharmaceutical approaches, **1–34**
Bipolar disorder, life expectancy in, 109
Blood pressure, body weight and, 112
Brain, aging of, drinking and, 252
      environmental exposures, 253
      head trauma and, 253
      lifestyle choices and, 251–252
      midlife vascular conditions and, 252
      occupation, 253
      smoking and, 252
   aging of, lifestyle choices and, 251–252
   lifestyle strategies for health of, combining, 257
      healthy diet, 254–255
      mental challenge/cognitive training, 255–256
      physical activity, 254
      promotion through technology, 256–257
      social connections, 253
      stress reduction, 253
Brief delay intervention, for PTSD, memory structuring, 83
      prolonged exposure therapy, 83
      stepped collaborative care, 84
      trauma-focused cognitive behavior therapy, 84

C

Childhood, depression in, epidemiology of, 35–36
Child parent psychotherapy (CPP), for children in foster care, 192
Children, protective factors for, **185–203**
Children in foster care, infusing protective factors for, **185–203**. See also *Illinois Department of Children and Family Services (DCFS)*.
Circadian rhythm improvement, for postpartum depression, 58–59
Cognition, healthy lifestyle effects on, **249–261**
Cognitive decline, National Institutes of Health State-of-the-Science conference and report on, 136–137
Cognitive training, for increase in brain reserve in later life, 134
Cortisol, for PTSD prevention following trauma, 87–88
Critical incident stress debriefing (CISD), for PTSD, 82

D

Dementia, **127–145**. See also *Alzheimer disease (AD)*.
   categories of, 127
   frontotemporal lobar, 128
   incidence of, 128–129

Parkinson's disease, 128, 130
pharmacological approaches in, acetylcholinesterase inhibitors, 141
    N-methyl-D-aspartate antagonists, 131
    vitamins, 131–132
prevalence of, 128–131
prevention of, biomarkers in, 129–130
    primary, public health, 129
    secondary, symptom reduction or progression, 129, 130
    tertiary, treatment to halt progression, 129
    timing of strategy for, 120
with Lewy bodies, 128
Dementia prevention, cognitive reserve and, 133–134
cognitive training for, 134
intellectual activities for, 133–134
Mediterranean diet for, 134–135
meta-analysis of evidence on cognitive decline and AD, 135–136
physical activity for, 132–133
social networks for, 135
Depression, behavioral vaccine model and, 168–169
    components of, 169–170
in adolescence. See *Adolescent depression.*
in later life. See *Older adults.*
Institute of Medicine and prevention, 168–169
Internet-based prevention of, **167–183**
life-course schedule for Internet-based behavioral vaccine, in adolescence and
    emerging adulthood, 171–172
    interventions for mothers, infants, and children, 170–171
    middle adult, 172–173
    older adult, 173
major depression, significance of, 168
prevention research in, conceptual framework for, 36–37
preventive interventions, need for, 168
technology approach to prevention of, 168
Diabetes mellitus, type 2, pharmacologic prevention of, 116–117
prevention of, 116

E

Evidence-based kernels, in public health prevention, 9–10
Evidence-based treatments, 10–11, 36
Exercise, in aging, 133

F

Family-based prevention program, for adolescents, 42–45
    clinician-facilitated intervention, 43–44
    cognitive behavioral, 43
    Family Bereavement Program, 44–45
    New Beginnings Program, 44
    public health interventions for families, 43
First episode of psychosis, duration of untreated, 96–97
    prior biological and psychosocial deficit processes in, 95–96

G

Genetics, definition of, 148
  gene-environment interaction, treatment of depression and, 155
  history of, 148–150
  in disease prevention and treatment, 153–158
    gene-environment interaction and, 155
  inheritance in, 149
  linkage studies of hereditary cancers, for screening, risk counseling and preventive
      treatment, 155–156
  predictive testing for disease, 155–156
  susceptibility testing for disease, 156
Genome-wide association study (GWAS), 149–150
  genetics, genomics and, 150–151
    sequencing for missing heritability, 152
  missing heritability and, in neuropsychiatric disorders, 151–152
  variation in DNA sequencing in, 151
Genomics, definition of, 148
  for treatment and prevention, **147–166**
  genome-wide association studies and, 149–152
  hereitability of major chronic diseases, 150
  history of, 148–150
  Human Genome Project, 149
  International HapMap Project, 149
    susceptibility variants in, 149
  origin of term, 149
  personal/consumer testing, 156–157
    implications of, 157
  pharmacogenomics and treatment response, 153–155
  public health, 160–161
  social, economic, and policy issues for, insurance companies and, 158–159
    pharmaceutical and biotechnology companies and, 158
    physicians and legislation, 159–160
Genomics biomarkers, in clinical care, 157
  in diagnosis, prognosis and, monitoring, 157–158

H

Healthy diet, for brain health, 254
  Mediterranean Diet, 134–135
Healthy lifestyle, cognition and, **249–261**. See also *Aging.*
High blood pressure, antihypertensive therapy for, 118
HIV infection, prevention programs for, CHAMP (Chicago HIV Prevention and Adolescent
    Mental Health Project), 225–226
    Familias Unidas (United Families), 224–225
    Keepin' it R.E.A.L., 224
    PATH (Parent-Preadolescent Training for HIV Prevention), 223–224
    SAAF Program (Strong African American Families Program), 224
  protective factors for, developing social and emotional skills, 221
    improving self-esteem, 221
    minimizing the effects of trauma, 223

providing access to ancient and modern technology, 220–221
rebuilding the village, 220
reestablishing the adult protective shield, 222–223
social connectedness, 221
risk factors for, community and context, 218–220
environmental, 219–220
family, 218
individual, 218
Homicide, youth. See *Youth homicide.*
Hyperlipidemia, adjunctive therapy for, 117–118
pharmacollogic treatment of, 117

I

Illinois Department of Children and Family Services (DCFS)
evidence-based treatments in, adaptation to local setting, 191–194
caseworkers and foster parents and, 193
child parent psychotherapy, 192
evaluation of, 192
psychological first aid, 193–194
trauma-focused cognitive-behavioral therapy, 192
future directions and, risky behavior trajectory in, 200–201
incorporating protective factors into prevention, 194–198
National Research Council, developmental framework in prevention recommendations,
200–201
protective factors, assumption of normal development and, 199–200
lessons learned regarding, 198–199
limitations, 198–199
research link between trauma, risk behaviors, and protective factors, 186–194
Strethening Families Through Early Care and Education strategy and, 194–195
Strengthening Families Illinois, addressing problems, 197
final model, 197–198
identification of relevant protective factors, 197–198
identifying specific problems in trauma treatment, 196–197
integration of protective factors with trauma-informed practices, 196–198
logic model in, 195–196
trauma, strengths, and risk behaviors and, prior to residential treatment, 188–191
while in residential treatment, 190–191
trauma-informed programs in, Child and Adolescent Needs and Strengths assessment
tool in, 187
level of care by strengths, 187–188
phases of, 186–187
strengths equivalence with protective factors, 187
Indicated prevention, defined, 39
evidence-based kernels in, 10–11, 450
in psychosis, 97, 102–103
in public health prevention, 10–11
in schizophrenia, 100
Internet-based programs for, 45
Indicated prevention programs, for adolescents, 45–46
for older adults, 69–71

Institute of Medicine (IOM), *Preventing Mental Disorders,* 36
Intellectual activities, for reduction of risk for cognitive decline or AD, 133–134
Internet, in adolescent depression prevention, 45
    research for older adults, 72
Internet-based behavioral vaccine, adolescent and emerging adulthood studies, CATCH-IT, 171–172
    MoodGym, 171
    problem-solving therapy, 171
    effectiveness of, comparable, 173–174
        duration of benefits and, 174
        moderators and mediators of, 174
        sociocultural relevance and, 174–175
    for mothers, infants, and children, Legend of the Snow Orchid site, 171
        Mothers and Babies Internet Project, 170–171
        Pennsylvania Optimism Study program, 171
    implementation of, delivery in, context of, 177
            mechanisms of, 176
        safety in, 177
    lifecourse schedule for, 170–173
    middle adult, Beating the Blues, 173
        BluePages, 172
        Color Your Life Cycle, 172
        Mood/Gym, 172
    motivational framework for, adherence and completion, 176
        peer-to-peer support, 175–176
        professional guidance, 175
    older adult, cognitive behavioral therapy, 173

L

Later life, depression in, **67–78**
Lifespan, Internet-based depression prevention, **167–183**
    Internet-based depression prevention over, **167–183**
    psychological protective factors across, **231–248**
Lifestyle intervention, for weight loss, in schizophrenia, 112–113
Lifestyle management, for brain health, 253–257
    in metabolic syndrome, for high blood pressure, 118
        for weight control, 111–113

M

Mediterranean Diet, cognitive decline of AD and, 134–135
Mental, emotional, and behavioral (MBE) disorders, behavioral vaccines for, **1–34**
    public health, consumer-focused approach to prevention of, common features of
        examples, 7–8
        evidence for, 5–8
        examples of, 6–7
        school-based violence prevention, 7
    public health approach to prevention of, consumer prevention product logic in, 4–5
        cost effectiveness and prevalence reduction with, 4–8
        cost offsetting consequences in, 5

parameters of, 3–4
rationale for, 2
vs. rationing of care, 3
Metabolic syndrome, abnormalities in, 110
criteria for, 110
inflammation in, 115
in schizophrenia, 111
in serious mental illness, **109–125**
integrated vs. nonintegrated care in, 119
integration of psychiatric and medical care in, 118–119
medical case management for, 119
lifestyle management in, for high blood pressure, 118
for weight control, 111–113
metabolic monitoring in, consensus guidelines for, 115–116
risk reduction in, antipsychotic choice for, 114
screening tools for, 110
secondary prevention of, switching antipsychotics for, 115
treatment of components of, hyperglycemia and type 2 diabetes mellitus, 116–117
hyperlipidemia, 117–118
hypertension, 118
LDL-C and triglyceride levels, 118
Metformin, in type-2 diabetes, 117
weight loss with, 112

N

N-methyl-d-aspartate antagonists, in AD, 131
Nutrition, for postpartum depression, 57

O

Obesity. See also *Weight.*
metabolic syndrome and, 111
Older adults, depression prevention in, cost of, 71
feasibility of, 71–72
future research for, 72–76
strategies for, 72–73
in adults on low income, 69
interventions for, promising, 73–74
measurement domains for, 74
methodologic challenges in, 75–76
objectives of, 70–71
of medical and psychosocial complications, 69–70
of recurrent episodes, 70
personalization of strategies in, 74, 76
protection from suicide in, 71–72
public health context and rationale for, 68–69
rationale for selective and indicated, 69
research needs for, efficacy trials, 72
improving rate of participation in primary care facilities, 72
Internet as opportunity in, 72

Older adults (*continued*)
     pathophysiological models, 72
    risk factors in, 69
    to protect health and life spans, 68
Opiates, for PTSD prevention, 85–86
Optimism, as protective factor, 234–235
  Pennnsylvania Optimism Program, 171

P

Pharmacogenomics, definition of, 153
  in psychiatry, 154
  pharmacogenomic medication, FDA label updates for, 153–154
  treatment response and, warfarin, 153
Physical activity, for brain health, 254
  for postpartum depression, 57–58
  for reduction of cognitive decline and AD, 132–133
Postpartum depression, **53–65**
  factors in, 53
  Mothers and Babies Internet Project for, 170
  prevention strategies, 55
  prevention strategies for, antidepressant medication, 55–56
    breastfeeding support, 59
    family planning, 59–60
    nutrition, 57
    physical activity, 57–58
    psychotherapy, 56
    sleep and circadian rhythm improvement, 58–59
    social support, 56–57
  protective factors for, 55
  risk assessment for, clinical, 54–55
    formal tools in, 60
    for secondary and tertiary prevention, 55
  risk factors and prevention interventions for, 60
Posttraumatic stress disorder (PTSD), **79–94**
  description of, 79–80
  future directions in, nightmare prevention strategies, 89–90
    psychological first aid, 88–89
    stepped clinical care, 88
  pharmacologic approaches to, α-1 adrenoreceptor agonists, 86
    cortisol administration following trauma, 87–88
    issues to consider in, 88
    opiate administration, 86–87
    propranolol, 85–86
    SSRIs, 88
  pretrauma interventions, for individuals at risk, 89
  psychosocial interventions for, brief delay, multiple session, 82–84
    comparison of, 83
    cost factor in, 84
    critical incident stress debriefing, 82
    debriefing, immediate, single-session, 82–84

timing of, 84
variables in, 81
theoretical perspectives on, cognitive dissonance in, 81
dual representation theory, 80
fear conditioning in, 81
stress hormone release and, 80–81
Propranolol, for PTSD prevention, 85–86
pilot studies of, 85–86
prophylactic use of, 85
Protective factors, for adolescent depression, 38
for children in foster care, **185–203**
for HIV infection, 220–223
for postpartum depression, 55
for youth homicide, 208–210
psychological. See *Psychological protective factors.*
Psychiatry, healthy lifestyle and cognition in, **249–261**
Psychological first aid (PFA), adaptation to child welfare, 193
for children in foster care, 193–194
for posttraumatic stress disorder, 88–89
for PTSD, 88–89
for workers, 193–194
Illinois Department of Children and Family Services, for children in foster care, 193–194
Psychological protective factors, across lifespan, **231–248**
future research, in enhancement of protective factors, 241
in mechanisms of protective factors, 240–241
in spirituality/religiosity, 241–242
future research in, 240–242
optimism, 234–235
personal control/mastery/self-efficacy, 235–236
positive attitudes toward own aging, 236–237
resilience, 232–234
spirituality/religion, 237–238
wisdom, 238–239
Psychosis. See also *Schizophrenia.*
alternative interventions, direct practice of neural substrate of cognition, 104
naturalistic study, 103–104
first episode, **95–107**. See *First episode of psychosis.*
indicated prevention in, Early Detection and Intervention for the Prevention of Psychosis
Project, 102–103
North American Prodromal Longitudinal Study, 103–104
North American studies, 102–104
indicated prevention of, Buckingham program in, 98
criticism of, 97
Danish National Schizophrenia Project, 99–100
Early Detection and Intervention Evaluation in, 98–99
efficacy trials of, 98–102
German Research Network on Schizophrenia, 99
Manchester cognitive therapy trial in, 98–99
Omega-3 fatty acids in, 101
Personal Assessment and Crisis Evaluation in, 98, 100
Portland Identification and Early Referral program, 98, 101–102

Psychosis (*continued*)
   Prevention through Risk Identification, Management, and Education, 98, 100–101
   psychosocial intervention, 102
   summary of studies of, 98, 102
Psychotherapy, for postpartum depression, 56
Public health prevention, behavioral vaccines in, definition of, 9–10
   economic impact of, 17–18
      cost-burden silo example, 19–20
      costs of risky behaviors, 18–19
      total annual cost burden, 19
   evidence-based kernels in, 9–10
      definition of, 9
      impact on selected, indicated, and universal prevention, 10–11
      potential reach of, 10–11
      Reach, Efficacy, Adoption, Implementation, and Maintenance formula for, 10
   of mental, emotional, and behavioral disorders, need for, 2
      vs. rationing approaches to, 3
   policy actions for, 11–12
      create cost-saving estimators, 14–15
      create third-party reimbursements, 12–13
      impact at population-level, 15–18
      impact estimators of, 15–18
      initiate public/private preventon mobilizations, 13–14
      unleash consumer access, 12
      use proven marketing campaign strategies, 14

   R

Rebuilding the village, 211, 220
Resilience, as psychological protective factor, 232–234
   for adolescent depression, 38, 41–42
   in prevention research, 232–234
Risk factors, for adolescent depression, nonspecific, 37–38
      specific, 37
   for depression in older adults, 69
   for HIV, 218–220
   for schizophrenia, 97

   S

Schizophrenia, biologic vulnerability in, environmental influences on, 96
   indicated prevention, Family-aided Assertive Community Treatment in, 100
   indicators and identifiers in, 97
   life expectancy in, 109
   lifestyle interventions for weight loss in, clinical trials of, 112–113
   metabolic syndrome in, 212–213
   prodromal phase in, 96
   risk factors for, 97
Selected prevention, defined, 39
   evidence-based kernels in, 10–11, 450
   in public health prevention, 10–11

Selective prevention programs, for adolescents, cognitive behavioral, 42
    Pennsylvania Resilience Program, 41–42
    school-based, 41–42
  for older adults, 69, 71
Selective serotonin reuptake inhibitors (SSRIs), for PTSD prevention, 88
Self-esteem, improving, 212–213, 221
Sleep improvement, postpartum depression and, 58–59
Social and emotional skills, improving, 213, 221
Social networks, protective against cognitive decline, 135
Social support, for postpartum depression, 56–57
Statins, for prevention of CVD, 118
Suicide, adolescent depression and, 36

  T

Technology, access to ancient and modern, 212, 220–221
Thiazolidinediones, in hyperlipidemia, 117
  in type 2 diabetes, 117
Trauma, cortisol administration following, 87–88
  minimizing the effects of, 213, 223
  research link between risk behaviors, protective factors and, 186–194
Trauma-focused cognitive behavioral therapy (TFCBT), for PTSD, 84
Trauma-focused cognitive-behavioral therapy (TFCBT), for children in foster care, 192

  U

Universal prevention, defined, 39
  in public health prevention, 10–11
Universal prevention programs, evidence-based kernels in, 10–11, 450
  for adolescents, cognitive behavioral, 40–41
    school-based, 39–40

  V

Violence prevention, public health approach vs. get tough approach for, 205–206
  school-based, 7, 210–211
Vitamins, in AD, 131–132

  W

Weight
  lifestyle management of
    behavioral strategies for, 112–113
    benefits of, 111–112
    guidelines for, 111
Weight gain, antipsychotic-induced, 112, 114
  prevention of, lifestyle management in, 111–113
    pharmacologic, 112

Y

Youth, HIV prevention in. See *HIV infection.*
Youth homicide, **205–216**
    developmental dynamics and, age at onset and, 207
        prevalence of psychiatric disorders and, 207–208
    evidence based violence prevention programs, school-based, 210–211
    neurodevelopment and, 208
        affect regulation in, 208
    principles of prevention and, access to ancient and modern technology, 212
        connectedness, 212
        from public health, 211
        improving self-esteem, 212–213
        increasing social and emotional skills, 213
        minimizing the effects of trauma, 213
        rebuilding the village, 211
        reestablishing the adult protective shield, 213
    protective factors, 208–210
    risk factors for, behavioral, 209
        biological, 208–209
        family-related, 209
        protective factors and, 208
        strength of, 209
    statistics for, gender and, 207
        race and, 206–207
        rates of, 206–207
    violence and, get tough vs. public health approach to, 205–206

Moving?

Make sure your subscription moves with you!

To notify us of your new address, find your **Clinics Account Number** (located on your mailing label above your name), and contact customer service at:

Email: journalscustomerservice-usa@elsevier.com

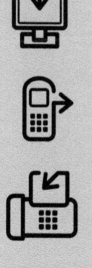

800-654-2452 (subscribers in the U.S. & Canada)
314-447-8871 (subscribers outside of the U.S. & Canada)

Fax number: 314-447-8029

Elsevier Health Sciences Division
Subscription Customer Service
3251 Riverport Lane
Maryland Heights, MO 63043

*To ensure uninterrupted delivery of your subscription, please notify us at least 4 weeks in advance of move.

Printed and bound by CPI Group (UK) Ltd, Croydon, CR0 4YY

03/10/2024

01040449-0020